PROLO YOUR PAIN AWAY!
Curing Chronic Pain with Prolotherapy
4ᵀᴴ EDITION

Ross A. Hauser, MD
&
Marion A. Boomer Hauser, MS, RD

Sorridi Business Consulting

Library of Congress Cataloging-in-Publication Data

Hauser, Ross A., author.
  Prolo your pain away! : curing chronic pain with
prolotherapy / Ross A. Hauser & Marion Boomer Hauser. —
Updated, fourth edition.
  pages cm
  Includes bibliographical references and index.
  ISBN 978-0-9903012-0-2

  1. Intractable pain—Treatment. 2. Chronic pain—
Treatment. 3. Sclerotherapy. 4. Musculoskeletal system
—Diseases—Chemotherapy. 5. Regenerative medicine.
I. Hauser, Marion A., author. II. Title.

RB127.H388 2016   616'.0472
                           QBI16-900065

Published by Sorridi Business Consulting
715 Lake Street, Suite 600, Oak Park, Illinois 60301

Printed in the United States of America

Scripture quotations are from: **Holy Bible, New International Version®, NIV®**
Copyrights © 1973, 1978, 1984, International Bible Society. Used by permission of
Zondervan Publishing House. All rights reserved.

ISBN 978-0-9903012-0-2

DEDICATION

This book is dedicated to our patients who have entrusted us with their health care. We are thankful that they have allowed us to help them achieve their hopes, dreams, and aspirations and help alleviate their pain and suffering. We love our patients and have been blessed many times over by their presence in our lives. It is with humble hearts that we dedicate this book to them.

We would not be able to perform the procedures that we provide in the manner in which we provide them, were it not for the presence of God in our lives. We are thankful to God for allowing the body to feel pain; for without that ability, we would have no way of knowing whether something was wrong.

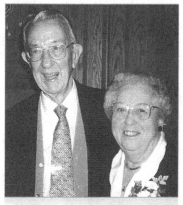

Dr. Gustav and Helen Hemwall

God's Son Jesus came to earth as the chief servant of all. Mark 10:43-45/ESV: "But it shall not be so among you. But whoever would be great among you must be your servant, and whoever would be first among you must be slave of all. For even the Son of Man came not to be served but to serve, and to give his life as a ransom for many." Because of this instruction from the Bible, we count it a blessing to be able to serve our patients. For that we are truly thankful.

Were it not for two of God's most faithful servants, Gustav and Helen Hemwall, we would not be writing this book today. Dr. Hemwall not only taught us the technique of Prolotherapy, having learned it from the inventor himself, George Hackett, MD, but he exemplified a life of service. He and Helen traveled to many countries servicing many of the poor and needy, as well as instructing other doctors in the technique of Prolotherapy. They have both passed away at the ages of 90 and 100 respectively. They are greatly missed. We are grateful for their legacy.

Providing Prolotherapy to our patients has been quite a blessing. We hope that you will find the contents of this book and the stories of changed lives something that provides you with hope for your particular pain or injury. ■

DISCLAIMER

The information presented in this book is based on the experiences of the authors, publishers, and editors, and is intended for informational and educational purposes only. In no way should this book be used as a substitute for your own practitioner's advice.

Because medicine is an ever-changing science, readers are encouraged to confirm the information contained herein with other sources. The authors, publishers, and editors of this work have used sources they believe to be reliable to substantiate the information provided. However, in view of the possibility of human error or changes in medical sciences, neither the authors, publishers, or editors, nor any other party who has been involved in the preparation or publication of this work warrants that the information contained herein is in every respect accurate or complete, and they are not responsible for any errors or omissions or for the results obtained from the use of such information. This is especially true, in particular, when an athlete or person in pain receives Prolotherapy and a bad result occurs. The authors, publishers, and editors of this book do not warrant that Prolotherapy is going to be effective in any medical condition and cannot guarantee nor endorse any certain type of Prolotherapy, solution used, or practitioner. It is the responsibility of the individual athlete or person who receives Prolotherapy to thoroughly research the topic and pick a particular practitioner whom he/she feels is qualified to perform the procedure.

As of this writing there is no certification available in Prolotherapy training. Any licensed medical (MD) or osteopathic doctor (DO) in the United States can perform Prolotherapy according to the laws. Naturopathic doctors (NDs) and Physician Assistants (PAs) may also provide Prolotherapy injections in some states. Practitioners should use and apply the technique of Prolotherapy only after they have received extensive training and demonstrated the ability to safely administer the treatment. The authors, publishers, editors, or any other people involved in this work, are not responsible if practitioners who are unqualified in the use of Prolotherapy administer the treatment based solely on the contents of this book, or if they receive training but do not administer it safely and a bad result occurs.

If Prolotherapy or any other treatment regimen described in this book appears to apply to your condition, the authors, publishers, and editors recommend that a formal evaluation be performed by a practitioner who is competent in treating pain and athletic injuries with Prolotherapy. Those desiring treatment should make medical decisions with the aid of a personal practitioner. No medical decisions should be made solely on the contents or recommendations made in this book. ■

TABLE OF CONTENTS

FOREWORD

By Marion A. Boomer Hauser, MS, RD, CEO

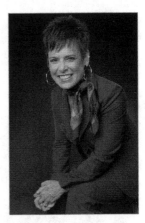

"Hope practiced here." When you arrive in our Caring Medical offices you will see that saying on the wall. Hope is what is missing for those who have been suffering with painful conditions or injuries that are keeping them from doing the things that they want to do. Mothers cannot care for their children. Workers cannot work. Athletes cannot participate in their sports. This occurs because they are unable to find long-term solutions to their pain or injuries. They lose hope. Prolotherapy provides hope.

Since learning about Prolotherapy in the 1990s and subsequently working together with Dr. Hauser and our team of extremely qualified, caring, and talented staff, I have seen many lives changed and hope restored. I am beyond passionate about Prolotherapy and living a healthy lifestyle. As a traditionally trained and practicing registered dietitian, I quickly learned that no one diet fits all. Thus, we developed the Hauser Diet and wrote a book about it! My passion IS still food! I love cooking, entertaining, and sharing meals with friends and family. If I could encourage all of our readers to do one thing related to diet, it would be to EAT REAL FOOD! Shop the perimeter of the grocery store. Read labels. Learn how to cook. Understand what you are putting into your bodies! As Hippocrates said, "Let your medicine be your food and your food be your medicine."

I am an avid athlete who loves participating in all sorts of outdoor activities and events. I have completed numerous 26.2 mile marathons, duathlons, triathlons and numerous shorter events such as 5Ks and 10Ks. I love cycling, swimming, strength training, snow shoeing, kayaking and hiking. I realize the importance of exercise for myself personally and have made it an active part of my life. Through all of this activity, I have sustained my share of sports injuries and have received Prolotherapy to nearly every area of my body!

I know what it feels like to be out with an injury that prevents you from doing what you love to do. Our goal is to get you back to doing those things YOU are passionate about. We want

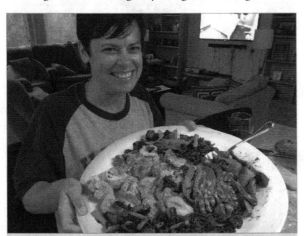

Never underestimate the power of food! Serving up fresh vegetables and protein gives the body what it needs to repair.

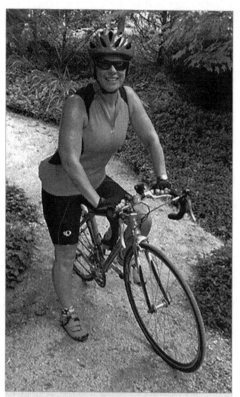

On a bike ride through one of the beautiful trails in Chicagoland. Fitness plays a large role in sports injury prevention and recovery!

you to live life to your fullest potential.

Patients come to see us at Caring Medical from all around the world. A day doesn't go by that we don't hear different languages being spoken in the waiting room; where people from all walks of life are discussing how Prolotherapy saved their lives. Some people may have minor irritating sports injuries, but others have life-altering, day-in-and-day-out chronic pain. We have been blessed to be able to provide a treatment that allows people to return to a fully functioning state.

As CEO of Caring Medical, I have worked very hard with our team of outstanding professionals to spread this word around the globe. We have dedicated ourselves to delivering exceptional service to our patients, even in cases where other practitioners have given up or only offered options that really didn't work, or worse yet, actually worsened their conditions. Many patients continue to suffer because traditional "pain management" or "sports injury treatments" do not work. Their care is driven by what insurance companies will cover, not by what cures the problem.

Since the original writing of this book in 1995, we have helped the Prolotherapy world change and improve. We are now able to offer additional treatment modalities that make the original Prolotherapy even better, including Cellular Prolotherapy and guidance options. My team and I have worked hard to provide you, our patients, with research that verifies our clinical results. We have spread the word about the life-changing effects of Prolotherapy through books, blogs, the *Journal of Prolotherapy,* and social media. A vast amount of work goes on behind the scenes to provide you with access to state-of-the-art medical information. I am

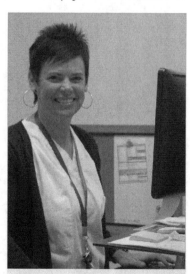

Work with heart! Seeing the joy in our patients after getting their lives back is worth all of the hard work.

blessed to head up this team of professionals! We will continue to press on in our quest to provide awesome service to our patients as well as provide you with the best quality and cost-effective services that we can.

Many people come to Caring Medical broken. Physically, emotionally, and spiritually broken. They have given up. They have been told to "live with the pain" or "wait until you are old enough for joint replacement surgery." In the meantime, they try various assortments of over-the-counter pain medications, then proceed to stronger medications, receive steroid injections, arthroscopies, and unsuccessful surgeries. Why? Because they have not found out about the regenerative, restorative treatment called Prolotherapy.

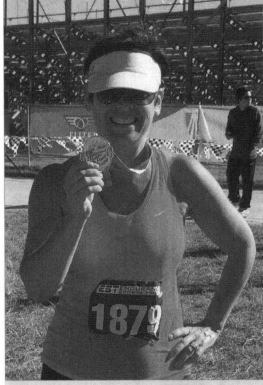

Happy to have completed another race after using Prolotherapy to overcome runner's knee.

This book has been written to give you hope and show you how a relatively simple, but highly effective treatment could be just what you have been looking for. ∎

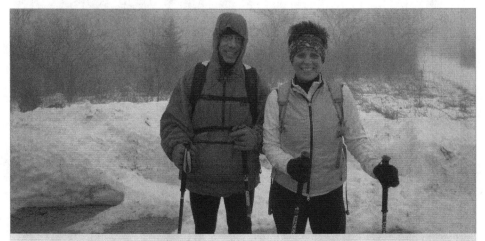

Snowshoeing through central Wisconsin. It is important to stay active, even through the winter months. Bundle up and get out there!

PREFACE: MY LIFE AS A PHYSIATRIST

By Ross A. Hauser, MD

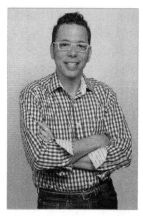

WHERE IT ALL STARTED

I became fascinated with pain during my Physical Medicine residency. I began accumulating articles on bizarre pain syndromes and obtained quite a collection. (Everyone needs a hobby, right?) What struck me most was the magnitude of the pain problem. It seemed as though everyone either had pain themselves or knew someone who was suffering from chronic pain. I also saw the lack of significant pain relief by modern treatments such as surgery, physical therapy, and anti-inflammatory drugs.

It appeared that the longer people had pain, the less likely such treatments were going to help cure their chronic pain. Pain clinics and pain programs do help some people, but have a poor cure rate. Pain programs teach people to live with their pain. The psychological aspect of the pain is addressed, but in many cases the cause is not determined.

When I began seeing pain patients during my residency training program in Physical Medicine and Rehabilitation, I thought they were a very difficult group of people to treat. They often appeared depressed, and traditional approaches to pain management did not seem to help. Then I said to myself, "How would I feel if I had pain day after day and no one could find a cure?" The families of many who suffer from pain often begin doubting the reality of their loved ones' pain. Many chronic pain patients who frequent pain clinics experience broken homes and lose their jobs because of the pain. It became evident to me that these patients' pain was indeed real and that pain pills and support groups did not cure the pain.

PROLOTHERAPY

A friend from church, Mrs. Wright, was experiencing terrible pain. I tried all the treatment modalities and

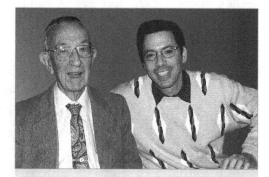

Dr. Hemwall and Dr. Hauser. Blessed to carry on Dr. Hemwall's Prolotherapy legacy.

gizmos I knew of, but without success. Mrs. Wright eventually received treatment from Gustav A. Hemwall, MD, the world's most experienced Prolotherapist. The Prolotherapy she received in her shoulder gave her a significant amount of relief. Mrs. Wright then encouraged me to learn about Dr. Hemwall's treatment.

In April 1992, I contacted Dr. Hemwall and he allowed me to observe him in his clinic. I was astonished to see him perform 30, 50, or 100 injections on a patient at one time! He called his treatment Prolotherapy. The only other time I had come across the term was when a fellow resident showed me a book on the treatment. I later discovered that Dr. Hemwall was one of the authors of that book.

During the next few months, I spent a considerable amount of time in Dr. Hemwall's office. People traveled from all over the world to be treated by this 84-year-old man. I have nothing against age, but to think that someone would travel from places like England, Mexico, Florida, and California to receive pain management was incredible. I learned that if someone suffers from pain and someone else has a technique that will help alleviate the pain, time and expense are minor considerations.

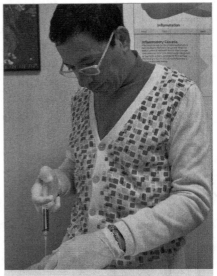

Dr. Hauser performing Cellular Prolotherapy for thumb arthritis.

It was clear that Dr. Hemwall was helping those whom traditional medicine had not helped. His average patient had been in pain for years and had tried it all: surgery, pain pills, anti-inflammatory medication, exercise, therapy, acupuncture, and hypnotism. Most patients had seen more than five physicians before consulting Dr. Hemwall. Almost all the patients I observed improved after one or two Prolotherapy treatments. People found relief from pain that had plagued them for years. Many said they wished they had known about Prolotherapy years ago.

Three months later, I began utilizing Prolotherapy in my medical practice as a treatment for chronic pain. In January 1993, I began working alongside Dr. Hemwall in his Prolotherapy practice. After Dr. Hemwall retired in 1996, he gave me the reigns to carry on his work. Since then, Marion and I have worked tirelessly to continue the Hackett-Hemwall technique of Prolotherapy at Caring Medical Regenerative Medicine Clinics, while adding in advancements such as cellular solutions, ultrasound and Digital Motion X-ray guidance.

JOINT INSTABILITY

Anyone picking up this book knows what it means to either have chronic pain or suffer alongside someone who has it. It is my hope and prayer that the "light bulb" will turn on as you read this book and understand what I have been saying for decades…*chronic pain is due to joint instability*. Plain and simple. *(See Figure 1.)*

Knee joint instability causes almost every diagnosis a person can have with the knee. Traditional treatments often don't work because they don't get at the root cause of these "diseases." Knee arthritis, meniscus tears, chondromalacia, and jumper's knee are some examples of ligament injury causing knee instability. The ligament injury leads to increased movement of the knee while running, for instance. This then causes increased pressure on the knee and its structures, leading to patellar tendon, meniscus and cartilage injury. The treatment of choice for these conditions is Prolotherapy, not anti-inflammatory medications, cortisone shots or surgery.

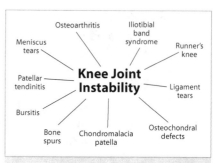

Figure 1. Conditions caused by knee joint instability.

One can go through each body part, as this book will cover many of them, and the scenario is the same. For example, consider the fact that cervical instability is what causes a number of conditions: degenerative arthritis in the neck, "pinched" nerves, post-concussion syndrome, vertigo, myofascial pain syndrome, and many others. As this book explains, the concept applies to the spine, hip, shoulder, ankle and every other joint in the body.

I am an avid athlete myself, having completed five ironman triathlons, a number of ultramarathons and marathons, as well as many other shorter running, cycling, and swimming events. I have sustained pretty much every injury imaginable from a debilitating pinched nerve in my neck to runner's knee and everything in between. I am passionate about helping people get back to doing the things they love to do. I understand what it is like to be side lined with an injury. I cannot even tell you how many times I have benefited from receiving Prolotherapy for the many injuries I have sustained over the years of hard training. It's life-saving! And I want that for you!

The research accumulating for this concept is overwhelming once you look

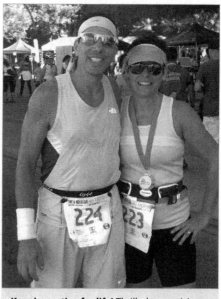

Keeping active for life! Thrilled to participate in the A-Mountain Half-Marathon in Tuscon. Such a fun event!

into it. This book is just to get your appetite going. As Prolotherapy continues to be established in areas around the world, it is exciting to see how other doctors and their patients are finding out what we have known for a very long time—No matter how bad your pain, how long you have had it, or how many surgeries you have gone through, you can always "Prolo Your Pain Away!" ■

1

WHY SHOULD YOU CONSIDER PROLOTHERAPY?

Prolotherapy is superior at curing chronic pain and, most importantly, getting people back to a happy and active lifestyle. Since this book may be your introduction to Prolotherapy, let us first present you with a case that may be very familiar to you. In fact, this person may be YOU! Your physical pain is standing between the activities you once enjoyed: golf, swimming, running. Eventually, it is standing between you and your ability to work or play with your children or grandchildren. Once you decide it is bad enough to seek a professional medical opinion, the patient's scenario goes something like this:

- Visits numerous allopathic and university specialists without success.
- Tries chiropractic treatments.
- Tries physical therapy.
- Tries massage therapy.
- Begins prescription anti-inflammatory medications.
- Moves to stronger prescription anti-inflammatory medications.
- Decides to get a cortisone shot.
- Receives a nerve block.
- And finally, receives SURGERY!

The end result of this scenario is that the patient continues to suffer with the painful condition for an even longer duration of time. Even worse, the patient has spent a lot of time and money with no resolution of the pain. What a terrible fate!

Why does this happen to millions of people? The answer: None of the treatments in this scenario actually fix the root cause of the patient's problem. What gives Prolotherapy patients a higher chance at permanently curing the pain is the fact that Prolotherapy is aimed to fix the root cause of the problem, ligament and tendon weakness resulting in underlying joint instability. Throughout this book you will learn in greater detail why and how this happens and how Regenerative Medicine works to cure pain, not just cover it up.

HOW DOES PROLOTHERAPY WORK?

The basic mechanism of Prolotherapy is simple. Prolotherapy solutions are injected into the painful areas, which produces local inflammation in the injected area(s). The localized inflammation triggers a wound-healing cascade, resulting in the deposition of new collagen. New collagen shrinks as it matures. The shrinking collagen tightens the ligaments that were injected and makes them stronger and more secure, thus stabilizing the unstable joint(s). Prolotherapy has the potential of being 100% effective at eliminating sports injuries and chronic pain, depending upon the technique of the individual Prolotherapist and the extent of the comprehensive healing program. One of the most important aspects of healing is injecting enough of the right type of solution into the entire injured and weakened area(s). If this is done, the likelihood of success is excellent.

A JOINT IS ONLY AS STRONG AS ITS WEAKEST LIGAMENT

Simply put, pain is due to weakness. In our experience, most neck, back, knee, and other musculoskeletal pains are due to weakness, specifically weakness in the ligaments and tendons, which in turn, leads to joint instability.

George S. Hackett, MD, grandfather of Prolotherapy, stated, "A joint is only as strong as its weakest ligament." He further stated, "Ligament relaxation is a condition in which the strength of the ligament fibers has become impaired so that a stretching of the fibrous strands occurs when the ligament is submitted to normal or less than normal tension."[1] This statement was made many years ago by Dr. Hackett, who believed chronic pain was simply due to ligament weakness in and around the joint. *(See Figure 1-1.)* Dr. Hackett coined the phrase "ligament and tendon relaxation," which is synonymous with ligament and tendon weakness, and subsequently developed the treatment known as Prolotherapy.

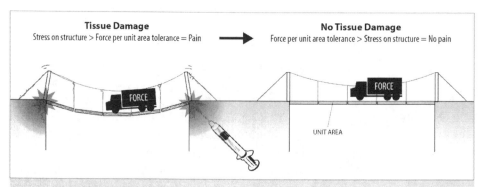

Figure 1-1: Why tissue damage occurs. Prolotherapy increases the force per unit area that a ligament and other joint structures can tolerate. When this tissue tolerance increases beyond the stress (force/ unit area) on this structure, no tissue damage occurs and thus no pain.

PROLOTHERAPY DEFINED

Webster's Third New International Dictionary defines Prolotherapy as "the rehabilitation of an incompetent structure, such as a ligament or tendon, by the induced proliferation of new cells."[2] Prolotherapy stimulates the repair of painful structures. These painful structures develop because God gave our bodies an alert system that notifies us when something is wrong. Prolotherapy stimulates structures to repair and strengthen, thus it can eliminate most structural musculoskeletal pain located anywhere in the body. When the body sustains significant force or trauma, an injury will occur either where the force is greatest or at the structures' weakest point(s). In the musculoskeletal system, the weak link in the system is typically located in the joints and the structures that hold them in place. The force is typically felt in the ligaments, especially if there is a rotatory component to the stress. Ligaments are injured at the point(s) where they attach to the bone(s) which is known in Prolotherapy circles as the fibro-osseous junction or in traditional medicine circles the enthesis (singular; plural is entheses). When we discuss proper Prolotherapy technique, we say that the needle touches the bone at the point where the ligament attaches to the bone; thus Prolotherapy injections are strengthening the entheses; with the exception of intra-articular joint injections which are given inside the joints.

ENTHESOPATHY

The enthesis is the point at which the connective tissue structures, such as a joint capsule, fascia, ligament, tendon, or muscle attach to the bone. Pathology (cause of disease) in the enthesis is called an enthesopathy. The term enthesopathy typically refers to a degenerated enthesis; though when modern medicine uses this term, they typically mean enthesitis. The problem occurs when allopathic physicians think every pain is due to inflammation and subsequently prescribe NSAIDs and corticosteroid shots. This book will discuss in more detail later how the body actually heals by the process of inflammation; thus anti-inflammatory medications not only do not treat the underlying cause of the condition, but make it worse by halting the healing process.

ENTHESITIS

A true systemic inflammatory condition causes a true enthesitis, which occurs in conditions such as chondrocalcinosis, diffuse idiopathic skeletal hyperostosis, ankylosing spondylitis, Reiter's syndrome, rheumatoid arthritis, psoriatic arthritis, and other spondyloarthropathies. There may be a limited role for anti-inflammatory medications in these conditions, but we can assure you that none of these conditions are caused by an "ibuprofen deficiency!" A comprehensive Natural Medicine assessment by a qualified practitioner is needed to cure these types of conditions. We review things in the patient's life that might be producing stress on the body, including the foods consumed, job, family relationships, and emotional state. *(See Chapter 18: Why You Don't Heal for more information.)*

A person with a systemic inflammatory condition is more likely to be taking anti-inflammatory or immune-suppressive medications. These medications make the patient less likely to heal a ligament or tendon injury when it occurs. Everyone sustains some kind of injury every once in a while, such as a sprained ankle. In these cases we still utilize Prolotherapy for people suffering with various spondyloarthropies such as ankylosing spondylitis and autoimmune diseases such as systemic lupus erythematosus or rheumatoid arthritis, however, we recommend that the underlying systemic inflammatory condition be treated using Natural Medicine methods.

THE ENTHESIS ORGAN

It is becoming clear through medical research that the area where a ligament and tendon attaches, the enthesis, should really be called "the enthesis organ."[3] This is a specialized area of the musculoskeletal system that contains fibrocartilage and other adjacent or congruous structures such as articular cartilage fat pads, bursae, or synovium.[4,5] This "organ" may be damaged like any organ of the body. In our experience, the entheses are typically damaged by medications. NSAIDs and corticosteroids are the most common culprits, but the medical literature contains many studies and case reports on various antibiotics damaging these structures, especially the quinolone antibiotics.[6-8] Most tendinopathies are actually enthesopathies; thus the injury occurs to the tendon where it attaches on the bone. *(See Figure 1-2.)* Steroid injections and other medications specifically have been shown to weaken this area.[7,8] Fortunately there is a treatment that is specifically designed to strengthen the entheses: Prolotherapy!

LIGAMENTS AND TENDONS

A strain is defined as a stretched or injured tendon. A sprain is a stretched or injured ligament. Blood flow is vital to the body's healing process and, because ligaments and tendons have naturally poor blood supply, incomplete healing may result after an injury to that structure.[9,10] This incomplete healing results in decreased strength of the area. *(See Figure 1-3.)* The ligaments and tendons, normally taut and thus strong bands of fibrous or connective tissue, become relaxed and weak. The weakened ligament or tendon then becomes the source of the chronic pain.

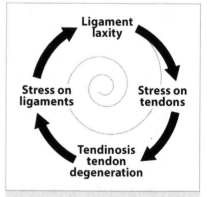

Figure 1-2: Relationship between ligament laxity and tendinosis. Note that the functioning of the tendons of a joint affects the ligaments and vice-versa.

Ligaments and tendons are bands of tissue consisting of various amino acids in a matrix called collagen. Tendons attach the muscles to the surface of the bone, enabling movement of the joints and bones. Ligaments attach one bone to another, thus preventing over-extension of bones and joints. *(See Figure 1-4.)*

Damage to ligaments and tendons will cause excessive movement of the joints, along with cracking sensations during movement. This results in joint instability, weakness, and chronic pain.

Many causes of chronic elbow pain exist, including tennis elbow (extensor tendonitis), annular ligament sprain, and biceps muscle strain. Since muscle, ligament, or tendon injury can all cause pain, a proper diagnosis is needed to permanently alleviate the pain. Tennis elbow is diagnosed when we observe weakness and pain with wrist extension and tenderness at the elbow where the extensor tendons attach. Annular ligament sprain is diagnosed when we palpate this ligament in the elbow and elicit a positive "jump sign." *(See Figure 1-5.)*

Another source of elbow pain is biceps muscle strain. When the biceps tendon is weak, resisted flexion (resisting the upward movement of the forearm) of the elbow is painful. Since the bicep muscle flexes at the elbow, carrying a box or turning a screwdriver may produce the painful symptoms associated with strain or weakness of this muscle. Since the extensor tendons, bicep muscle, and annular ligament all attach to the bone in the elbow,

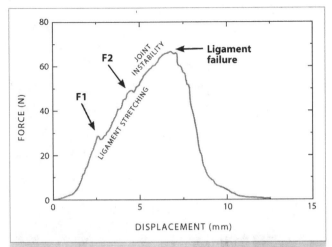

Figure 1-3: Typical results of a ligament elongation to failure test. Once the ligament is injured, it then takes very little force on it to cause joint instability and total ligament (joint) failure. F1 and F2 show two subcatastrophic injuries that cause elongation to the ligament. A person could have symptoms anywhere from F1 to the point where the ligament completely tears (ligament failure). Prolotherapy, during this period, can tighten the ligament so joint stability is recovered. Once a ligament is completely torn, surgery is generally needed.

Adapted form Figure 5. Winkelstein BA, et al. The cervical facet capsule and its role in whiplash injury. *Spine.* 2000;25(10):1238-1246.

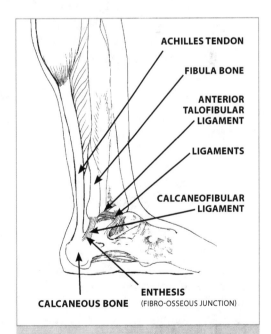

Figure 1-4: Anatomy of the foot.
The enthesis or fibro-osseous junction is the area where ligaments and tendons attach to the bone.

good palpatory skills are necessary for proper diagnosis. Prolotherapy is given at the enthesis or fibro-osseous junction where the positive "jump sign" is elicited. Prolotherapy causes proliferation, or growth of tissue at this point. Prolotherapy to the ankle in *Figure 1-6* shows how new ligament tissue is stimulated to grow. Prolotherapy will strengthen the muscle, tendon, or ligament tissue at the enthesis, which is needed to alleviate pain.

JOINT INSTABILITY: THE MISSING DIAGNOSIS IN MOST CHRONIC PAIN CASES

Ligaments function primarily to maintain smooth joint motion, restrain excessive joint displacement, and provide stability across the joint. *(See Figure 1-7.)* For example, ligaments of the knee provide passive stability, guide the motion of the femur and tibia, define contact mechanics between the femur and tibia, and restrain excessive motion to prevent dislocation.[11] When the forces to which ligaments are subjected are too great, failure occurs, resulting in drastic changes in the structure and physiology of the joint. Ligamentous injuries can result in joint laxity, which presents as looseness or instability of the joint; this can occur at almost every joint in the body. *(See Figure 1-8.)*

Ligaments are the primary passive joint stabilizers whereas muscles are the active joint stabilizers. Mechanical laxity refers to an excess in the range of motion in the joint due to loss of integrity of the ligaments and other soft tissues which contribute to joint stability. Functional instability refers to

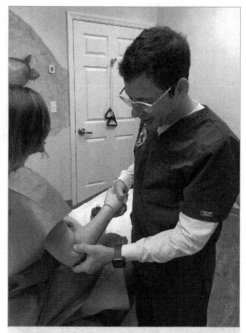

Figure 1-5: Examining the elbow for tenderness. Dr. Hauser eliciting a positive "jump sign" while palpating the annular ligament.

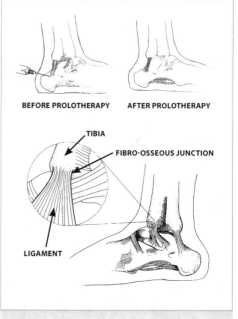

BEFORE PROLOTHERAPY   AFTER PROLOTHERAPY

TIBIA

FIBRO-OSSEOUS JUNCTION

LIGAMENT

Figure 1-6: Prolotherapy of the ankle. Prolotherapy stimulates the growth of new ligament tissue in the ankle.

a sense of instability or giving out of the joint experienced in the course of daily activities or strenuous exercise. It is possible to have functional joint instability from muscle weakness alone; thus functional instability may or may not be associated with mechanical laxity.[12]

Ligament injuries and degeneration (ligamentosis) are among the most common causes of joint instability, and the resultant pain. They create disruptions in the balance between joint mobility and

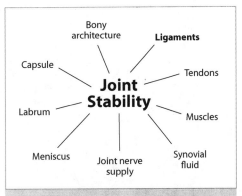

Figure 1-7: Structures involved in joint stability. The **major** structures involved in joint stability are the ligaments.

joint stability, causing abnormal force transmission through the joint, which results in damage to structures in and around the joint, including the cartilage, nerves, bone, and others. To properly identify and correct the root cause of most musculoskeletal pain, understanding the function of the ligaments and how to restore them is absolutely necessary.

If joints move too much, the bones may compress or pinch nerves or blood vessels, resulting in permanent nerve damage. Weakened structures are strengthened by the growth of new, strong ligament and

Possible Signs and Symptoms of Ligament Injury:

- Balance difficulties
- Decreased joint motion
- Dizziness
- Joint cracking
- Joint instability
- Muscle spasm
- Numbness
- Pain
- Swelling
- Vertebral subluxations
- Weakness

Figure 1-8: Ligament injury can produce diverse symptomatology.

tendon tissue induced by the Prolotherapy injections. This is illustrated in a relatively common back condition called spondylolisthesis. A weak area of bone, in conjunction with stretched ligaments, allow vertebrae to slip and pinch a nerve, resulting in terrible back pain and radiating pain down the leg. Incomplete healing and lower functional integrity of the new ligament tissue may result in ligament laxity, joint instability, and secondary muscle weakness, which predispose the joint to osteoarthritis.[13] Prolotherapy strengthens the weakened areas, relieving the pinched nerve and eliminating the chronic pain. *(See Figures 1-9A &1-9B.)*

THE ROLE OF PROLOTHERAPY

Prolotherapy permanently strengthens tissue. Strengthening weakened structures restores joint stability and produces permanent pain relief. Prolotherapy addresses structural weakness the same way a screwdriver addresses a loosened screw within

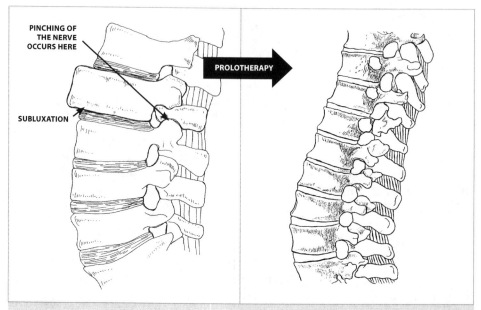

Figure 1-9A: Spondylolisthesis – slippage of the vertebrae. Weakened ligaments lead to spondylolisthesis and pinching of the nerves.

Figure 1-9B: Proper vertebral alignment after Prolotherapy. Prolotherapy strengthens the ligaments and joints that support the vertebrae to move into proper alignment and relieves nerve pinching.

a hinge. Just like the motion of a door relies on the hinge, our joints rely on taut ligaments. *(See Figure 1-10.)* If a cabinet door becomes wobbly, for instance, the hinge is addressed and any loosened screws are simply tightened with a screwdriver. Thus, proper motion is restored and the door remains in good condition. If the screws are not tightened, the hinge continues to loosen, allowing the cabinet door to begin hitting the adjacent door. Eventually, this wears out the finish on the cabinet doors, warps and splinters the wood, and puts added stress on adjacent hinges. All of this can be avoided by simply tightening the original loosened screws with a screwdriver. In our bodies, Prolotherapy stimulates the tightening of ligaments the same way a screwdriver tightens screws, in order to avoid further joint degeneration. This concept is discussed more in *Chapter 13.*

REFERRED PAIN

Prolotherapy effectively eliminates pain because it addresses the source of the pain: the enthesis, an area rich in sensory nerves.[14,15] When a weakened ligament or tendon is stretched, the sensory nerves become irritated, causing local and referred pain throughout the body. These referred pain patterns of ligaments were outlined in Dr. Hackett's early observations after he performed more than 18,000 intraligamentous injections to 1,656 patients over a period of 19 years.[16]

A referred pain occurs when a local ligament injury sends pain to another area of the body. Dr. Hackett described the referral patterns of the ligaments involving the hip, pelvis, lower back, and neck. Many physical therapists, chiropractors, family physicians, and orthopedists may be unaware of ligament referral pain patterns. From the illustrations, note that the hip ligaments refer pain to the big toe. The sacroiliac ligaments refer pain to the lateral foot, which causes the symptoms resulting in a common misdiagnosis of "sciatica." Pain traveling down the back into the leg and foot is usually from ligament weakness in the sacroiliac joint, not pinching of the sciatic nerve. Patients who are misdiagnosed with "sciatica" are often subjected

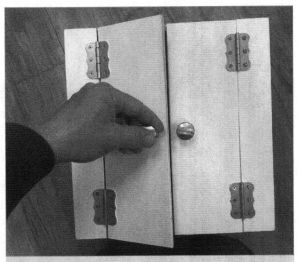

Figure 1-10: The force with normal opening of a cabinet door is primarily felt at the hinge. That is why it is the *weak link* in the door frame-hinge-cabinet kinetic chain. Structures typically breakdown at their connection points.

to numerous tests, anti-inflammatory medicines, and surgical procedures with unsatisfactory results. Prolotherapy eliminates the local ligament pain, as well as the referred pain, and is curative in most cases of sciatica.

Ligament injuries may cause crushing severe pain because the ligaments are full of nerves, some of the nerve tissue being free nerve endings.[14,15] Movement may aggravate the damaged nerve in the ligament and produces a shock–like sensation, giving the impression that a nerve is being pinched. It is a nerve-type pain that is due to a ligament stretching, not a nerve pinching. When a weak ligament is stretched, the nerves inside the ligament often send shock–like pain to distant sites, as in sciatica pain. If the ligament is strengthened with Prolotherapy, the nerves in the ligaments do not fire, thereby relieving the pain.

Among Prolotherapists, it is well known that an injury in one segment of the body can affect other distant body parts, especially in regard to ligament injury. For example, when dye is injected into the nerves of the ligaments of the lower neck, the dye will travel four segments above and four segments below the initial injection site. The dye may be seen in the autonomic (sympathetic) nerves in these areas.[17] This implies that ligament laxity at one vertebral level could manifest pain, muscle tension, adrenal, or automatic dysfunction four segments above or below the actual injury site. This is one of the explanations as to why ligament pain is often diffuse and can take on a burning quality.

Knowledge of referral pain patterns, along with a complete patient medical history, allows us to make accurate diagnoses of specific weak ligaments. We may examine a back pain patient with pain radiating down the leg to the knee. This reveals that the source of the pain is likely the sacroiliac ligaments, and pain radiating to the big toe reveals the source is in the hip area. *(See Figures 1-11 & 1-12.)*

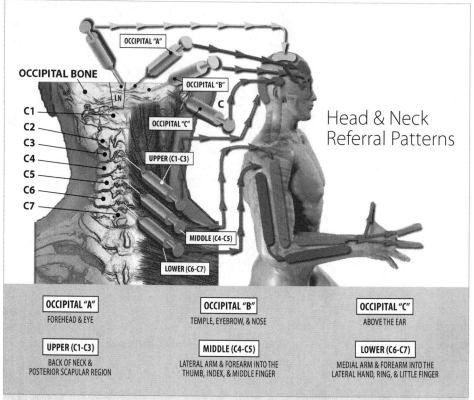

OCCIPITAL "A"	OCCIPITAL "B"	OCCIPITAL "C"
FOREHEAD & EYE	TEMPLE, EYEBROW, & NOSE	ABOVE THE EAR

UPPER (C1-C3)	MIDDLE (C4-C5)	LOWER (C6-C7)
BACK OF NECK & POSTERIOR SCAPULAR REGION	LATERAL ARM & FOREARM INTO THE THUMB, INDEX, & MIDDLE FINGER	MEDIAL ARM & FOREARM INTO THE LATERAL HAND, RING, & LITTLE FINGER

Figure 1-11: Prolotherapy: diagnosis and treatment all in one. Prolotherapy injections can reproduce localized and referral pain patterns, thus confirming the diagnosis for both the patient and physician. The elimination of pain is, of course, an added bonus.

PROLOTHERAPY FOR PAIN AND INJURY

Prolotherapy is so successful because it repairs the root cause of chronic pain, which is most commonly ligament laxity (weakness) leading to joint instability. Signs of ligament laxity and joint instability are the following:

- Balance difficulties
- Chronic pain
- Chronic subluxation
- Cracking sound when the joint is moved
- Decreased joint motion
- Grinding sensation when the joint is moved
- Muscle spasms
- Numbiness or burning sensations
- Pain aggravated by movement
- Positive "jump signs"
- Referral pain patterns
- Subluxations
- Swelling
- Temporary help from physical therapy, massage, or chiropractic manipulation
- Tenderness in areas upon palpation
- Weakness

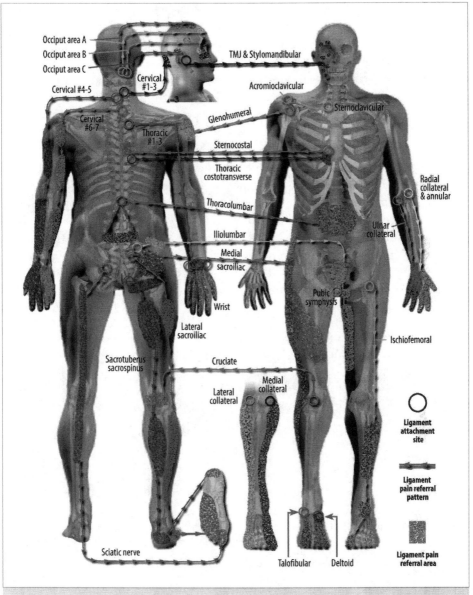

Figure 1-12: Hackett-Hemwall ligament referral patterns. Ligament laxity can cause localized pain as well as refer to distant sites.

Prolotherapy helps strengthen chronically weak ligaments and relieves all of these symptoms. The typical patient seen at Caring Medical is a person with chronic pain, who when examined reports tenderness where a structure such as a ligament inserts onto the bone. This is an enthesopathy, which may be more appropriately termed a "focal insertional disorder." This means that the main problem causing the patient's pain is weakness at the enthesis of the ligament, causing subtle joint instability.

The treatment for this condition is to provide Prolotherapy injections to stimulate the repair or strengthening of the enthesis. *(See Figure 1-13.)*

If the area is appropriately treated with Prolotherapy, not only is the chronic pain eliminated, but the joint instability is corrected. Often when a patient presents to Caring Medical with so-called knee arthritis, but wants to avoid knee replacement surgery, we get out the MRI: My Reproducibility Instrument. The thumb (aka the MRI) can press right onto the entheses of the pes anserine tendons, for example, and cause the person to jump off the examination table. Injecting with Prolotherapy solution containing extra procaine (Novocaine®) into that area will effectively eliminate just about all of the pain. Even in some cases of end stage arthritis, the actual pain stems from an enthesopathy, not from the articular cartilage. Remember, articular cartilage has no nerve endings, whereas ligaments have plenty of nerve endings and they fire when the ligament is under too much stretch or tension, thus producing pain! *(See Figure 1-14.)* Nociceptors are sensory nerve endings that signal actual or potential tissue damage. In summary, Prolotherapy works by permanently strengthening the ligament, muscle, and tendon attachments to the bone—the entheses. Because the cause of pain is addressed, Prolotherapy is often curative.

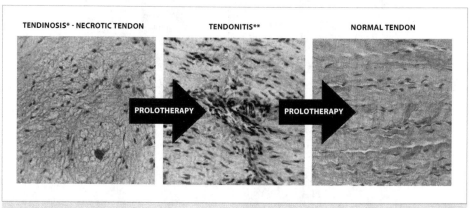

Figure 1-13: The histology of how Prolotherapy heals. While corticosteroid injections cause tendon cell death, Prolotherapy injections at entheses cause the proliferation of cells with the goal of making new stronger ligament and tendon attachments.

Used with permission from *Overuse Injuries of the Musculoskeletal System*—Marko M. Peling, CRC Press, 1993, Boca Raton, FL.
*Biopsy of tendon of athlete with "overuse injury"
**Biopsy of tendon showing tendonitis. This is what occurs immediately after Prolotherapy.

COMPREHENSIVE PROLOTHERAPY AT CARING MEDICAL: HACKETT-HEMWALL PROLOTHERAPY

The Prolotherapy technique we use at Caring Medical Regenerative Medicine Clinics is called Comprehensive Prolotherapy or Hackett-Hemwall Prolotherapy. This type of Prolotherapy incorporates the teaching and techniques of doctors George S. Hackett, MD, and Gustav A. Hemwall, MD, two of the pioneers in the field. *(See Chapter 21 that discusses the details of their work.)* This technique involves

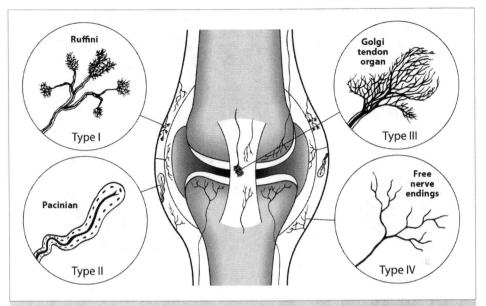

Figure 1-14: The ligament is the sensory organ of the joint. It tells the brain what is happening with the joint, such as too much force. There are various ligament joint receptor types. Type I, II, and III receptors are mechanoreceptors. Type IV receptors are nociceptors.

Adapted from: Freeman MAR, et al. The innervation of the knee joint. An anatomical and histological study in the cat. *J Anat (Lond).* 1976;101:505. And, Polacek P. Receptors of the joints. Their structure, variability and classification. *Acta Fac. Med. Uni. Brun.* 1966;23:1:107.

using a simple and safe base solution containing dextrose as the primary proliferant, along with an anesthetic (such as procaine or lidocaine), that is given into and around the entire painful/injured area(s). Many injections are given during each treatment, versus just a few injections. Most treatments are provided every 4 to 6 weeks to allow time for growth of new connective tissues. Some more urgent cases may be treated more frequently. When stronger proliferants or Cellular Prolotherapy *(See Chapter 3)* is used, the treatments may be provided every 6-8 weeks. The average person requires 3-6 visits total, some more, some less. The treatments are typically performed without imaging, x-ray guidance or conscious sedation. In our office we offer both ultrasound and Digital Motion X-ray (DMX) guidance (a type of fluoroscopy) for cases that warrant these modalities. However, a true Prolotherapist should be highly skilled at anatomical based treatments if they are adept at the treatment.

WHY COMPREHENSIVE PROLOTHERAPY IS SUCCESSFUL

The major cause of degenerative arthritis, chronic pain, and injury is joint instability. Most structural chronic painful conditions involve ligament laxity. *(See Figure 1-15.)* Most tendinopathies are caused by joint instability and ligament laxity. To cure these conditions, it is typically best to treat all or most of the ligaments of an unstable joint if that joint and/or its surrounding structures are painful to palpation. Many injections are needed to produce enough of a healing reaction to

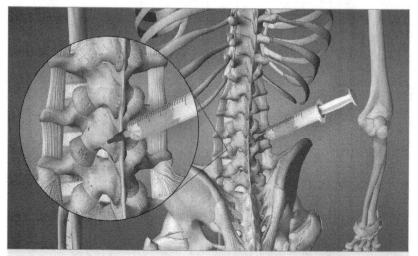

Figure 1-15: Prolotherapy of the lower back. Injured capsular, sacroiliac and other ligaments can be thickened and strengthened with Prolotherapy.

restore proper joint function to an unstable painful joint. It is a lot like spot welding.

Because the solutions are safe and well-tolerated, many joints and structures can be treated at the same visit. The neck, thoracic, and low back facet joints can also be thoroughly and safely treated without the need of fluoroscopy, which keeps costs down.

With a comprehensive approach, we utilize many different types of Prolotherapy solutions, individualizing each treatment according to the patients' unique needs. The solutions are changed depending on the individual patient and the amount of inflammatory reaction required to produce sufficient healing and new collagen growth. We use natural ingredients that can be added to the dextrose-based solutions, such as minerals, fatty acids, and hormones; and of course, cellular proliferants such as blood, PRP (platelet rich plasma), bone marrow, and stem cells.

Comprehensive Prolotherapy is typically well-tolerated and does not require use of narcotic medications or NSAIDs, and certainly not steroid injections. Most patients receive treatments and are able to return to work the same or next day. Immediately following Prolotherapy treatments, we ask our patients to refrain from vigorous exercise for at least 4 days. After that, the patients are allowed to let their bodies be their guides.

Results speak for themselves! We have documented our patient results in many published papers which we will review in more detail throughout this book. Suffice it to say, we can unequivocally state that Prolotherapy is effective at producing pain relief in greater than 90% of the patients. ■

CHAPTER

CHAPTER

2

PROLOTHERAPY, INFLAMMATION, & HEALING: WHAT'S THE CONNECTION?

Inflammation is the key to healing. The body depends on inflammation to heal itself. Yet modern medicine does everything it can to halt the inflammatory process. You may be asking yourself "why?" Let us explain further.

INFLAMMATION SHOULD BE THE HERO, NOT THE ZERO!

The following statement comes from a well-known sports medicine book that has gone through five printings. "In spite of the widespread use of NSAIDs, there is no convincing evidence as to their effectiveness in the treatment of acute soft tissue injuries."[1]

How did modern medicine get so off track to the point where they are prescribing treatments that actually stop healing instead of **help healing**? It is hard to believe that all around the world, the typical medical advice for a simple ankle sprain is basically flat out wrong! After an injury to a joint, the treatment should be MEAT (Movement, Exercise, Analgesics, and Therapy) versus RICE (Rest, Ice, Compression, and Elevation.) *(See Figure 2-1.)*

Modern medicine makes the error of treating ligament injuries the same as muscle injuries. Muscles are very vascular structures as evidenced by the fact that they are beefy and red; whereas the white structures of the body, including the tendons, ligaments, fibrocartilage (menisci and labrum)

RICE vs. MEAT

MODALITY	RESULT	MODALITY	RESULT
REST	Decreased joint nutrition	**M**OVEMENT	Increased joint nutrition
ICE	Decreased blood flow	**E**XERCISE	Increased blood flow
COMPRESSION	Decreased pain control	**A**NALGESIC	Increased pain control
ELEVATION	Incomplete healing	**T**REATMENT	Complete healing

Figure 2-1: RICE vs. MEAT. The RICE treatment leads to incomplete healing of soft tissue whereas MEAT encourages complete healing.

and articular cartilage have little or no blood supply. Muscles can undergo the RICE treatments and feel immediately better and avoid compromised healing because of the large influx of healing cells available, despite the non-healing aspects of the RICE protocol. The white structures are not so lucky and over time research has shown that the RICE protocol, NSAIDs and corticosteroid shots inhibit healing.

THE ATHLETE EXAMPLE

Many athletes, professional, Olympic, or even high school or children, will badly sprain an ankle or tear their meniscus in the knee, or sustain some other type of injury while playing a sport. As the athlete lays wincing in pain, the medical personnel faithfully administer the RICE (Rest, Ice Compression and Elevation) treatment. Many athletes suffer ligament sprains when they are injured during play. Ligaments are the supporting structures of the musculoskeletal system that connect the bones to each other. A stretched or weakened ligament is defined as a sprain. In order to heal these injuries, the body produces an inflammatory response designed to bring blood flow and nutrients to the weakened area. However, the modern medical treatment protocol stops that process right in its tracks, actually decreasing ligament strength. *(See Figure 2-2.)*

NATURE'S PROLOTHERAPY: JOINT SWELLING

When athletes twist their knees during soccer or basketball games, for example, and suffer meniscal and/or

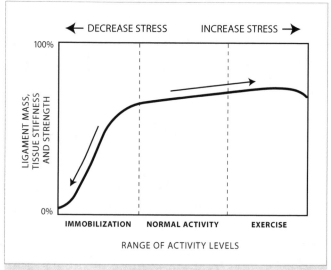

Figure 2-2: The response of ligaments to different levels of stress and motion. Ligaments (and tendons) weaken in response to immobilization, but increase in strength to moderate stresses and motion.

Adapted from: Jung HJ, et al. Role of biomechanics in the understanding of normal, injured, and healing ligaments and tendons. Sports Med Arthrosc Rehabil Ther Technol. 2009;1:9.

ligament tears, the inflammation that results is nature's Prolotherapy; an attempt by the body to heal the injuries as quickly as possible. Immediately after the injury, the athlete has one of two choices: eliminate the chemistry that is causing the joint swelling or eliminate the cause of the joint swelling.

The MEAT protocol, including Prolotherapy, stimulates the repair of the structures that are causing the joint instability. This offers a long-term cure of the problem and resolution of the joint swelling. Unfortunately, modern medicine's attempts to ease pain using RICE and NSAIDs is effective at decreasing the short-term pain, but does so at the cost of creating long-term pain by stopping the inflammatory healing cascade that is needed to heal the injury. Realize that even the creator of the RICE protocol, Gabe Mirkin, MD, states that inflammation is necessary for healing and that RICE can delay healing.[2]

When the body suffers a muscle, ligament, tendon, cartilage or fibrocartilage (meniscus, labrum) trauma, substances including prostaglandins and cytokines are released from the injured tissues and cells to promote the inflammatory healing cascade; in effect, this is **nature's Prolotherapy.**

What does the body want to do after an injury? Heal, of course! Go to any medical textbook, website on healing, or exercise physiology text and you will find that the normal inflammatory healing cascade must be stimulated not hampered, in order for the body to heal after trauma or an athlete to improve in athletics.

Research even in the 1990s revealed that NSAIDs delay and hamper the healing in all of the soft tissues, including muscles, ligaments, tendons, and cartilage. Anti-inflammatories can delay healing and delay it significantly, even in muscles with tremendous blood supply. In one study on muscle strains, piroxicam essentially wiped out the entire inflammatory proliferative phase of healing (days 0-4). At day 2, there were essentially no macrophages (cells that clean up the area) in the area and by day four after the muscle strain, very little muscle regeneration was observed compared to the normal healing process. The muscle strength at this time was only about 40% of normal.[3]

THE BIOLOGY OF PROLOTHERAPY:
THE INFLAMMATORY CASCADE

All human ailments, including ligament and tendon injury, involve inflammation. Inflammation is defined as the reaction of vascularized, living tissue to local injury.[4] The first stage of inflammation is the actual injury. Inflammation is the body's reaction to a local injury. Healing an injured area is dependent on the blood supplying inflammatory cells to repair the damaged tissue, which explains why vascularized, living tissue is crucial to the repair of any injured area. Vascularization refers to the blood supply to an area. Poor blood flow proportionately reduces healing.

Chronically weak ligaments and tendons are a result of inadequate repair following an injury and occur because of poor blood supply to the area where ligaments and tendons attach to the bone, the fibro-osseous junction (also known as the enthesis.).[5-7] **(See Figure 2-3.)** Due to the poor blood supply, the immune cells necessary to repair the affected area cannot reach the injury. Inadequate healing is the result. Nonsteroidal anti-inflammatory drugs (NSAIDs) and ice treatments decrease the blood flow even further, thus hampering the body's capability to heal the injured tissue.

Healing of an injured tissue, such as a ligament, progresses through a series of stages: inflammatory, fibroblastic, and maturation.[5,6,8] The inflammatory stage is characterized by an increase in blood flow, transporting healing immune cells to the area, often resulting in painful swelling. Swelling tells the body, especially the brain, that an area of the body has been injured. The immune system is activated to send immune cells, called polymorphonuclear cells, also known as "polys," to the injured area and remove the debris. *(See Figure 2-4.)* Other immune cells, including the monocytes, histocytes, and macrophage cells, assist in the cleanup. The macrophages and polys begin the process of phagocytosis whereby they engulf and subsequently destroy debris and any other foreign matter in the body.

A day or two after the initial injury, the fibroblastic stage of healing begins. The body forms new blood vessels, a process called angiogenesis, because of factors released by the macrophage cells. Fibroblasts are formed from local cells or

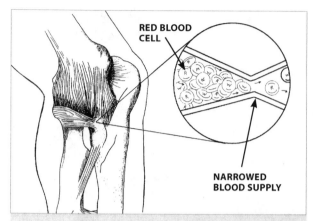

Figure 2-3: Poor blood supply at the fibro-osseous junction (enthesis). The fibro-osseous junction has poor blood supply compared to other structures such as muscles.

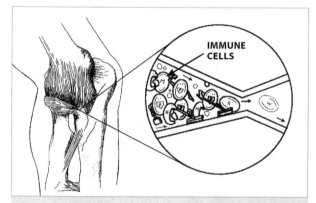

Figure 2-4: Immune system activity at the fibro-osseous junction (enthesis) immediately after an injury. Responding to an injury, the immune system activates to remove debris.

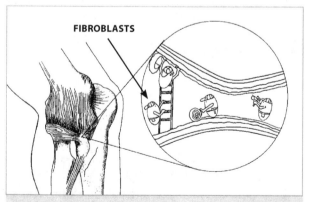

Figure 2-5: Immune system growing tissue at the fibro-osseous junction (enthesis). Fibroblasts forming new collagen tissue which makes the ligament and tendon strong.

other immune cells in the blood. They are the carpenters of the body that form new collagen tissue, the building blocks of ligaments and tendons. *(See Figure 2-5.)* Collagen is responsible for the strength of the ligament and tendon. The fibroblastic stage continues for approximately four to six weeks after the injury. Consequently, Prolotherapy treatments are typically administered every four to six weeks, allowing maximal time for ligament and tendon growth.[9]

The maturation phase of healing begins after the fibroblastic stage and may continue for 18 months after an injury. During this time the collagen fibers increase in density and diameter, resulting in increased strength. *(See Figure 2-6.)*

Anything that decreases inflammation is detrimental to the healing process of soft tissue injury. NSAIDs, for example, should only be prescribed when inflammation is the cause of the problem. In the case of soft tissue injury, inflammation is the cure for the problem. Prolotherapy injections stimulate ligament and tendon tissue growth, which only occurs through the process of inflammation. *(See Figure 2-7.)* Inflammation is the key to the treatment of human ailments. Those who suffer from chronic pain have a choice: Anti-inflame the pain to stay or inflame your pain away with Prolotherapy.

RICE VS MEAT: THE PROOF IS IN THE RESEARCH

RICE generally involves resting or immobilizing the joint for some time because of an injury. Patients are often taped, braced, casted, or told to rest because their injuries will not heal. Nothing could be worse for the articular cartilage throughout the joints of the body than this. The articular cartilage can only receive nourishment from the synovial fluid when it is pushed into the joint by weight-bearing and loading. The cartilage has no blood supply of its own. Moving, exercising, and loading the joint will allow the nourishment to get into the articular cartilage and the waste products to get out. There is only one effect of RICE and immobilization on cartilage—it is not good.

Basic animal research has shown that in as little as six days of immobilizing a joint, pressure necrosis of the articular cartilage can occur with subsequent degenerative arthritis.[10] Another study showed that prolonged immobilization, as occurs with casting, can lead to degeneration of the articular cartilage even in non-contact areas secondary to the adhesion of synovial membrane to the joint surface, which would not happen if the joints were moved. Subsequent use of such immobilized joints also led to degenerative arthritis.[11]

As expected, immobilization causes a reduction in chondrocyte synthesis.[11] The chondrocytes cannot be nourished without movement, so their ability to make collagen and proteoglycans for the articular cartilage declines with immobility. Studies have confirmed that simple immobilization causes a thinning of articular cartilage and, specifically, a decrease in the glycosaminoglycan and chondroitin sulfate.[10,11]

The Biology of Prolotherapy

Inflammatory Cascade.

After tissue damage by injury, the body attempts to heal the area by mediating this cascade. When the body is unable to heal itself, which is often the case when avascular (no or little blood supply) tissues such as ligaments, tendons, cartilage and fibrocartilage (meniscus and labrum) are injured, Prolotherapy is utilized to stimulate healing.

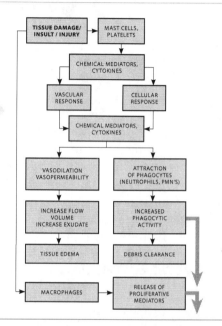

Proliferation Cascade.

Prolotherapy stimulates healing via inflammation. After Prolotherapy solutions are injected into the injury site, a cellular reaction takes place in which various cells including fibroblasts, endothelial cells and myofibroblasts form new blood vessels and ultimately lay down collagen which enhances tissue repair and strength.

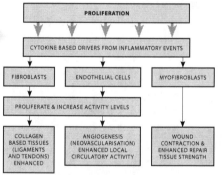

Tissue Remodeling Cascade.

The final phase of healing is tissue remodeling. For many months after an injury or Prolotherapy, tissue continues to remodel. The new tissue that results looks and functions very closely to the original tissue before the injury. Once the tissue strength approaches that of the normal parent tissue, pain resolves.

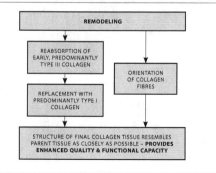

Figure 2-6: The biology of Prolotherapy.

MOVEMENT HEALS

Exercise, on the other hand, has a dramatic effect of increasing chondrocyte synthesis.[12] This would be expected since exercise enhances the ability of the chondrocytes to receive nutrients and eliminate waste. Exercise has the following beneficial effects:

- Enhances the nutrition and metabolic activity of articular cartilage.
- Stimulates pluripotential mesenchymal cells to differentiate into articular cartilage.
- Accelerates healing of both articular cartilage and periarticular tissues, such as tendons and ligaments.[13]

The above was all proven by the many studies done by Dr. Robert Salter at the University of Toronto. Dr. Robert Salter is the father of the theory that a limb must be continuously moved after an injury. He found that the healing rate was six times greater comparing movement and exercise with immobility in patients with articular cartilage defects.[10] Articular cartilage injuries which are rested have an over 50% chance of causing compromised range of motion of the limb at one year. Cartilage-damaged limbs that are exercised had completely normal motion. Articular cartilage defects in rabbits that were immobilized caused 50% of them to develop arthritis at one year. None had visible evidence of arthritis in the exercised group.[14]

Dr. Salter showed that 80% of articular cartilage fractures healed with exercise and movement, where none healed in the immobilized group. In an interesting study on infected joints, the researchers showed that continuous passive motion of the joint had a striking and statistically significant protective effect on prevention of progressive degeneration of the articular cartilage, when compared with the effects of

PROLOTHERAPY STIMULATES INFLAMMATION

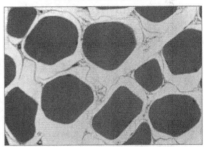

NORMAL MUSCLE TISSUE

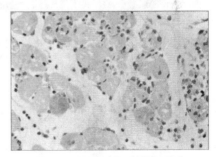

MUSCLE TISSUE 48 HOURS AFTER PROLOTHERAPY: Injections with 12.5% dextrose in 0.5% xylocaine. Notice the massive inflammatory reaction—the basis of Prolotherapy.

Figure 2-7: Prolotherapy stimulates inflammation. Prolotherapy stimulates the natural healing mechanisms of the body via inflammation. Slides prepared by Gale Bordon, MD, from K. Dean Reeves, MD. Used with permission.

immobilization.[15] Dr. Salter felt the possible explanations for these findings were the following:

- Prevention of adhesions (scar tissue).
- Improvement of nutrition of the cartilage through increased diffusion of synovial fluid.
- Enhancement of clearance of lysosomal enzymes and purulent exudate from the infected joints (removal of the bad stuff).
- Stimulation of living chondrocytes to synthesize the various components of the matrix.

Dr. Salter showed by x-ray and clinical findings that the animals that received exercise did much better than the ones who were immobilized. This same statement could be said about Prolotherapy.

One of the great things about Prolotherapy is that movement is encouraged during the treatment course. Those patients who lead an active lifestyle are particularly thankful for that. Those who are sedentary use this as an opportunity to change their lifestyles in order to maximize healing. Joint injuries requiring the patients to limit weight-bearing, require adaptation of the rehabilitation programs, but not complete rest by any means. We utilize a number of exercises that are non-weight-bearing, but get the patients moving and even increase their heart rates so that fitness can be maintained, or achieved if the patients were previously sedentary (often due to the injury.) Running on the elliptical machine, stationary cycling, swimming, and fluid (pool) running are activities that we utilize with our patients in these circumstances. Because we are athletes ourselves, we know the importance of daily physical activity for overall health and well being. We provide individualized physical activity and rehabilitation programs for all of our Prolotherapy patients at Caring Medical and work closely with them to achieve their goals, adapting the workouts as needed.

Continuous passive motion exercise was also shown to heal or clear a hemarthrosis (blood in the joint) twice as fast as immobilized limbs.[16] This is significant for patients who have massive bruising of a joint. The notion that the area must be iced and compressed to decrease swelling is outdated. Ice and compression will decrease swelling, but will also compromise healing. Bleakley reported that ice seemed to be more effective at limiting swelling and decreasing pain in the short-term, immediately after injury; however the long-term effects on tissue repair seemed to indicate that evidence is limited and outcome has not been shown to improve with use of ice post injury.[17] Yes, there is a better way. The best way to resolve swelling is to use the MEAT treatment. This involves exercise and proteolytic enzymes, which help clean out the damaged tissue. Exercise or passive motion by a physical therapist or on your own at home is tremendously effective at helping resolve the bleeding and edema but will also aid the healing process.

Dr. Salter summarized his first 18 years of basic research on the biologic concept of continuous passive motion (CPM) exercise with the following conclusions:

- CPM exercise is well tolerated.
- CPM exercise has a significant stimulating effect on the healing of articular tissues, including cartilage, tendons, and ligaments.
- CPM exercise prevents adhesions and joint stiffness.
- CPM exercise does not interfere with the healing of incisions over the moving joint.
- The time-honored principle that healing tissues must be put to rest is incorrect: indeed—it is this principle that must be put to rest rather than the healing soft tissues.
- Regeneration of articular cartilage through neochondrogenesis both with and without periosteal grafts is possible under the influence of CPM exercise.[13]

Dr. Salter wrote those words in the 1980s, yet there are still people with injuries around the world doing the RICE protocol today. Putting injured tissues to rest hurts the healing process. Animals continue their activities after an injury, therefore they heal well after an injury. Human beings need to do the same. It is time for a paradigm shift from the RICE to MEAT protocol to encourage healing of soft tissue and cartilage injuries. Exercise is vital to this process. His work continues to be validated years later. Here are a few more studies that show motion is helpful.

JOINT SWELLING PRODUCES HEALING

Let's face it, most traumatic injuries to the body actually heal on their own! How do they heal? They go through the inflammatory cascade, just as if the body received Prolotherapy! Why? Because the body has its own type of Prolotherapy which is the inflammation that occurs after an injury. The stimulus for healing with basic Prolotherapy is the D-glucose (dextrose) that is injected and with Cellular Prolotherapy it is the patient's own blood, platelets, bone marrow, or lipoaspirate. *(See Figure 2-8.)* What most people do not realize is that the initial trauma releases these same substances to the injury site. When cells burst open from the trauma, D-glucose and cytokines are released from inside the cell, platelets change their shape to stop the bleeding and release growth factors such as platelet-derived growth factor and fibroblastic growth factor and the arachidonic acid from the lipid layer of the cells eventually is turned into various prostaglandins. This inflammatory reaction sends a signal to the brain that a four-alarm injury is occurring in this location and we need resources! Soon the resources arrive on the scene, but along with them comes pain! Remember, pain is a blessing because it tells the body there is a problem that needs to be fixed. The best course of action is to let the body fix it. *(See Figure 2-9.)*

The Science Behind Prolotherapy

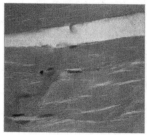

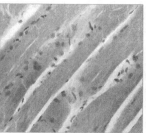

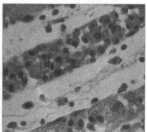

Normal muscle tissue (prior to Prolotherapy).

Photos compliments of K. Dean Reeves, MD. Slides made by Gale Bordon, MD, and given to various members of the Prolotherapy Association in the 1960s. Dr. Bordon's research into the histology of Prolotherapy was presented at the annual Clinical Symposium of the Prolotherapy Association, June 16, 1968, Bellevue Hotel, San Francisco, California. Used with permission from Yvonne Bordon.

Muscle tissue 96 hours after an injection with 12.5% dextrose and 0.5% xylocaine. Note the high concentration of fibroblasts, indicative of a good inflammatory reaction. This is the basic Hackett-Hemwall Prolotherapy solution.

Muscle tissue 96 hours after an injection with 12.5% dextrose and an equal amount of 1% xylocaine, 2.5% phenol, and 12.5% glycerine. The inflammatory reaction is substantial in comparison with the middle photo. This is the Prolotherapy solution known as P2G.

Figure 2-8: The science behind Prolotherapy. Prolotherapy stimulates the body to repair the painful area. The various solutions, when injected into the injured area, induce the normal inflammatory cascade to help heal such tissues as ligaments, tendons, discs, and cartilage.

AREN'T ALL TYPES OF ARTHRITIS DUE TO INFLAMMATORY PROCESSES?

Osteoarthritis is simply not rheumatoid arthritis. Rheumatoid arthritis is a systemic inflammatory condition and treatment involves use of medications that inhibit tumor-necrosis factor such as Enbrel® and Humira® (or generics etanercept and adalimumab) which have been shown to enhance quality of life and slow the arthritic process. However, to think osteoarthritis is the same process is delusional. Consider the fact that in rheumatoid arthritis you went from giving patients high dose steroids and methotrexate (chemotherapy drug) to these tumor–necrosis factor inhibitors. Anything would be an improvement from having to take a chemotherapy drug! Rheumatoid arthritis is a systemic disease affecting the whole body. Osteoarthritis or a single joint disease develops because the person injures his knee and swelling results in that individual joint. Osteoarthritis might develop if the condition goes untreated and bony overgrowth starts in order to try to stabilize the unstable joint. This is a localized single joint

The Many Benefits of Joint Swelling
- Promotes joint stability immediately after injury.
- Alerts the body of an injury.
- Stimulates the healing cascade.
- Cushions the articular cartilage.
- Evenly distributes pressure in joint.
- Promotes stability in joint upon reinjury.
- Important signal to gauge activity level and treatment.
- Indicates level of healing.

Figure 2-9: The many benefits of joint swelling.

disease! Does it make sense to offer drug treatments that are passed throughout the entire body; whether an NSAID or cytokine inhibitor? It does not make any sense.

In rheumatoid arthritis, which involves joint swelling, an increase in cytokines, such as tumor-necrosis factor and interleukin-1, occurs in the joint fluid. Therefore, modern medicine uses drugs to block these substances thinking that the joint swelling will be reduced and hopefully the amount of articular cartilage breakdown will also be reduced. In rheumatoid arthritis this has been successful, except the articular cartilage still breaks down. You see, the advent of these medications, though more sophisticated, is still producing the same old story: modern therapeutics believing the savior for joint pain is going to be a **drug**, when clearly the cause of the disease and the propagation of the joint swelling is joint instability! Treatment should be geared **at repairing the cause of the joint swelling, not the chemistry of the joint swelling!**

Halting joint swelling with a drug makes no sense. The RICE protocol and NSAIDs can stop a joint from swelling for the short-term. Use of more sophisticated drugs such as interleukin-1 blockers or corticosteroid injections (or for that matter, interleukin injection blockers) just limit joint swelling for a longer period of time, but you leave the joint vulnerable to further injury and degeneration. In a knee ligament injury, such as the medial collateral ligament (MCL), forces on the joint are concentrated on the medial side. Swelling helps to disperse the forces on the joint in an attempt to protect the joint structures, including the medial cartilage. By taking NSAIDs and applying the RICE technique, the protective swelling mechanism cannot help disperse the force on the knee joint. Therefore, the medial cartilage deteriorates faster. Taking anti-inflammatories while maintaining athletics and activities can become a devastating combination. Without the joint swelling, stretching the ligaments, which then activates nerve endings within the ligament, the body has no idea that the joint is breaking down. So as your joint is breaking down, you feel no pain because you have taken these medications. What will be the long-term result? Pain from progressive aggressive osteoarthritis.

FROM BEGINNING TO END,
ENHANCE VS INHIBIT THE HEALING CASCADE

Joints need motion without stress after injury. Many of our patients do deep water running, which is one of the best ways to get motion without stress. Some swim in a pool or cycle. As the injury heals they progress to more advanced exercises. We tell our patients to feel the injured joint before and after exercise and compare it to the uninjured side. Heat is indicative of joint swelling. When the joint swells from inflammation, it will feel warm compared to the uninjured side; thus joint swelling is a great indication to guide not only exercise and activity, but also therapies.

Immediately after an injury heat is produced in the joint. As a Prolotherapist, this is helpful to guide the therapy. Injection solutions can be modified to stimulate healing, but not promote more pain and swelling. Once the heat is eliminated from the joint, then more "inflammatory" solutions can be used. Our patients can receive Prolotherapy immediately after injuries. As for more severe injuries, Prolotherapy can speed up healing many-fold, and our athletes typically do not want to be out of competitions for months, so they come in for Prolotherapy treatments right away. This is especially true for meniscus and labrum tears. The earlier a patient starts treatment, the quicker he gets back on the field!

Swelling in the joint is also a guide as to how much exercise to do and how to proceed. We ask our athletes to check the temperature of the injured joint before, during, and immediately after exercise. If the joint becomes hotter during the exercise, this means that the exercise is causing the joint to move into an unstable position, producing joint swelling (the body's attempt to stabilize the joint) and thus, this particular exercise is inhibiting, not stimulating healing. These same guidelines are given after Prolotherapy. It is definitely possible for an athlete to experience setbacks just because of pushing the exercise too much after an injury. After an injury or after Prolotherapy do not push exercise to the point where the joint feels hot. New heat sensations in the joint means the joint is swelling because the activity or exercise put the joint in a compromised, unstable position which will inhibit, not help healing! So you can see, receiving treatments that stop joint swelling could have major devastating effects on joints that would clearly promote osteoarthritis, not slow its progression!

Joint swelling indicates that the joint is unstable. The injured person has two choices: change the chemistry that is causing the joint swelling or treat the cause of the chemical changes which cause the joint instability. Prolotherapy treats the cause. Without treating the joint instability, even if modern medicine comes up with a medication concoction that blocks 80 of the 100 substances that cause joint swelling, there will still be 20 left because the cause of the joint swelling will remain. The best way to approach life is to always solve the underlying cause of the problem vs a band-aid approach. Medications for joint instability are just a bunch of band-aids. These band-aids, even if seemingly successful at slowing the degenerative cascade, (though this is not true in most cases), allow the underlying disease process to continue. The joint instability is never resolved. With the body's protective mechanism gone (joint instability), the person puts too much pressure on the joint and this leads to progressive, aggressive joint degeneration which will ultimately lead to further medication and procedures including surgeries such as joint replacements.

For the independent thinker who says, "I don't want joint replacement in my future," Prolotherapy is the best treatment option because it gets at the root cause of the joint swelling which is joint instability caused by injury to one of the white structures, including the ligaments, meniscus, or labrum. Once the injured joint structures are repaired, joint swelling is eliminated. Once the joint swelling is eliminated, the patient can exercise without hesitancy for the rest of his life. This gives peace of mind and where there is peace of mind, there is health.

ANTI-INFLAMMATORY MEDICATIONS AND STEROID INJECTIONS: THE WORST TREATMENTS FOR HEALING!

As we have been reiterating in this chapter, the body heals by the process of inflammation. Taking medications that stop inflammation will subsequently stop the body from healing. Arthritis is one of the most common conditions causing pain. Interestingly enough, the reason arthritis forms in the first place is because an injured area did not heal. The pain of the initial injury may have been relieved by taking a medication that blunted the symptoms, but the injured tissue remained injured, as manifested by decreased strength. Exercise alone does not cause arthritis. Only injury causes arthritis. In a study where dogs were exercised for one year carrying jackets weighing 130% of their body weight, all knee joints were inspected for evidence of joint injury and degeneration at the completion of the study. Articular cartilage surfaces from the medial tibial plateau were examined by light microscopy, the cartilage thickness was measured, and intrinsic material properties were determined by mechanical testing. No joints had ligament or meniscal injuries, cartilage erosions, or osteophytes. Light microscopy did not demonstrate fibrillations in the cartilage. Furthermore, the tibial articular cartilage thickness and mechanical properties did not differ between the exercised group and non-exercised group. These results show that a lifetime of regular weight-bearing exercise in dogs with normal joints did not cause alterations in the structure and mechanical properties of articular cartilage that might lead to joint degeneration.[18] Exercise is healthy and does not cause injury if properly performed. If an injury occurs, it is important to treat it until it is completely healed. The worst things for healing an injury are to take anti-inflammatories and receive cortisone injections. These are the main reasons so many people have articular cartilage problems.

NSAIDS

Ibuprofen became available over the counter in 1984. People have been reaching over the counter ever since then. Sales of over-the-counter pain relievers were $2.67 billion dollars in 1994. There are numerous studies showing the deleterious effects of anti-inflammatories, such as ibuprofen, on healing. Ibuprofen, the prototype anti-inflammatory medication, has been shown to have an inhibitory effect on bone healing, remodeling, resorption, and metabolism.[19-22] Ibuprofen has also been shown to have a tremendous dose-dependent suppressive effect on articular cartilage healing.[23] As ibuprofen doses increase, healing of the articular cartilage decreases.

Not only is there no evidence that NSAIDs favorably modify the progression of joint breakdown in patients with osteoarthritis or cartilage injury, several NSAIDs, for example, acetylsalicylic acid (aspirin), fenoprofen, tolmetin, and ibuprofen, have been shown to inhibit the synthesis of proteoglycans by normal cartilage.[16,24,25] Because proteoglycans are essential for the elasticity and compressive stiffness of articular cartilage, suppression of their synthesis as a consequence of NSAID administration must have adverse consequences. **(See Figure 2-10.)**

NSAIDs inhibit cyclooxygenase, the enzyme involved in the synthesis of prostaglandins which aid in the inflammatory healing response. NSAIDs have the additional effect of inhibiting the enzymes involved in proteoglycan biosynthesis. Aspirin and ibuprofen, in concentrations that can be achieved in joint tissues, inhibit glucuronyltransferase, an enzyme responsible for the elongation of chondroitin sulfate chains on the proteoglycan complex.[26,27] NSAIDs inhibit the synthesis of proteoglycans that are being made by the chondrocytes to heal the articular cartilage damage.[28] The only result that can be obtained from NSAIDs in a patient with articular cartilage damage is a guarantee to produce more damage. This is exactly what is seen. **(See Figure 2-11.)**

When animals with anterior cruciate ligament injuries were given NSAIDs the amount of articular cartilage damage that occurred over time was accelerated at a wicked rate. The proteoglycan concentration of the cartilage matrix was also suppressed significantly.[26,29]

In 1967, Dr. H. Coke was the first medical doctor to suggest that NSAIDs might accelerate bone destruction.[30] More reports confirmed his suspicions shortly thereafter.[31] In a retrospective study of patients with osteoarthritis of the hip,

The Effect of NSAIDs on Joints

- Acceleration of radiographic progression of osteoarthritis.
- Decreased joint space width.
- Increased joint forces/loads.
- Increased risk of joint replacement.
- Inhibition of chondrocyte proliferation.
- Inhibition of collagen synthesis.
- Inhibition of glycosaminoglycan synthesis.
- Inhibition of prostagalandin synthesis.
- Inhibition of proteoglycan synthesis.
- Inhibition of synthesis of cellular matrix components.

Figure 2-10: NSAIDs taken long-term have a negative effect on joint physiology and ultimately lead to degenerative arthritis.

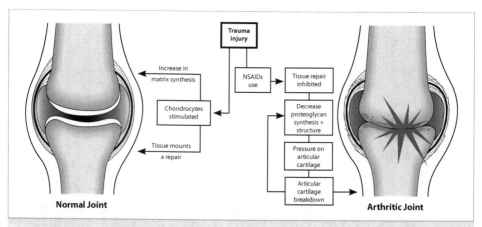

Figure 2-11: The pathogenesis of osteoarthritis accelerated by NSAIDs. NSAID use inhibits the body's repair processes, leading to decreased proteoglycan and extracellular matrix content and function, which ultimately leads to articular cartilage breakdown.

a variety of NSAIDs were considered to have contributed to destruction of the hip joint, as confirmed by x-ray studies.[32] Another study confirmed that the stronger the NSAIDs, the faster the arthritic changes occurred.[33] This is why people who start on the anti-inflammatory train need stronger and stronger medications. The NSAIDs accelerate the degenerative process. *(See Figure 2-12.)*

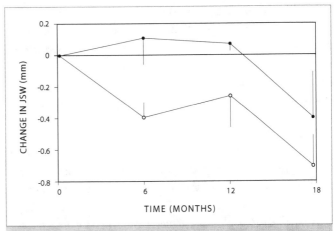

Figure 2-12: Graph of the mean (SD) change in joint space width at each 6-month visit in knees with late stage osteoarthritis (joint space width <50% of that in normal healthy knees) in patients receiving either diclofenac (○) or placebo (●).

Source: Buckland-Wright JC, et al. Quantitative microfocal radiography detects changes in OA knee joint space width in patients in placebo-controlled trial of NSAID therapy. *J Rheumatol.* 1995;22:937-43.

In an interesting study involving 20 rheumatology clinics in the United Kingdom, patients were placed in a placebo group or in a group that received daily indomethacin. Radiographic analysis was done yearly with an average length of follow up being three years. By the third year of the study, the results were so dramatic demonstrating the acceleration of the degeneration of the articular cartilage in the osteoarthritic knee patients that this part of the study had to be stopped. There were more than twice as many patients showing deterioration in the indomethacin group as the placebo.[34]

NSAIDs also have adverse effects on bone healing. Interactions occur between prostaglandin metabolism, inflammatory proteins, and bone metabolism. Systemic as well as local source of inflammation appear to be actively involved in both bone formation and resorption. NSAIDs can actually harm bone fracture healing and have a negative impact on bone resorption.[35]

CONTINUED EVIDENCE AGAINST USING NSAIDS

Just as older studies revealed the ill effects of using NSAIDs for the management of soft injuries, a paper published in 2012 showed that there is little evidence in support of using NSAIDs for pain reduction in soft tissue injuries. Potential side effects are a serious cause for concern.[36]

Ibuprofen is often prescribed after tendon repair. This study showed that early administration of ibuprofen in the postoperative period was detrimental to tendon healing. Thus this shows that ibuprofen should also not be used when treating acute tendon injuries.[37]

In our extensive review of the use of NSAIDs in osteoarthritis (OA), the results are overwhelming against their long-term use.[38] We found that in human studies, NSAIDs have been shown to accelerate the radiographic progression of OA of the knee and hip. For those using NSAIDs compared to the patients who do not use them, joint replacements occur earlier and more quickly and frequently. We noted that massive NSAID use in osteoarthritic patients since their introduction over the past forty years is one of the main causes of the rapid rise in the need for hip and knee replacements, both now and in the future.

While it is admirable for the various consensus and rheumatology organizations to educate doctors and the lay public about the necessity to limit NSAID use in OA, we recommended that the following warning label be on each NSAID bottle:

> *The use of this nonsteroidal anti-inflammatory medication has been shown in scientific studies to accelerate the articular cartilage breakdown in osteoarthritis. Use of this product poses a significant risk in accelerating osteoarthritis joint breakdown. Anyone using this product for the pain of osteoarthritis should be under a doctor's care and the use of this product should be with the very lowest dosage and for the shortest duration of time.*

If NSAID use continues, then most likely the exponential rise in degenerative arthritis and subsequent musculoskeletal surgeries, including knee and hip replacements as well as spine surgeries, will continue to rise as well. One research team confirmed that NSAID use increases the risk of getting a hip replacement due to primary osteoarthritis by 50% during a two year period.[39]

For the athlete or the physically active person, the RICE treatment is a scary prospect. It devastates the natural healing response. People are often given NSAIDs along with RICE, which further suppresses the local inflammatory reaction that is needed to heal the injured tissues. Instead of recommending Prolotherapy for continued complaints of pain, the usual course of treatment is perhaps the most potent of all anti-healing therapies: the cortisone shot.

WANT NO BONE? TAKE CORTISONE!

Receiving a cortisone shot is one of the quickest ways to lose strength at the ligament-bone junction (fibro-osseous junction or enthesis). Cortisone and other steroid shots have the same detrimental effects on articular cartilage healing.[40] *(See Figure 2-13.)*

Corticosteroids, such as cortisone and prednisone, have adverse effects on bone and soft tissue healing. Corticosteroids inactivate vitamin D, limiting calcium absorption by the gastrointestinal tract and increasing the urinary excretion of calcium. Bone also shows a decrease in calcium uptake, ultimately leading to weakness at the fibro-osseous junction (enthesis). Corticosteroids also inhibit the release of Growth Hormone, which further decreases soft tissue and bone repair.

Ultimately, corticosteroids lead to a decrease in bone, ligament, and tendon strength.[41-46]

Corticosteroids inhibit the synthesis of proteins, collagen, and proteoglycans, particularly cartilage, by inhibiting the production of chondrocytes, which are the cells that comprise the articular cartilage. *(See Figure 2-14.)* The net catabolic effect (weakening) of corticosteroids is inhibition of fibroblast production of collagen, ground substance, and angiogenesis (new blood vessel formation). The result is weakened synovial joints, supporting structures, articular cartilage, ligaments, and tendons. This weakness increases the pain, and the increased pain leads to more steroid injections. Cortisone injections should play almost no role in injury care or pain management.

Although anti-inflammatory medications and steroid injections reduce pain, they do so at the cost of

> ### Known Effects of Intraarticular Corticosteroids on Articular Cartilage
>
> - Deleterious effects more serious in animals with the greatest number of injections.
> - Higher doses leads to worse deterioration.
> - Destruction worsened with time and exercise.
> - Inhibition of synthesis and deposition of chondroitin sulfate and glycosaminoglycan.
> - Breakdown of proteoglycans and collagen.
> - Decrease of protein and matrix synthesis.
> - Matrix hyaline appearance becomes fibrous.
> - Clumping of collagen.
> - Alteration in chondrocyte cell shape.
> - Chondrocyte cytotoxicity enhanced.
> - Loss of chondrocytes.
> - Surface deterioration including edema, pitting, shredding, ulceration and erosions.
> - Inhibition of articular cartilage metabolism.
> - Articular cartilage necrosis.
> - Thinning of articular cartilage.
> - Decrease of cartilage growth and repair.
> - Formation of articular cartilage cysts.
> - Articular cartilage destruction.

Figure 2-13: Known effects of intraarticular corticosteroids on articular cartilage.

destroying tissue. In a study conducted by Siraya Chunekamrai, DVM, PhD, steroid shots were given to horses with a substance commonly used in humans. The injected tissue was examined under the microscope. The steroid shots induced a tremendous amount of damage including chondrocyte necrosis (cartilage cell damage), hypocellularity (decreased number of cells) in the joint, decreased proteoglycan content and synthesis, and decreased collagen synthesis in the joint. All of these effects were permanent.[47]

Dr. Chunekamrai concluded, "The effects on cartilage of intra-articular injections of methylprednisolone acetate (steroid) were not ameliorated at eight weeks after eight weekly injections, or 16 weeks after a single injection. Cartilage remained biochemically and metabolically impaired."[47] In this study, some of the joints were injected only one time. Even after one steroid injection, cartilage remained biochemically and metabolically impaired. Other studies have confirmed similar harmful effects of steroids on joint and cartilage tissue.[48,49] A cortisone shot can permanently damage joints. Prolotherapy injections have the opposite effect— they permanently strengthen joints. *Figure 2-15* explains the monumental difference between cortisone and Prolotherapy injections.

Corticosteroids are often used to treat tendon injuries but may also be associated with tendon ruptures and impaired healing. This study by Scutt revealed that

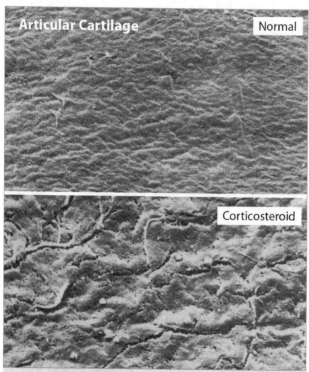

Figure 2-14: Electronmicroscopy of articular cartilage after saline injections versus corticosteroid injections. Articular cartilage injected with saline has a normal, smooth appearance (top), whereas corticosteroid injected cartilage has obvious fissuring and is in the process of deteriorating (bottom).

Pictures originally from the *Journal of Anatomy*, volume 127, Oct. 1978, pages 393-402. Article title: Effects of intraarticularly administered corticosteroids and salicylates on the surface structure of articular cartilage.

dexamethasone (steroids) reduced both cell number and collagen synthesis in tenocyte culture in a concentration-dependent manner by both direct effect on tenocyte proliferation and collagen accumulation, as well as by changing the recruitment of tendon progenitor cells. In other words, the steroid injections stopped the healing process.[50]

In another study performed on knees, researchers found that dexamethasone (steroid injections) caused a paradoxical effect on the injured tendons it was supposed to treat by causing non-tenocyte differentiation of hTSCs, depleting the stem cell pool and leading to the formation of non-tendious tissues such as fatty and cartilage-like tissues, making the tendons more susceptible to rupture.[51]

In a review study by Coombes, corticosteroid injections reduced pain in the short-term compared with other interventions, but this effect was reversed at intermediate and long-terms in treating epicondylagia.[52]

Single intraarticular injections for sacroiliac pain using steroids showed a short-term positive response but long-term response was not provided.[53]

Dexamethasone significantly decreased cell viability, suppressed cell proliferation, and reduced collagen synthesis in cultured human tenocytes (tendon cells).[54]

Unfortunately, many people suffering with chronic pain look for quick relief without thinking about the long-term, potentially harmful side effects that could occur such as those clearly outlined in the aforementioned papers. The problem with cortisone is that immediate pain relief is possible, but in reality it may be permanently reducing the ability to remain active. For example, athletes often receive cortisone shots in order to be able to play. They then go onto the playing field with severe injuries that required cortisone shots to relieve the pain. Because they feel no pain, they play as if the injury does not exist. The injury will, unfortunately, never heal because of the tremendous anti-healing properties of cortisone. The athlete is, therefore, further injuring himself by playing. The same goes for the chronic pain sufferer who is trying to return to normal function.

Cortisone is dangerous because it inhibits just about every aspect of healing. Cortisone inhibits prostaglandin and leukotriene production, as already discussed. It also inhibits chondrocyte production of protein polysaccharides (proteoglycans), which are the major constituents of articular ground substance.[55] Behrens and his colleagues reported a persistent and highly significant reduction in the synthesis of proteins, collagen, and proteoglycans in the articular cartilage of rabbits who received weekly injections of glucocorticoids. They also reported a progressive loss of endoplasmic reticulum, mitochondria, and Golgi apparatus as the number of injections increased.[55]

Cortisone Versus Prolotherapy

	Cortisone	Prolotherapy
Capillary dilation	Decreased	Increased
Blood flow	Decreased	Increased
Migration of immune cells to area	Decreased	Increased
Phagocytic activity (clean up)	Decreased	Increased
Leukocyte numbers in area	Decreased	Increased
Capillary proliferation (new blood vessels)	Decreased	Increased
Fibroblast proliferation	Decreased	Increased
Deposition of collagen	Decreased	Increased
Collagen strength	Decreased	Increased
Protein synthesis	Decreased	Increased
Tissue strength	Decreased	Increased

Figure 2-15: Cortisone versus Prolotherapy. There really is no comparison.

THE ROLE OF EXERCISE IN INJURY: RESEARCH WITH EXERCISE AND CORTISONE

Exercise has the opposite effect of cortisone. Exercise has been shown to positively affect articular cartilage by increasing its thickness, enhancing the infusion of nutrients, and increasing matrix synthesis.[56-59] However, the effects of both exercise and cortisone in combination can be detrimental.

An excellent study pointing out the dangers of an athlete exercising after receiving cortisone was conducted by Dr. Prem Gogia and associates at the Washington University School of Medicine in St. Louis. Animals were divided into three groups: **1.** Group One received a cortisone shot only. **2.** Group Two received a cortisone shot and exercised, and **3.** The Control Group received no treatment. This study was done in 1993 and was the first study to look at the effects of exercising after receiving cortisone shots. The authors did this study because it was common practice in sports medicine to give an athlete with an acute or chronic injury a cortisone shot. Athletes were typically returning to full-intensity sports activities within a few hours to one or two days after receiving the shot.

The animals receiving the cortisone shots showed a decrease in chondrocytes. When they exercised in addition to the cortisone shot, the chondrocyte cell count decreased by a full 25%. Degenerated cartilage was seen in all the cortisone–injected animals, but severe cartilage damage was seen in 67% of the animals that exercised and also received cortisone. The cortisone and exercise group also showed a significant decline in glycosaminoglycan synthesis compared to the other groups. The authors concluded, "The results suggest that running exercise in combination with intra-articular injections results in damage to the femoral articular cartilage."[59] *(See Figure 2-16.)*

SUMMARY

The body heals by the process of inflammation. Taking medications, using RICE, or injecting cortisone all block the natural inflammatory healing response of the body. Prolotherapy induces inflammation at the points where the injections were given, causing healing inflammatory cells to rush to the white, poor blood supply areas to help heal them. Prolotherapy is the only treatment that we know of that can stimulate healing in this area. Soft tissue injuries are not systemic problems, thus it makes no sense to take systemic medications. Let your body do what it is meant to do—heal. If you find you need assistance with the healing, consider Prolotherapy to do the job safely and effectively! ■

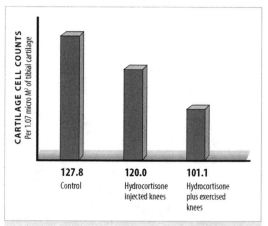

Figure 2-16: Cartilage cell counts decline with cortisone plus exercise. Hydrocortisone injections in the knee combined with exercise is a deadly combination for cartilage cells.

CHAPTER

CELLULAR PROLOTHERAPY

Hackett-Hemwall dextrose Prolotherapy stimulates repair of a painful area. The primary proliferant, dextrose, sets off the healing cascade in the injected area, attracting immune cells to the degenerated structure for the purpose of repair and healing. In some painful conditions, cellular proliferants are needed for the desired healing effect. These cases can be treated with Cellular Prolotherapy, which utilizes a person's own (called "autologous") growth factors and stem cells as the primary proliferant, delivering them directly to the injured area. As with all types of Prolotherapy, the goal is to assist the body in repair of the injured structures with tissues that are functionally, structurally, and mechanically equivalent to the pre-injured or pre-damaged tissue, along with elimination of pain and the return to full activities and sports.

CELLULAR PROLOTHERAPY ADDRESSES LOCALIZED CELLULAR DEFICIENCY

In degenerative diseases, such as osteoarthritis, the frequency and potency of an individual's mesenchymal stem cells may be depleted, along with a reduced proliferative capacity and ability to differentiate.[1,2] *(See Figure 3-1.)* Mesenchymal stem cells can self-renew and differentiate (or change)

TISSUE	CONDITION(S)
Cartilage	Osteoarthritis, osteochondral defect
Subchondral bone	Osteoarthritis
Ligament	Ligament sprains, joint instability, ligamentosis, enthesopathies
Meniscus	Meniscus degeneration, tears
Tendon	Tendinosis
Aged/damaged connective tissue	Myofascial pain, myalgias, non-healed painful connective tissues
Labrum	Labral degeneration, tears

Figure 3-1: Conditions and tissues with cellular deficiencies. Cellular Prolotherapy provides the cells and growth factors that these tissues and conditions lack, to aid in their healing.

into a variety of cell types including osteoblasts (bone cells), chondrocytes (cartilage cells), myocytes (muscle cells), fibroblasts (ligament and tendon cells), and others, homing in on injured tissue and initiating repair.[3-10] *(See Figure 3-2.)* Growth factors are also an important part of the repair process. These small proteins direct critical cellular functions such as cell division, matrix synthesis, and tissue differentiation. When activated, these growth factors augment stem cell proliferation and angiogenesis, which enhances musculoskeletal healing.[11,12] The mesenchymal stem cells and growth factors delivered during Cellular Prolotherapy beneficially alter the microenvironment of the injured area.

In one peer-reviewed article from Tokyo Medical and Dental University on articular cartilage defects in rabbits, the authors showed that direct mesenchymal stem cell injections stimulated articular cartilage repair. The authors were not trying to

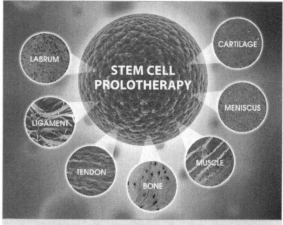

Figure 3-2. Conquer chronic pain with Stem Cell Prolotherapy. The mesenchymal stem cells used in Cellular Prolotherapy are able to differentiate into cells types such as labrum, ligament, tendon, bone, muscle, meniscus, and cartilage.

prove that direct bone marrow injection stimulates articular cartilage defects to heal, because they used the direct mesenchymal stem cell injection as a control. The study went as follows: full-thickness osteochondral defects (5mm x 5mm wide, 3mm deep) were created in the trochlear groove of the femurs in adult rabbits. The defect was filled with synovial mesenchymal cells suspension and then as controls, some of the cells were directly injected into the joint or nothing was done at all. They were examining the results of directly filling the defect compared to just injecting mesenchymal stem cells intra-articularly versus doing nothing at all. In total 36 rabbits' knees were examined macroscopically, histologically, as well as under the microscope with fluorescent dye (the mesenchymal stem cells were tagged with a dye to identify them.) The knees were examined at 12 weeks and 24 weeks. In the control group of animals where nothing was done, the articular cartilage defect remained, but in the intra-articular group as well as the group of animals where the mesenchymal stem cells were placed directly on the wound, the defects were completely covered by new articular cartilage tissue. In the directly placed group, the regenerated cartilage matrix was well developed. In other words, at 6 months, the intra-articular stem cell therapy group was regenerating articular cartilage, but it wasn't at the level of the normal cartilage, whereas when the stem cells were placed directly on the wound, the process was taking place at a faster rate.[13]

What does this mean? It means that if you inject stem cells into a joint with an articular cartilage defect, the stem cells do adhere to the wound and start regenerating cartilage. You can place the stem cells on the wound or you can inject them into the joint. *(See Figure 3-3.)*

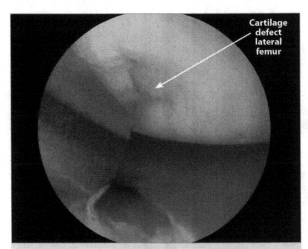

Cartilage defect lateral femur

Figure 3-3: Arthroscopy showing extensive knee degeneration. Comprehensive Prolotherapy provided tremendous pain relief for this patient.

TYPES OF CELLULAR PROLOTHERAPY AT CARING MEDICAL

AUTOLOGOUS BLOOD INJECTION (ABI)

ABI involves the injection of the patient's own blood into an area of the body for the purposes of healing. A blood draw is the easiest place to obtain reparative cells. The blood carries many healing elements including the platelets filled with growth factors and stem cells; however, the amount of stem cells is much greater in bone marrow and adipose tissue versus blood components. We and others have used ABI successfully in tendinopathies of the rotator cuff and epicondyle (elbow extensor tendon), as well as joint subluxations, including the tempomandibular joint.[14-18]

PLATELET RICH PLASMA (PRP) PROLOTHERAPY

Platelet Rich Plasma (PRP) has gained in popularity over recent years, particularly for athletic injuries and tendon degeneration (tendinosis). Platelets secrete numerous growth factors and other bioactive substances that contribute to healing through their initiation and regulation of the body's inflammatory wound–healing cascade.[19] *(See Figure 3-4.)* In addition to facilitating the inflammatory cascade, concentrated platelets also promote the migration, proliferation, and differentiation of mesenchymal and stromal repair cells to the area of injury.[20,21] PRP consists of a simple blood draw from the patient, plasma separation (which means the blood is centrifuged), and application of the plasma rich in growth factors (injecting the plasma into the afflicted joint.) *(See Figure 3-5.)*

High-density Platelet Rich Plasma (HD-PRP) is defined as autologous blood with concentrations of platelets at equal

Platelet-Derived Growth Factor (PDGF)	Attracts immune system cells to the area and stimulates them to proliferate. Has been shown to enhance ligament and tendon healing.
Transforming Growth Factor- β (TGF- β)	Secreted by and affects all major cell types involved in healing. Similar affects as PDGF.
Vascular Endothelial Growth Factor (VEGF)	Helps new blood vessel formation, thereby increasing vascularity in injured areas.
Fibroblast Growth Factor (FGF)	Promotes the growth of the cells involved in collagen and cartilage formation.

Figure 3-4. Various growth factors found in platelets and their actions.

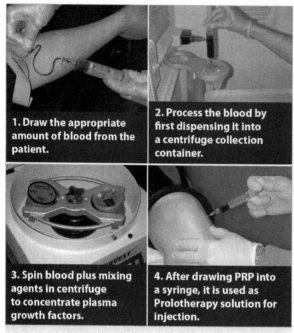

1. Draw the appropriate amount of blood from the patient.

2. Process the blood by first dispensing it into a centrifuge collection container.

3. Spin blood plus mixing agents in centrifuge to concentrate plasma growth factors.

4. After drawing PRP into a syringe, it is used as Prolotherapy solution for injection.

Figure 3-5: Platelet Rich Plasma (PRP) injection technique.

or greater than four (4) times circulating baseline levels, and which increases the important bioactive protein load (growth factors) in a direct correlative fashion.[22] Cell ratios in average circulating whole blood contain only 6% platelets. In true high-density PRP preparations, the concentration achieved is 94%.[21] An average patient platelet count is 250,000 platelets/dl. Four times this is 1 million platelets/dl, which is considered the desired benchmark for "therapeutic PRP."[23] In our experience, PRP has been an incredible addition to a Prolotherapist's arsenal for tendinosis, meniscal tears, labral tears, and other sports injuries. PRP Prolotherapy is typically given every 1-2 months for 3-6 visits.

STEM CELL PROLOTHERAPY

This term describes using autologous adult pluripotent mesenchymal stem cells (MSCs) from an individual's bone marrow or adipose (fat) tissue, as the "proliferating" solution. An interesting observation made about MSCs is the ability to "home in" and help repair areas of tissue injury.[24] Stem Cell Prolotherapy is typically done for more advanced cases of joint degeneration, including osteochondral defects, or where dextrose Prolotherapy and/or PRP Prolotherapy have not fully resolved a problem. *(See Figure 3-6.)* With Stem Cell Prolotherapy a stem cell niche (microenvironment which favors healing) is moved from one tissue in which these niches are abundant (adipose or bone marrow) into one where they are scarce (a non-repairing connective tissue).[25] Stem cells are activated by specific cues within this localized environment to either self replicate or differentiate. From these niches, the tissues, and ultimately the body, can maintain function and replace cells that have been damaged or have died. The niche is a physiologically segregated area of the tissue wherein stem cells are restrained from commitment to extensive proliferation and differentiation and where the stem cells are housed throughout life.[26,27] Of particular interest is the observation in degenerative diseases, such as osteoarthritis, that an individual's adult stem cell frequency and potency may be depleted, with reduced

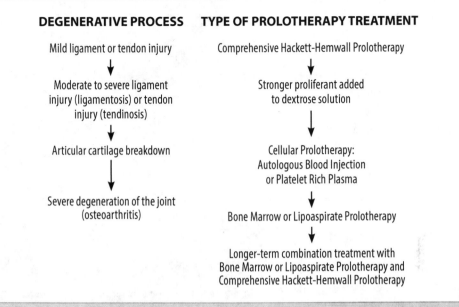

DEGENERATIVE PROCESS

Mild ligament or tendon injury
↓
Moderate to severe ligament injury (ligamentosis) or tendon injury (tendinosis)
↓
Articular cartilage breakdown
↓
Severe degeneration of the joint (osteoarthritis)

TYPE OF PROLOTHERAPY TREATMENT

Comprehensive Hackett-Hemwall Prolotherapy
↓
Stronger proliferant added to dextrose solution
↓
Cellular Prolotherapy: Autologous Blood Injection or Platelet Rich Plasma
↓
Bone Marrow or Lipoaspirate Prolotherapy
↓
Longer-term combination treatment with Bone Marrow or Lipoaspirate Prolotherapy and Comprehensive Hackett-Hemwall Prolotherapy

Figure 3-6: Applying the various types of Prolotherapy solutions. When soft tissue injuries are not treated early on with traditional Prolotherapy, the degenerative process continues, requiring the use of Cellular Prolotherapy to repair the damaged tissue and resolve the pain.

proliferative capacity and ability to differentiate.[1,2] It has been suggested that addition of these missing stem/stromal cell elements might help these degenerative conditions.

Studies have demonstrated such improvement with adult stem cell therapy by the successful regeneration of osteoarthritic damage and articular cartilage defects.[28,29] In 2003, Murphy et al. reported significant improvement in medial meniscus and cartilage regeneration with autologous stem cell therapy in an animal model. Not only was there evidence of marked regeneration of meniscal tissue, but the usual progressive destruction of articular cartilage, osteophytic remodeling and subchondral sclerosis commonly seen in osteoarthritic disease was reduced in MSC-treated joints compared with controls.[30] In 2008, Centeno et al. reported significant knee cartilage growth and symptom improvement in a human case report using culture expanded autologous MSCs from bone marrow.[31] In 2011, Albano and Alexander used autologous adipose cells as a living bioscaffold and stem cell source to repair a torn patellar tendon.[32] The number of treatments varies depending on the condition and prior treatment regime, along with clinical protocols in the recent medical literature.[33,34] Stem Cell Prolotherapy is typically given every month to few months.*

---

* The various nomenclature for the specific types of heterogeneous cells in these injections includes stromal or undifferentiated stromal cells.

LIPOASPIRATE
PROLOTHERAPY (ADSC)

While bone marrow has historically been used as a source of MSCs, adipose (fat)-derived stem/stromal cells (AD-SCs) have been shown to have nearly identical fibroblast-like morphology and colonization (CFU-F), immune phenotype, successful rate of isolation, and differentiation capabilities.[6,35,36] Autologous bone marrow stem cell volume is limited, but adipose tissue represents a large reservoir of stem cells. Research also supports as much as 500 to 1000 times as many mesenchymal and stromal vascular stem-like cells in adipose as compared to bone marrow.[26,37,38] AD-SCs have been

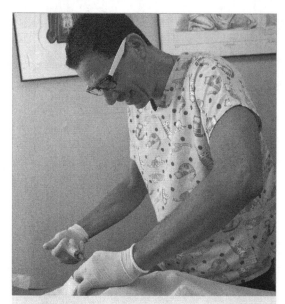

Dr. Hauser performing a lipoaspiration procedure. This patient came to Caring Medical because he suffered from chronic meniscal tear and knee degeneration. Since receiving Cellular Prolotherapy he has been able to return to tennis and all other activities.

shown, in multiple studies, to improve wound healing and stimulate fibroblast proliferation, migration and collagen secretion, thereby increasing connective tissue tensile strength and healing. Multiple human and animal investigations have clearly demonstrated the in vitro ability of AD-SCs to differentiate into, and repair, musculoskeletal connective tissues including ligament,[7] tendon,[6,39,40] cartilage,[41-43] disc,[44] muscle,[45-47] nerve tissue,[27,48,49] bone,[50-52] hematopoietic-supporting stroma,[53-55] to actively participate in tissue homeostasis, regeneration, and wound healing.[56-58] Lipoaspirate Prolotherapy is typically given every 1-3 months and usually requires 4-7 sessions. This is slightly more than average compared to traditional dextrose Prolotherapy because these cases are more advanced.

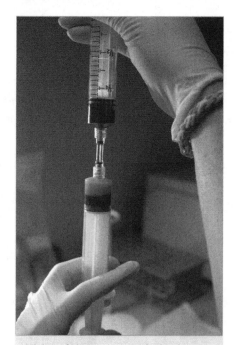

Mixing of Lipoaspirate with Platelet Rich Plasma. Once the solutions are mixed together, they are used as the proliferant in Lipoaspirate Prolotherapy.

BONE MARROW PROLOTHERAPY

The primary current use of adult stem cells in orthopaedic therapies are those derived from the bone marrow. In orthopaedic therapies, bone repair and regeneration is driven by the implanted bone marrow MSCs (BMSCs) that either engraft directly into the bone or are recruited from the marrow to the bone.[59-60] Human studies have documented enhanced treatment outcomes for nonunion fractures, avascular necrosis (osteonecrosis) and spinal fusions with the utilization of BMSCs.[62-65] The FDA has already approved the use of bone marrow stem cells for use in orthopaedics and many companies have products that help separate and thus concentrate the BMSCs from plasma and red blood cells. Centrifugation can concentrate BMSCs up to seven times the normal levels seen in whole marrow without losing cell viability, functionality and ability to osteogenically differentiate.[59,66-68] Initial research found that using whole bone marrow increased fusion rates in nonunion fractures 28%, but with centrifuged marrow, healing increased to 70%.[59] Others have documented the facilitation of healing with increased BMSC's counts.[62,63] Cell counts in the literature for concentrated marrow have ranged from 16.4 x 106 cells/ml to as high as 2.2 x 109 cells/ml in successful fusions or healings in orthopedic procedures.[61,62] Numerous publications

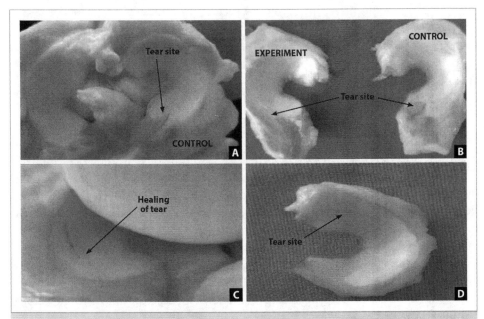

Figure 3-7: Histology of meniscus tear healing by autologous bone marrow aspirate. (A) Appearance of meniscus in the control group after dissection of knee ligaments. **(B)** Increase in synovial tissue and vascularization at the femoral and tibial surface of the meniscus in the experiment (treated with bone marrow aspirate) and control groups. **(C)** Appearance of the meniscus and healing in the experiment (treated) group at the postoperative 16th week macroscopically. **(D)** Healing meniscal tissue with bridging between the rims of tear site in the treated group.

Adapted and used with permission from: Duygulu F, et al. Effects of intra-articular administration of autologous bone marrow aspirate on healing of full-thickness meniscal tear: an experimental study on sheep. *Acta Orthop Traumatol Turc.* 2012;46(1):61-67. Figures 1 & 2.

have demonstrated the benefits of concentrated bone marrow for the regeneration of various structures of the skeletal system including bone, cartilage, and connective tissues.[42,69-76] **(See Figure 3-7.)** With the exception of a few studies, bone marrow-derived mesenchymal stem cells have an enhanced potential for chondrogenic differentiation as compared to adipose stem cells.[77-82] Proponents of bone marrow-derived stem cells note the large number of human studies and the fact that bone marrow contains the necessary MSCs and growth factors that are needed for use in orthopedic medicine.[83-87] Bone Marrow Prolotherapy, like Lipoaspirate Prolotherapy is typically given every 1-3 months and usually requires 4-7 sessions.

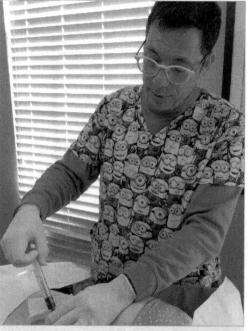

Dr. Hauser performing a bone marrow aspiration for Bone Marrow Prolotherapy for a patient who has struggled with osteoarthritis. In our clinic, we find this is an excellent alternative to surgery that gets patients back to activities and sports quickly.

RESULTS WITH CELLULAR PROLOTHERAPY FOR OSTEOARTHRITIS

At Caring Medical, this autologous solution, whether whole blood, PRP, bone marrow, or lipoaspirate, is used as part of the comprehensive Hackett-Hemwall Prolotherapy treatment. Cellular Prolotherapy is generally utilized for severe degenerative arthritis, significant articular cartilage injury, and in patients whose musculoskeletal problems have not fully resolved with dextrose Prolotherapy. Any condition that is helped by dextrose Prolotherapy can also be helped by Cellular Prolotherapy including cartilage injuries, ligament and tendon injuries, ligament and tendon degeneration (ligamentosis and tendinosis), joint instability, ligament laxity, labral tears, meniscal tears, osteoarthritis, osteochondral defects, severe joint degeneration, avascular necrosis in a bone, and more.

If one studies the pathophysiology of osteoarthritis, the following principles become evident:

- As stem cell counts decline with aging, the incidence of osteoarthritis increases.
- Degenerative joints have catabolic physiology.
- Anabolic factors necessary for healing are lacking in degenerative joints.
- Joint instability is a significant risk factor for joint degeneration.

- The degree of joint degeneration directly correlates with the amount of articular cartilage breakdown.
- Meniscus and synovium degeneration play a significant role in osteoarthritis.
- Much of the symptomatology of osteoarthritis can be attributed to the degenerated tissue structures around the joint and the decline in joint fluid.

To have a significant chance to reverse or stop the progression of osteoarthritis, the physiology of the joint has to change from degenerative to regenerative. That process of regenerating a joint is precisely what Prolotherapy is. Whether Prolotherapy is done with dextrose, hormones, natural extracts, or autografts (such as platelet rich plasma, bone marrow or lipoaspirate injections), the principle is the same: stimulate the damaged, injured, weakened, or degenerated structure to repair itself and regenerate.

This is what is needed for healing to occur in a degenerated joint:

1. Chondrocytes stimulate articular cartilage regeneration.
2. Fibrochondrocytes stimulate menisci tissue to regenerate.
3. Synoviocytes proliferate to normalize the amount of joint fluid that serves as nutrition for the meniscus, articular cartilage and other joint structures.
4. Fibroblasts cause a strengthening and tightening of the ligaments and entheses around the joint.

The net goal is to produce articular cartilage, ligament, meniscus and joint capsular tissue that is able to withstand the forces a person puts on them and then to replenish the joint fluid sufficiently to cushion the joint effectively. If you receive only cartilage cell injections into your knee, you are still going to have bone on bone. Unless there is some meniscus tissue present and enough joint fluid produced by the synoviocytes, bones will still hit and rub, even with articular cartilage present. Furthermore, if there is instability in the joint or the knee cap does not track correctly, the joint will continue to degenerate and the condition will worsen.

END STAGE ARTHRITIS

We published a paper in *The Open Arthritis Journal* in 2014 where we treated 24 end stage arthritis patients with *in situ* (direct) unfractionated whole bone marrow (WBM) taken from the patients' tibias. The WBM was injected directly into their arthritic joints immediately after it was removed from their tibias. The patients also received comprehensive Hackett-Hemwall dextrose Prolotherapy all around the joints. Eighteen of the 24 patients were told by surgeons prior to receiving Prolotherapy that their joints needed surgery, including 14 who were told they required knee or hip joint replacements. All of the patients were trying

Prolotherapy as a last resort prior to surgery. These were difficult cases!

The results with WBM injections in these arthritic joints were incredible! *(See Figure 3-8.)* Not only did the direct bone marrow injections eliminate their pain at rest, but it eliminated pain they felt with activity as well. Prior to receiving direct bone marrow injections, the average pain level was 6.33 (0 to 10 scale), while after direct bone marrow injections (average of 3-4 bone marrow treatments) pain declined to 0.46 (nearly 0!) These are the best results ever published in a peer-review journal that we know of for end stage arthritis.[88] We obtained the same results in another case study published.[89]

THE POWER OF CELLULAR PROLOTHERAPY

Using bone marrow or lipoaspirate as a Prolotherapy proliferant for arthritis and degenerative joint disease is successful because the body has tremendous regenerative capabilities. Cellular Prolotherapy takes advantage of this by injecting the progenitor (stem) healing cells into areas that are deficient in cells, such as in cases of bone-on-bone arthritis. This is discussed in greater detail, including before and after x-rays, in *Chapter 13.*

Bone Marrow Prolotherapy Study Results	
Total patients	24
Average age	64.9
Prior recommendation for surgery by other doctor	18 (75%)
Pain at rest before Prolotherapy	4.58
Pain at rest after Prolotherapy	0.25
Pain with ADLs before Prolotherapy (activities of daily living)	5.88
Pain with ADLs after Prolotherapy (activities of daily living)	0.38
Pain during exercise before Prolotherapy	6.33
Pain during exercise after Prolotherapy	0.46
Patients with knee osteoarthritis	13 (54%)
Patients with hip osteoarthritis	8 (33%)
Patients with other arthritis (back, toe, ankle)	3 (13%)

Figure 3-8: Caring Medical's Bone Marrow Prolotherapy study results.
Data from Hauser RA, et al. Treating osteoarthritic joints using dextrose Prolotherapy and direct bone marrow aspirate injection therapy. *The Open Arthritis Journal.* 2014;7:1-9.

SUMMARY

Caring Medical is one of the clinics that uses Cellular Prolotherapy as an alternative to surgery for patients with articular cartilage defects, as well as meniscal and labral defects, severe chondromalacia, degenerated discs, and advanced osteoarthritis. While these advanced cellular solutions have provided outstanding patient results, it is important to remember the principles of treating chronic pain with Prolotherapy. The underlying cause of most chronic pain is joint instability. In order for the patient to receive the full benefit, we combine Comprehensive Prolotherapy to the surrounding joint structures as well. In our opinion, future studies will confirm these findings that the treatment of choice for arthritis and joint degeneration is not joint replacement surgery, but Prolotherapy, including Cellular Prolotherapy! ∎

4

PROLO YOUR BACK PAIN AWAY!

Each year 65,000 patients are disabled with conditions associated with back pain, and an estimated 80% of people will suffer from back pain at some point in their lives. This is one of the most common reasons people come to us for Prolotherapy. Unfortunately, by the time we see many of these

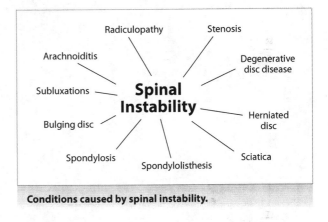

Conditions caused by spinal instability.

patients, they have already been through a failed back surgery, been prescribed numerous pain medications, received hours of physical therapy, and countless spinal adjustments. How can this be?

There is some consensus in the medical community on how to treat acute low back pain, but treatment of chronic pain presents many challenges and little agreement on standard of care. Nonsteroidal anti-inflammatory drugs and antidepressants provide some short-term benefit, but no published data warrant their long-term use.[1] Manipulative therapy, physiotherapy, and massage therapy studies have also shown only temporary benefit.[2,3] Long-term results on more invasive therapies, such as intradiscal electrothermal therapy (IDET) or surgery, have been poor.[4,5] Some believe the poor results for the treatment of chronic low back pain stem from the fact that too much emphasis has been placed on pain arising from the intervertebral discs and not enough on chronic low back pain originating from the sacroiliac joint and ligaments.[6,7]

The most common cause of unresolved chronic back pain is spinal instability. In the instance of low back pain, injury to the sacroiliac ligaments typically occurs from bending over and twisting with the knees in a locked, extended position. This maneuver stretches the sacroiliac ligaments, placing them in a vulnerable position. Remember that because the ligaments are white (poor blood supply), they are very unlikely to heal on their own, especially in chronic back pain, yet are incredibly important for spinal stability and movement. *(See Figure 4-1.)* Thus, spending a lot of time and money on therapies that work the surrounding *muscles* is only going to produce a temporary benefit. This should come as no surprise as you understand the principles of Prolotherapy. Patients with back pain frequently complain about muscle tightness, spasms, or feeling like the SI might "give out." They focus so much on the muscles (workout harder, stretch more, get more massage, etc...), that they forget why the muscles got that way is due to overcompensation for the lack of stability in the ligaments that hold the lumbar spine and sacroiliac joints in place.

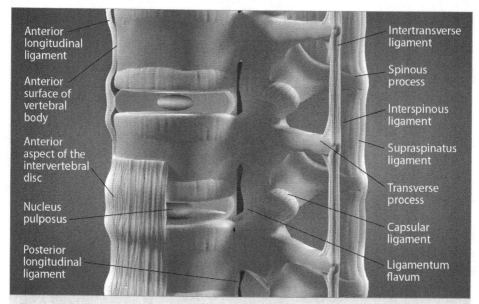

Anterior longitudinal ligament

Anterior surface of vertebral body

Anterior aspect of the intervertebral disc

Nucleus pulposus

Posterior longitudinal ligament

Intertransverse ligament

Spinous process

Interspinous ligament

Supraspinatus ligament

Transverse process

Capsular ligament

Ligamentum flavum

Figure 4-1: The ligamentous complex of the lumbar spine. If there is too much motion in the ligaments at the facet joints causing spinal instability, undue pressure can be exerted onto the disc and potentially lead to problems such as disc herniations and degeneration.

MECHANICAL AND FUNCTIONAL SPINAL INSTABILITY

Instability begins when the stabilizing structures of the spine, especially the ligaments can no longer hold adjacent bones together. When present, this is termed mechanical instability. The term functional instability is used when the mechanical instability causes symptoms with a certain function or activity. *(See Figure 4-2.)* Many people are walking with mechanical instability but are asymptomatic because the force required to perform current normal activities is not beyond the tissue strength. Problems arise when the mechanical instability worsens when patients overdo an activity or start a new exercise program. Thus the patient may have symptoms only when performing a certain activity, such as back pain with running. From the patient's perspective, pain symptoms do not exist during any other activities. This is called functional spinal instability with running and mechanical instability of the entire low back.

Functional instability, or symptomatic instability with movement, occurs with mechanical failure of the spinal ligaments and the subsequent excessive motion of adjacent bones. This can be caused by trauma, disease, surgery, or any combination thereof to one or more regions of the spine.

LIMITATIONS OF MRI AND X-RAYS

Most medical physicians rely too heavily on diagnostic tests, especially for low back problems.

Symptoms of Spinal Instability

- Condition is progressively worsening.
- Difficulty with unsupported sitting and better with supported backrest.
- Frequent bouts or episodes of symptoms (recurrence, not first episode).
- Frequent episodes of muscle spasms.
- Giving way or back giving out, feeling of instability.
- Greater pain returning to erect position from flexion.
- History of painful catching or locking during trunk motions.
- Long-term, chronic disorder.
- Need to frequently crack or pop the back to reduce symptoms.
- Pain during transitional activities.
- Pain increased with sudden, trivial, or mild movements.
- Rotational symptoms, different symptoms on different days.
- Temporary relief with back brace or corset.
- Worse with sustained postures or a decreased likelihood of reported static position that is not painful.

Figure 4-2: Symptoms of spinal instability.
Modified from: Biely S, et al. Clinical instability of the lumbar spine: diagnosis and intervention. *Orthopedic Practice.* 18;3:06. Table 1.

Consequently, many who suffer from low back pain do not find relief. The typical scenario is as follows: A person complains to a physician about low back pain that radiates down the leg. The physician orders x-rays and an MRI. The scan reveals an abnormality in the disc—such as a herniated, bulging, or degenerated disc. Unfortunately for the patient, this finding usually has nothing to do with the pain.

In the 1980s, modern medicine developed a high-tech diagnostic tool to look at vertebrae, nerves, and discs on film—the MRI scan. People were subjected to various treatments and surgeries for abnormalities found on the scan in the hopes of curing their pain. Very few people were cured. But all received hefty bills for the tests and surgeries.

Fifty consecutive patients undergoing open lumbar microdiscectomy for herniated discs - MRI was 72% sensitive, 68% specific and 70% accurate in detecting containment status of lumbar herniated discs. The authors concluded that MRI alone may provide insufficient or inaccurate information upon which to base surgical/technical decisions in about 30% of cases, and that other methods should be considered.[8]

Ten years of using MRI technology passed before research was conducted on the MRI findings of the lower back of people who had no pain symptoms.[7,8] Scott Boden, MD, found that nearly 100% of the people he tested who were over 60 years of age with no symptoms had abnormal findings in their lumbar spines (lower backs) on MRI scans. Thirty-six percent had herniated discs, and all but one had degeneration or bulging of a disc in at least one lumbar level. In the age group of 20 to 39, 35% had degeneration or bulging of a disc in at least one lumbar level.[7]

In a study published in *The New England Journal of Medicine* in 1994, Maureen Jensen, MD, and associates, studied MRI scans of the lumbar spine in 98 asymptomatic people. Only 36% had a normal scan, 64% had abnormal findings overall, and 38% had abnormal findings in more than one lumbar vertebral level. The conclusion was, "Because bulges and protrusions on MRI scans in people with low back pain or even radiculopathy may be coincidental, a patient's clinical situation must be carefully evaluated in conjunction with the results of MRI studies."[9] In other words, physicians should begin listening with their ears and poking with their thumbs! X-ray studies should never take the place of a good history and physical examination. Unfortunately for many, x-ray findings have nothing to do with their pain.

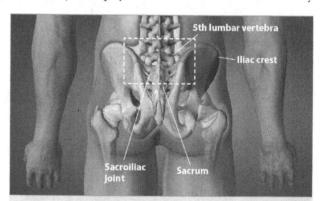

Figure 4-3: **Almost all chronic pain in the lower back occurs in a six-by-four inch area.** Pain in the lower back occurs in the area where the lumbar vertebrae join the sacrum and iliac crest.

DIAGNOSIS OF LOW BACK PAIN

Low back pain is one of the easiest conditions to treat with Prolotherapy. Ninety-five percent of low back pain is located in a six-by-four inch area, the weakest link in the vertebral-pelvis complex. At the end of the spine, four structures connect in a very small space, which happens to be the six-by-four inch area. The fifth lumbar vertebra connects with the base of the sacrum. This is held together by the lumbosacral ligaments. The sacrum is connected on its sides to the ilium and iliac crest. This is held together by the sacroiliac ligaments. The lumbar vertebrae is held to the iliac crest and ilium by the iliolumbar ligaments. This is typically the area treated with Prolotherapy for chronic low back pain. *(See Figure 4-3.)*

The diagnosis of ligament laxity in the lower back can be made relatively easily. Typical referral pain patterns are elicited, as previously described in **Chapter 1**. The sacroiliac ligaments refer pain down the posterior thigh and the lateral foot.[10,11] The sacrotuberous and sacrospinous ligaments refer pain to the heel. The iliolumbar ligament refers pain into the groin or vagina. Iliolumbar ligament sprain should be considered for any unexplained vaginal, testicular, or groin pain.

The first step in determining ligament laxity or instability is by physical examination.[12] The examination involves maneuvering the patient into various stretched positions. If weak ligaments exist, the stressor maneuver will cause pain.

Do this simple test at home: Lie flat on your back and lift your legs together as straight and as high as you can, then lower your legs. If it is more painful to lower your legs than to raise them, laxity in the lumbosacral ligaments is likely. The next step is palpating various ligaments with the thumb to elicit tenderness. A positive "jump sign" indicates ligament laxity.

TREATMENT OF LOW BACK PAIN

Low back pain conditions have been one of the most well-studied in the Prolotherapy arena.[13] In one of the original papers by George S. Hackett, MD, he noted 82% of people treated for posterior sacroiliac ligament relaxation considered themselves cured and remained so 12 years later.[10] You can read more about some exciting studies in our literature review on dextrose Prolotherapy in the *Journal of Prolotherapy*.[14] In our own published research, 145 patients with chronic low back pain were interviewed an average of 12 months after their last Prolotherapy treatment. These patients, who had been in pain an average

Prolotherapy Study Results for Back Pain			
Demographics	**All Back Patients**	**No Other Treatment Option**	**Surgery Only Option**
Total number of patients	145	55	26
Avg. months of pain	58	53	60
# of pain meds used before Prolotherapy	1	0.9	1.1
# of pain meds used after Prolotherapy	0.3	0.3	0.4
Pain level before Prolotherapy	5.6	7.1	6.0
Pain level after Prolotherapy	2.7	3.1	2.1
Stiffness level before Prolotherapy	6.1	7.0	6.1
Stiffness level after Prolotherapy	2.6	3.1	2.0
Greater than 50% pain relief	96%	89%	96%
Athletic ability > 30 minutes of exercise before Prolotherapy	19%	30%	12%
Athletic ability > 30 minutes of exercise after Prolotherapy	78%	81%	90%
Prolotherapy changed life for the better	97%	94%	81%

Figure 4-4: Summary of results of Hackett-Hemwall dextrose Prolotherapy back study.

of four years and ten months, were treated quarterly with Hackett-Hemwall dextrose Prolotherapy. This included a subset of 55 patients who were told by their medical doctor(s) that there were no other treatment options for their pain and a subset of 26 patients who were told by their doctor(s) that surgery was their only option. In these 145 low backs, average pain levels decreased from 5.6 to 2.7 after Prolotherapy (scale of 1-10); 89% experienced more than 50% pain relief with Prolotherapy; more than 80% showed improvements in walking and exercise ability, anxiety, depression and overall disability; 75% were able to completely stop taking pain medications.[15] *(See Figure 4-4.)*

HERNIATED AND DEGENERATED DISCS

A person with a degenerated, bulging, or herniated disc must realize that this may be a coincidental finding and unrelated to the actual pain he or she is experiencing. A degenerated disc is one that is losing water and flattening. *(See Figure 4-5.)* This is a usual phenomenon that occurs with age. It is also normal for a disc to bulge with bending. A herniated disc occurs when the annulus fibrosus no longer holds the gelatinous solution in the disc. The result is a weakened disc. The annulus fibrosus is basically a ring of ligament tissue. What is the best treatment to strengthen ligament tissue? That's right... Prolotherapy.

Why did the disc degenerate in the first place? Degeneration of a disc begins as soon as the lumbar ligaments become loose and cause spinal instability, allowing the vertebral segments to move excessively and cause pain. The body attempts to correct this by tensing the back muscles.

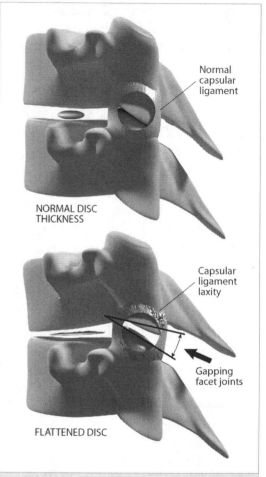

Figure 4-5: Untreated capsular ligament laxity results in flattening of the disc, which is termed degenerative disc disease. This progressive flattening of the intervertebral disc then increases the force on the facet joints with normal activity; worsening instability from capsular ligament injury.

Visits to a chiropractor or medical doctor typically begin at this time. The hypermobile vertebral segments add strain to the vertebral discs. Eventually these discs cannot sustain the added pressure and begin to flatten and/or herniate. The lumbar ligaments then work harder because the discs no longer cushion the back. A dismal, downward path of pain is the end result. *(See Figure 4-6.)*

Prolotherapy is the treatment of choice for spinal instability. It strengthens the lumbar vertebral ligaments and prevent the progressive degeneration that occurs with age to the intervertebral discs.

A patient with chronic low back pain is typically treated with Prolotherapy injections into the insertions of the lumbosacral, iliolumbar, and sacroiliac

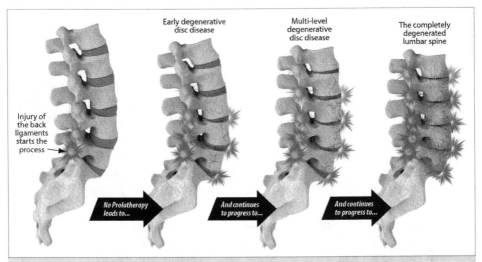

Figure 4-6: The progression of degeneration of the lower back. An initial injury to the spinal ligaments causes the start of spinal instability. The process progresses to involve more spinal segments. The completely degenerated lumbar spine is the final consequence of not resolving spinal instability.

ligaments. The initial assessment may reveal that the chronic low back pain and referred leg pain may be caused by a referred pain from other areas such as the pubic symphysis, hip joint, ischial tuberosity, sacrospinous, and sacrotuberous ligaments. Therefore, these areas are also examined.

Off-centered low back pain is often caused by a posterior hip sprain or osteoarthritis of the hip. The hip joint often refers pain to the groin and down the leg to the big toe. Prolotherapy is very effective in this area, often alleviating the necessity for hip replacement surgery. Some patients benefit from a combined low back and hip treatment course if there is noted weakness, instability, and/or pain in both the low back and hip. Hip pain is discussed more in **Chapter 8**.

SPINAL STENOSIS

Bone spurs form as a result of microinstability of the spine, as the body attempts to stabilize the unstable spine, which can eventually narrow the spinal canal and cause resultant spinal stenosis. **(See Figure 4-7.)** Spinal stenosis is defined as a specific type and amount of narrowing of the spinal canal,

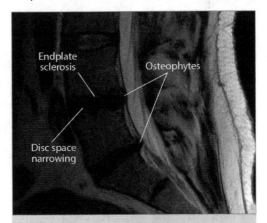

Figure 4-7: MRI showing lumbar spondylosis. Joint instability is the best explanation for degenerative radiographic findings, including endplate sclerosis, disc space narrowing and osteophytes. Osteophytes (bone spurs) are the body's attempt to limit motion in order to stabilize the spine. If left unchecked, the bone spurs can compress nerves and the spinal cord.

nerve root canals, or intervertebral foramina and can be either congenital or developmental or be acquired from degenerative changes.[16] Some evidence suggests that disc degeneration, narrowing of the spinal canal, and degenerative changes in the facets and spinal ligaments all contribute to spinal stenosis.[17]

The hallmark symptom of spinal stenosis is neurogenic claudication, which is neurologically-based pain that occurs upon walking; other common symptoms include sensory disturbances in the legs, low back pain, weakness, and pain relief upon bending forward. Segmental instability is thought to be a source of the low back pain. No association has been found between the severity of pain and the degree of stenosis, although patients who are symptomatic tend to have narrower spines than asymptomatic patients. Studies have found that diagnosing spinal stenosis with 10 mm as the sagittal diameter alone produces false positive rates approaching 50%.[18,19] Making a diagnosis of spinal stenosis based on the absolute size of the spinal canal also has its drawbacks since it does not indicate whether or not there is impingement or distortion of either the spinal cord or nerve roots. Impingement or encroachment of the spinal cord by bone is called myelomalacia; impingement of the spinal nerve roots is called radiculopathy.

Something has to be responsible for the back pain or leg pain in diagnosed cases of spinal stenosis. Most people will refer to some motion, often one of combined flexion and rotation that they performed before developing certain positional symptoms. For instance, symptoms that are worse with one position or motion (eg, walking or standing) then improve with spinal flexion (eg, sitting). This indicates that the spinal ligaments are loose and causing symptoms based on the patient's position. This is why giving Comprehensive Prolotherapy to stabilize the ligaments is often the ideal treatment, even in patients who have been diagnosed with spinal stenosis.

POSITIONAL PAIN RESPONDS TO PROLOTHERAPY

For some this concept of Prolotherapy helping spinal stenosis is difficult to grasp. "Doctor, I don't see how Prolotherapy is going to open up the space?" We can think of spinal stenosis as two different disorders, one needs surgery and the other Prolotherapy. There is SSAR and SSWA which stand for Spinal Stenosis At Rest and then Spinal Stenosis With Activity. *(See Figure 4-8.)* Surgery is needed for SSAR but Prolotherapy resolves SSWA. They are differentiated on symptoms and a test called electromyography/nerve conduction studies (EMG/ NCV). The patient who has severe pain, especially nerve irritation down the leg at rest has a narrowing off the space for the nerves that is not affected by activity. It means that there just is never enough room for the nerve, even at rest. In these instances, a lot of nerve damage or irritation is present on an EMG/NCV test. This patient would be referred for a surgical decompressive surgery, where the surgeon makes more room for the nerve. Any residual pain after the surgery can then be treated with Prolotherapy. However, almost all the cases of spinal stenosis fall into the second

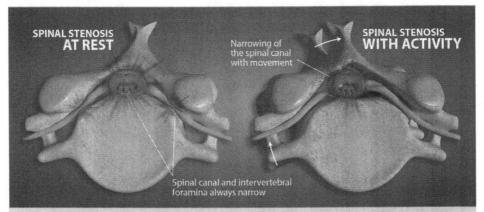

Figure 4-8: Spinal stenosis at rest (SSAR) vs. spinal stenosis with activity (SSWA). With SSAR, the spinal cord and nerves are always getting compressed because there is not enough room in the spinal canal and intervertebral foramina. This can only be fixed with decompressive surgery. With SSWA, there are no symptoms at rest because there is enough room for the spinal cord and nerve root; however, with activity, one or both of these can get narrowed and then the person experiences pain down the leg when standing or walking. In SSWA, the excessive movement of bones is narrowing the spinal cord space and/or intervertebral foramina because of ligament weakness. This type of spinal stenosis can be effectively treated with Prolotherapy.

category, SSWA. These are patients who have no symptoms when they are sitting and laying recumbent and resting. But upon standing or walking for too long, they develop back pain, buttock pain and pain down the leg. In other words, the symptoms are only precipitated with movement or change in position. This means that the nerves have enough room at rest, but the room for the nerve is decreased with standing or walking. The symptoms are dependent on position. Positional pain is a hallmark feature of conditions that respond to Prolotherapy, in the spine and any joint of the body! *(See Figure 4-9.)*

PINCHED OR COMPRESSED NERVES

If you have ever experienced a pinched nerve or lumbar radiculopathy, you know the pain is excruciating. Burning pain zooming down an extremity can cause such blinding pain, it will stop anyone in their tracks. But even in cases of acute pain, we have to ask why this problem started in the first place. The answer is ligament laxity, which causes the vertebrae to slip out of place and pinch the nerve. In our office, these cases are often seen as needing a two-part solution. First, we have to work to get the patient out of acute pain. Nerve blocks utilizing a 70.0% Sarapin and 0.6% lidocaine solution are often given, in addition to Prolotherapy. The nerve block provides initial pain relief, so the person is able to rest and repair while the Prolotherapy begins to work. Upon nerve relaxation, the vertebrae will realign and the nerve compression will cease. Even in cases of such extreme pain as a pinched nerve, the pain is typically positional. This means that it gets more intense when a person gets into certain positions. For example, if someone has unbearable pain upon sitting or kneeling, but is relieved somewhat while standing or lying

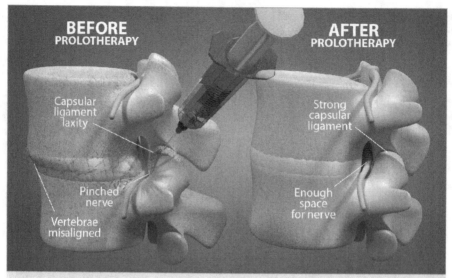

Figure 4-9: Prolotherapy treatment of spinal stenosis. Prolotherapy, by tightening the capsular ligaments, causes improvement of the vertebral alignment thereby increasing the space for neurologic or nerve tissues including the spinal cord and nerve root.

flat, this means certain positions are causing the vertebrae to slip and pinch on the nerve. This also should be the point where someone is picking up the phone for a Prolotherapy treatment. In our in-house analysis of consecutive patients treated for radiculopathy with Prolotherapy, the average starting pain level in patients treated for lumbar radiculopathy was 6.3 and ending pain level was 2.5 (VAS 0-10). In this same radiculopathy data, we looked at cervical radiculopathy patient outcomes as well. They were equally impressive with an average starting pain level of 5.6 and an ending pain level of 1. Prolotherapy proved to be an excellent nonsurgical option for the unrelenting pain characteristic of radiculopathy. Whether the spine or other joints, positional pain is indicative of joint instability and an ideal application for Prolotherapy! *(See Figure 4-10.)*

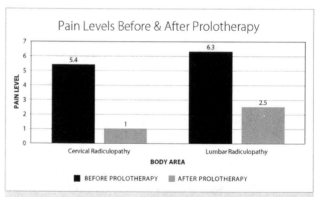

Figure 4-10: Results of comprehensive Hackett-Hemwall Prolotherapy to resolve cervical and lumbar radiculopathy in patients who were surgical candidates but did not want to undergo surgery.* Prolotherapy is a very successful nonsurgical option to resolve cervical and lumbar radiculopathy.

*The in-house results from Caring Medical Regenerative Medicine Clinics represent 17 consecutive patients diagnosed with cervical radiculopathy and 23 patients with lumbar radiculopathy. The average age of patients was 53. The average number of Prolotherapy treatments was 5.7. At the time of follow-up, the average length of time since the last treatment was 27 months. Three patients in each group did end up undergoing surgery. Out of the 40 total patients, 37 would recommend Prolotherapy to others.

THE ROLE OF SURGERY

Except in a life-threatening situation or impending neurologic injury, surgery should always be a last resort and performed only after all conservative treatments have been exhausted. Pain is not a life-threatening situation, although it can be very anxiety-provoking, life-demeaning, and aggravating. Pain should not be an automatic indication that surgery is necessary. Conservative treatments such as vitamins, herbs, massage, physical therapy, chiropractic/osteopathic care, medications, and, of course, Prolotherapy should precede any surgical intervention. Conservative care for back pain is complete only after treatment with Prolotherapy.

It is not uncommon for patients to say that surgery has been recommended to resolve their painful back conditions. Reasons for surgery may be herniated discs, compressed nerves, spinal stenosis, severe arthritis, and intractable pain. Such conditions may have nothing to do with the problem causing the pain. As previously discussed abnormalities noted on an MRI scan, such as a pinched nerve or herniated disc, rarely are the reasons we find for someone's chronic back pain. We find at Caring Medical that spinal instability due to ligament weakness is the number one reason for chronic low back pain, and this diagnosis is not made by an MRI.

Surgery is fraught with many potential risks, one being the required anesthesia. General anesthesia greatly stresses the body and complications may occur while under, including kidney and liver failure or a heart attack. A significant percentage of anesthesia-related deaths result from the aspiration (swallowing) of food particles, foreign bodies like dentures, blood, gastric acid, oropharyngeal secretions, or bile during induction of general anesthesia.[20] Other possible complications include damage to the mouth, throat, vocal cords, or lungs from the insertion of the anesthesia tube. If you have ever seen anyone after anesthesia, you know it's no Sunday picnic!

Even back in early 1981, as new and more effective methods of conservative treatments were being used (including Prolotherapy), the need for surgery was decreasing. Bernard E. Finneson, MD, pointed out in a survey of surgical cases that "80% that should not...have been brought to surgery." It is quite possible that with the widespread use of Prolotherapy this percentage would be even higher.[21]

PROLOTHERAPY VERSUS SURGERY

In 1964, John R. Merriman, MD, compared Prolotherapy versus operative fusion in the treatment of instability of the spine and pelvis and wrote, "The purpose of this article is to evaluate the merit of two methods of treating instability of the spine and pelvis, with which I have been concerned during 40 years as a general and industrial surgeon...The success of either method depends on regeneration of bone cells to provide joint stabilization, elimination of pain and resumption of activity...Ligament and tendon relaxation occurs when the fibro-osseous attachments to bone do not regain their normal tensile strength after sprain and lacerations, and when the attachments are weakened by decalcification from disease, menopause and aging."[22] *Figure 4-11* describes Dr. Merriman's results. The idea of using Prolotherapy as an alternative to surgery has always been one of our goals for patients searching for a more conservative route to end their back pain. We put this to the test in a study that we published in the *Journal of Prolotherapy*. You can read more about this study, reporting on 34 patients who utilized Prolotherapy as an alternative to a variety of surgeries, including spinal fusion, in **Chapter 19.**

AREAS AFFECTED	RESPONSE TO PROLOTHERAPY (PHYSIOLOGIC TREATMENT)	RESPONSE TO FUSION OPERATION (MECHANICAL TREATMENT)
NEW BONE	PROMPT	RETARDED
LIGAMENTS	STRENGTHENED	EXCISED (REMOVED)
TENDONS	STRENGTHENED	INCISED (CUT)
SPINOUS PROCESS	STRENGTHENED	SACRIFICED
JOINT MOTION	PRESERVED	ABOLISHED
PAIN	ELIMINATED	MAY CONTINUE
LOSS OF TIME	NEGLIGIBLE	CONSIDERABLE
RESULTS	80-90% CURES	VARIABLE

Figure 4-11: Dr. Merriman's study results.

Dr. Merriman summarized that conservative physiologic treatment by Prolotherapy after a confirmed diagnosis of ligamental and tendinous relaxation was successful in 80-90% of more than 15,000 patients treated.

FAILED BACK SURGERY SYNDROME

Many people only become aware of Prolotherapy after they have undergone a surgical procedure for back pain. Although the pain may not be as severe as it was before the surgery, most people continue to experience significant back pain after surgery. Why? Because the back surgery involved removing supporting structures, such as a lamina, facet, or disc, thus weakening surrounding segments.

Prolotherapy injections to the weakened segments in the lumbar vertebrae often result in definitive pain relief in post-surgery pain syndromes. *(See Figure 4-12.)* Back pain is commonly due to several factors and surgery may have eliminated only one. It is possible, for example, to have back pain from a lumbar herniated disc and a sacroiliac joint problem. Surgery may address the herniated disc problem but not the sacroiliac problem. In this example, Prolotherapy injections to the sacroiliac joint would cure the chronic pain problem.

Unfortunately, it is common for a person to have lumbar spine surgery for a "sciatica" complaint diagnosed from an "abnormality" on an MRI scan. The "sciatica" complaint was a simple ligament problem in the sacroiliac joint and the MRI scan finding was not clinically relevant—it had nothing to do with the

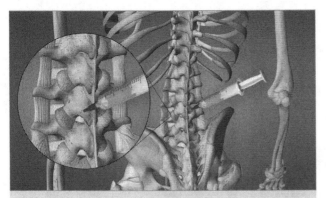

Figure 4-12: Prolotherapy of the lower back. Injured capsular, sacroiliac and other ligaments can be thickened and strengthened with Prolotherapy.

pain problem. For the majority of people who experience pain radiating down the leg, even in cases where numbness is present, the cause of the problem is not a pinched nerve but sacroiliac ligament weakness. *(See Figure 4-13.)*

Ligament laxity causing sacroiliac joint instability is the number one reason for "sciatica,"

or pain radiating down the side of the leg, and is one of the most common reasons for chronic low back pain.[6] This can easily be confirmed by examining these ligaments and producing a positive "jump sign." *(See Figure 4-14.)* Ligament weakness can cause leg numbness. Most people sense pain when they have ligament weakness, but some people experience a sensation of numbness. Doctors typically believe nerve injury is the only reason for numbness, a reason so many people believe they have a sciatic nerve problem. In reality, it is a sacroiliac ligament problem. The referral patterns of the sciatic nerve and the sacroiliac ligaments are similar.

In this scenario, it is unfortunate that thousands of dollars were spent on surgery and post-operative care. Had Prolotherapy treatments been performed on the pain-producing structure, this could have been avoided.

PAIN FROM SCOLIOSIS

Scoliosis is a lateral curvature of the spine of 11 degrees or more. An estimated 500,000 adults in the United States have symptomatic scoliosis.[23] Scoliosis is usually discovered during adolescence and is called idiopathic scoliosis, a fancy term meaning the doctor has no idea what caused the scoliosis.

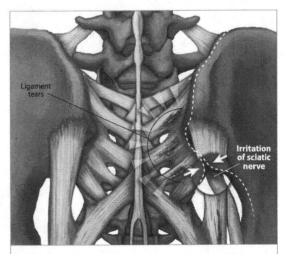

Symptoms:
- Crepitation with movement
- Loss of motion
- Loss of muscle strength
- Low back pain
- Muscle spasms
- Numbiness down leg
- Popping
- Referral leg pain

Figure 4-13: Sacroiliac instability. Arrows signify excessive joint motion. Sacroiliac instability can irritate the sciatic nerve and refer pain down the leg.

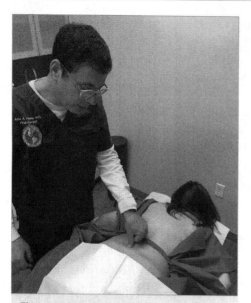

Figure 4-14: Dr. Hauser using his "MRI" to reproduce the patient's pain and confirm joint instability during a consultation.

In common language, scoliosis means that the spine is crooked. The spine is held together by the same thing that holds all the bones together, ligaments. The patient often experiences pain at the site where the spine curves. At the apex of this curve, the ligaments are being stretched with the scoliosis, and localized ligament weakness is one of the etiological bases for it. *(See Figure 4-15.)*

Traditional treatments for scoliosis, especially during adolescence, include observation, bracing, and surgery.[24-26] Observation of a crooked spine does not sound very helpful, bracing has been shown to decrease the progression of mild scoliosis, and surgery involves placing big rods in the back to stabilize the spine. Surgery is generally utilized for severe scoliosis when bracing has failed to stop the progression.

Scoliosis pain produces common patterns depending on where the scoliosis is located. These pain patterns are reproduced by palpating the ligaments over the scoliotic segments of the spine. A positive "jump sign" will be elicited, ensuring the diagnosis. Prolotherapy treatments over the entire scoliotic segment are effective at eliminating the pain of scoliosis. It has the added benefit of causing the ligaments to strengthen, which will help stabilize the segment. If the scoliosis is progressing quickly, then bracing would be necessary in addition to Prolotherapy. For these reasons, Prolotherapy should be a part of comprehensive scoliosis management.

BACK PAIN FROM PREGNANCY

During pregnancy, a woman's body secretes a hormone called relaxin, which causes ligaments to loosen allowing the baby to pass through the birth canal. Ligament laxity is normal during pregnancy. The baby's position in the pelvic region during pregnancy, the lax ligaments to allow delivery, and the mother carrying her baby on her hip after the baby is born all contribute to a resultant sacroiliac laxity and lower back pain.

In 1942, William Mengert, MD, wrote, "It is now generally accepted that the overwhelming majority of backaches and sciaticas during pregnancy are due to pelvic girdle relaxation."[27] The average mobility of the joint is increased by 33%, leading to lax ligaments in people experiencing back pain from the sacroiliac joint.[28]

Womens' hips are not wide for carrying a baby on them, but are wide to get a baby out! A woman should not carry a baby on her hip. Many months are required after pregnancy for the sacroiliac joints to regain normal strength. It is imperative not to place any undue stress on the hips during this time. This causes additional stress on the sacroiliac joints. Often the sacroiliac joints are already loose and painful during pregnancy. The addition of carrying a child on the hip after pregnancy does not give the sacroiliac joint a chance to heal, often resulting in back pain.

Prolotherapy is an excellent treatment for back pain caused by pregnancy. Prolotherapy strengthens joints to relieve back pain but does not interfere with the birthing process. It can make pregnancy much more bearable. Prolotherapy is the treatment of choice for chronic low back pain that may occur during or linger after pregnancy if other conservative treatments have proven unsuccessful. If the area becomes damaged or weakened through another pregnancy or other event, a "touch up" treatment can be done.

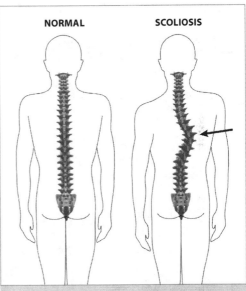

Figure 4-15: Normal and scoliosis posterior views. This shows the spine with a right thoracic scoliosis, which is often the site of pain (arrow) because this is where the force per unit area is greatest with this condition.

COCCYGODYNIA

Acute coccygodynia is most often caused by trauma to the coccyx and its surrounding structures, usually due to falling while in the half-seated position. The coccyx itself is a bony structure attached to the end of the sacrum and is composed of three to five segments. The first and second segments may be separated by an intervertebral disc, but more commonly the segments are fused. The mobility, however, between the first and second segments predisposes this segment of the coccyx to fracture and dislocate.[29]

On the other hand, chronic coccygodynia is most commonly due to faulty posture while sitting, or trauma to the coccyx during childbirth. Sitting in the slouched position puts stress on the coccyx rather than on the ischial tuberosities. *(See Figure 4-16.)* Other possible causes for coccygeal pain are chronic infection and dysfunction of the musculature of the pelvic floor.

People without a spinal cord injury, who experience rectal pain, typically elicit a positive "jump sign" when the sacrococcygeal ligament is palpated. Prolotherapy to this ligament is curative in most cases. Some patients may also have laxity in the sacroiliac joint, which requires treatment to resolve the chronic rectal pain.

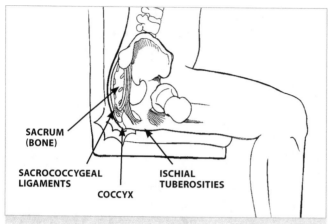

Figure 4-16: Why sitting can cause chronic rectal pain. The weight of the body in the sitting position puts strain on the coccyx and sacrococcygeal ligaments.

The presentation of symptoms of coccygodynia in people without spinal cord injury and the dysesthetic syndrome that occurs in people with a spinal cord injury are almost identical.

Traditional medical treatments for burning rectal pain include various medications, physical therapy, seat cushions, and psychological support. These treatments typically provide only temporary benefits. Prolotherapy injections, which strengthen the supporting structures of the sacrococcygeal joint, eliminate chronic rectal pain because they address the root cause of the problem. Chronic rectal pain from coccygodynia occurs because of a weakness in the sacrococcygeal joint or a weakness between one of the coccygeal segments. Prolotherapy to strengthen the ligamentous support of the weakened area cures chronic rectal pain from coccygodynia.

SUMMARY

In summary, Prolotherapy is the ideal treatment for chronic back pain due to spinal instability. Some telltale signs that you have spinal instability include chronic muscle spasms, pain that shoots down the legs intermittently, your spine cracks and pops, and you feel the need to manipulate your spine or receive frequent adjustments and massages. The true source of pain is due to ligament weakness. The causes can be many, such as traumatic or over time due to poor posture or overuse. Either way, it is a ligament problem. Prolotherapy strengthens ligaments and eliminates chronic back pain in conditions such as degenerated discs, herniated discs, spondylolisthesis, post-surgery pain syndromes, arachnoiditis, and scoliosis. The most common cause of chronic low back pain and "sciatica" is laxity of the sacroiliac ligaments. Prolotherapy should be tried before any surgical procedure is performed for chronic back pain. Because Prolotherapy is an extremely effective treatment for chronic low back pain, and it permanently strengthens the structures that are causing the pain, many people are choosing to Prolo their chronic back pain away! ■

CHAPTER

5

PROLO YOUR HEAD & NECK PAIN AWAY!

As with pain in all other body parts, neck, headache, and facial pain are almost always caused by weakness in a soft tissue structure. Ligament weakness in the neck accounts for the majority of chronic headaches, neck, ear, and mouth pain. Because Prolotherapy stimulates the growth of the weakened ligament causing the pain, many people obtain

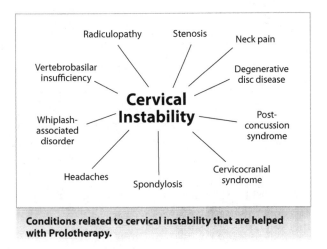

Conditions related to cervical instability that are helped with Prolotherapy.

permanent pain relief with this treatment. What this chapter will explain is not just how Prolotherapy helps with common headache and neck pain, but also how it helps bizarre symptoms that are due to cervical instability, such as dizziness, visual disturbances, eye pressure, mouth pain, sinus congestion, tinnitus, and more.

CAPSULAR LIGAMENT LAXITY CAUSES CERVICAL INSTABILITY

The capsular ligaments are the main stabilizing structures of the facet joints in the cervical spine and have been implicated as a major source of chronic neck pain.[1] Such pain often reflects a state of instability in the cervical spine and is a symptom common to a number of conditions such as disc herniation, cervical spondylosis, whiplash injury and whiplash associated disorder, post-concussion syndrome, vertebrobasilar insufficiency, and cervicocranial syndrome. When the capsular ligaments are injured, they become elongated and exhibit laxity, which causes excessive movement of the cervical vertebrae. In the upper cervical spine (C0-C2), this can cause symptoms such as nerve irritation and vertebrobasilar insufficiency with associated vertigo, tinnitus, dizziness, facial pain, arm pain, and migraine headaches. In the lower cervical spine (C3-C7), this can cause muscle spasms, crepitation, and/ or paresthesia in addition to chronic neck pain. In either case, the presence of excessive motion (hypermobility)

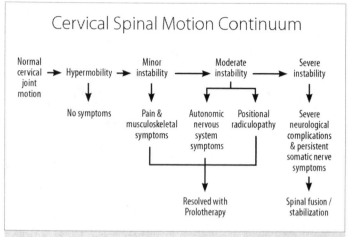

Figure 5-1: Cervical spinal continuum and role of Prolotherapy.
When spinal instability causes symptoms such as pain, dizziness, tinnitus, vertigo, sinusitis, vision changes, swallowing difficulty, as well as pain and tingling down the arm that comes and goes, the treatment of choice is Prolotherapy. Severe spinal instability such as what occurs with fracture necessitates spinal fusion for stabilization.

between two adjacent cervical vertebrae and these associated symptoms is described as cervical instability. *(See Figure 5-1.)* The instability continues to worsen and cause additional symptoms until the area is stabilized. If fusion surgery has been recommended, an opinion from a Prolotherapist who specializes in complicated neck cases should be sought. Prolotherapy can prevent the need for cervical spine fusion, and alleviate the symptoms by restoring ligament strength and normal motion.

CREEP

Ligament weakness in the neck can occur suddenly, such as after a whiplash injury during a car accident, but it more commonly occurs slowly over time. This is known as "creep" and refers to the elongation of a ligament under a constant or repetitive stress.[2] *(See Figure 5-2.)* Excessive tension on the capsular ligaments can cause upper cervical instability and related neck pain.[3] Capsular ligament tension is increased during abnormal postures,

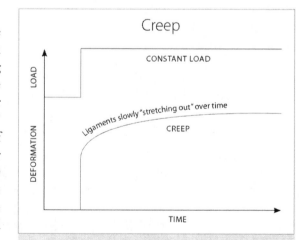

Figure 5-2: Ligament laxity graph. When subjected to a constant stress, ligaments display Creep behavior—a time-dependent increase in strain or the fact that ligaments slowly "stretch out" over time.

causing elongation of the capsular ligaments, with magnitudes increased by up to 70% of normal.[4] Such excessive ligament elongation induces laxity to the facet joints, which puts the cervical spine more at risk for further degenerative changes and instability. Therefore, capsular ligament injury appears to cause upper cervical instability because of laxity in the stabilizing structure of the facet joints.[5]

HEADACHE PAIN

Migraine headaches tend to take over a family. If one member is "out" with a migraine headache, another member is helping them cope. Anyone who has experienced a migraine headache or has seen a loved one suffer through a migraine attack knows it is a most unpleasant experience.

Typical medical management of migraine headaches involves the avoidance of various foods like chocolate, tyramine-containing cheese, and alcoholic beverages.[6] Various medications are used in an attempt to abort the migraine once it has started. Prophylactic medications, such as Propranolol, are used in an attempt to prevent the dreaded migraine. Unfortunately, a migraine headache is not due to a Propranolol deficiency. Neither is it an aspirin, ibuprofen, acetaminophen, imitrex, or Elavil® deficiency. Migraine headaches have a cause and that cause can be determined by a careful examination. The cause of migraine headaches can nearly always be found by a good listening ear and a strong thumb. (**See Figure 5-3.**)

CAUSES OF MIGRAINES

Sometimes a person has other factors, in addition to ligament weakness in the neck, associated with initiating the migraines, including food sensitivities, hormone deficiencies, and yeast infections. In these instances, Prolotherapy must be combined with Natural Medicine techniques, such as elimination of allergic foods from the diet, natural hormone supplementation, or yeast infection treatment, to obtain completely curative results.

If the migraine headaches occur at a particular part of a woman's menstrual cycle, a hormonal abnormality is likely

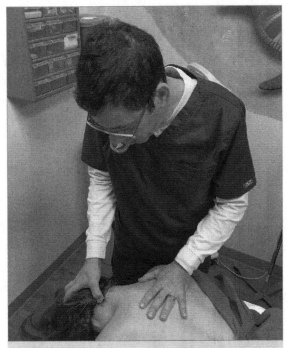

Figure 5-3: Dr. Hauser using his "MRI" during an exam to reproduce the patient's pain symptoms.

involved. The hormonal abnormality is usually due to a low progesterone level during the second half of the menstrual cycle. Giving natural progesterone during this part of the menstrual cycle will often relieve the problem.

If the migraine headaches occur when eating particular foods, during particular times of the year, or when exposed to certain scents, an allergic component to the migraines should be investigated. Migraine headaches are a common symptom of food allergies. Eliminating the suspect food from the diet will likely solve the migraine problem. In addition, there are times when a person's protein/fat/carbohydrate ratio is off. Eating according to one's individual Diet Type can be a helpful piece to the puzzle to alleviate migraine headaches.

TREATMENTS FOR MIGRAINES

Current traditional drugs for migraine headaches, such as ergotamine, fiorinal, sumatriptan, zolmitriptan, and other medications, provide only temporary relief. The patient dependent on these drugs for headache relief lives in fear of the next migraine attack. Patients describe their migraine headaches as similar to having one half of their head hit repeatedly with a baseball bat.

From an anatomical perspective, cervical instability is the culprit in the majority of non-hormone or diet-related headaches and migraines. Upon palpation along the base of the head, and through the neck, tenderness or pain indicates weakness at the ligament attachments, the pain sensors of the body. Often patients also tell us that they have a lot of "knots" in their neck all the time, and for years they just attributed it to stress. While stress can certainly be a contributing factor to healing, the structures are tight for a reason. The muscles in the neck are trying to keep a 10 pound head balanced on the small, upper cervical vertebra. Like balancing a bowling ball on an espresso cup without a little assistance. Normally, the ligaments provide the stability needed to turn the head, side to side, up or down, and safely return back to a neutral position. With cervical ligament damage, the muscles have to kick into high gear, without rest, in order to stabilize the head. The muscles and ligaments are screaming for relief in the form of a crushing headache. Thus, Prolotherapy to the cervical ligament attachments makes the most sense for long-term success against headaches and migraines.

CARING MEDICAL'S PUBLISHED RESEARCH ON HEADACHE AND NECK PAIN

For 10 years, we ran a charity clinic in southern Illinois for the underserved who did not otherwise have access to Prolotherapy. Patients were seen quarterly, and the only treatment that many of them had available was the Prolotherapy we offered, or possibly some pain medication. Due to limited funds, many were not able to do testing for food allergies or hormone levels. Therefore, we had a very clear picture of just how powerful Prolotherapy could be, even when given months apart, instead of the more ideal 4-8 weeks. Fifteen total patients were included in the study for either tension headaches (8) or migraine headaches (7). All participants had at least monthly headaches prior to Prolotherapy and 67% reported headache intensity of 10 out of 10 (on a scale of 1-10), and the other 33% reported at least an 8 out of 10. After Prolotherapy, 47% had no headaches and 100% experienced at least some relief in regard to headache intensity and frequency.[7]

In another study based in the same charity clinic, we reported on 98 patients seen at the quarterly clinic who were treated for neck pain. Prior to Prolotherapy, the average length of neck pain complaints was 4.9 years. In a subgroup of 43 patients, they had been previously told by another doctor that there were no other treatment options available. Within that subgroup alone, their average pain levels fell from 7.5 to 2.7 (scale of 1-10). As a whole, pain and stiffness levels dropped significantly from 5.6 and 6.7 to 2.3 and 2.4, respectively. In this study, the average number of treatments received was 4.2.[8]

A retrospective study of 21 patients, with the primary complaint of neck pain and cervical instability, was conducted in our office. Following a series of Prolotherapy treatments, patient-reported assessments were measured using questionnaire data, including range of motion (ROM), crunching, stiffness, pain level, numbness, and exercise ability. The assessments were conducted between one and 39 months post-treatment (mean = 24 months). Ninety-five percent of patients reported that Prolotherapy met their expectations in regards to pain relief and functionality. Significant reductions in pain at rest, during normal activity, and during exercise were reported. A mean of 86% of patients reported overall sustained improvement, while 33% reported complete functional recovery. Thirty-one percent of patients reported complete relief of all recorded symptoms. No adverse events were reported.[9]

BARRÉ-LIEOU SYNDROME ALSO KNOWN AS CERVICOCRANIAL SYNDROME (HEADACHE WITH CHRONIC SINUSITIS/ ALLERGIES)

In 1925, Jean Alexandre Barré, MD, a French neurologist, and in 1928, Yong-Choen Lieou, a Chinese physician, each independently described a syndrome with a variety of symptoms thought to be due to a dysfunction in the posterior cervical sympathetic nervous system.[10] The posterior cervical

Symptoms that characterize cervicocranial syndrome:

- Chest pain
- Clicking in the neck
- Ear pain
- Facial pain
- Headache
- Hoarseness
- Light headedness
- Loss of voice
- Memory problems
- Migraine headaches
- Neck pain
- Recurrent disturbed vision
- Severe fatigue
- Sinus congestion
- Thinking impairment
- Tinnitus
- Vertigo
- Symptoms often increase with neck motion

Figure 5-4: Cervicocranial syndrome symptoms are very similar to those of post-whiplash or post-concussion syndrome. The good news is that Prolotherapy to the cervical spine resolves the underlying cause of these syndromes, mainly cervical instability and many of the symptoms above, over time.

sympathetic syndrome became known as Barré-Lieou syndrome and cervicocranial syndrome. The posterior cervical sympathetic nervous system is a group of nerves located near the vertebrae in the neck.[11,12] *(See Figure 5-4.)*

Other symptoms may include dysesthesias of the hands and forearms (painful pins-and-needles sensation), corneal sensitivity, dental pain, lacrimation (tearing of the eyes), blurred vision, facial numbness, shoulder pain, swelling of one side of the face, nausea, vomiting, and localized cyanosis of the face (bluish color).

A reasonable question to ask is: How can one disorder cause all of these problems? The answer lies in understanding the function of the sympathetic nervous system, which is part of the autonomic nervous system. The autonomic nervous system operates automatically. That is why it is called the autonomic nervous system. It keeps your heart pumping, your blood flowing through your blood vessels, your lungs breathing, and a myriad of other activities that occur in your body all the time, every day of your life. The sympathetic nervous system is part of the autonomic nervous system. It is activated when the body is "on alert." For instance, if you are being robbed your body shifts into "fight-or-flight mode." Your heart rate, blood pressure, and breathing rate dramatically increase. The blood vessels shift blood away from the intestines into the muscles, enabling you to run or fight the offender.

The posterior-cervical sympathetic nervous system signals the sympathetic part of the autonomic nervous system that controls the head, neck, and face area. In cervicocranial syndrome, the posterior cervical sympathetic system is underactive because the vertebrae in the neck are pinching the sympathetic nerves. **(See Figure 5-5.)**

What symptoms are produced in the face, head, and neck when the sympathetic nervous system is not working well in these areas? The primary symptom is a headache, since headaches are caused by dilation of blood vessels, as in cervicocranial syndrome.

Another symptom of cervicocranial syndrome is tinnitus (ringing in the

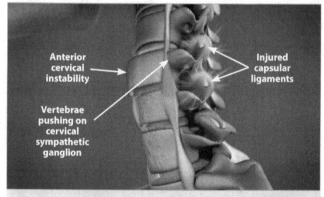

Figure 5-5: Anterior cervical instability. Injury to the capsular ligaments, allows excessive anterior cervical movement, causing cervicocranial syndrome. Symptoms can include dysphagia, tongue numbness, blurred vision, tinnitus, vertigo, dizziness, neck pain, and migraine headaches.

ears). A decrease in sympathetic output to the inner ear will cause an accumulation of fluid in the inner ear. When fluid accumulates in the inner ear, as is often the case with an upper respiratory infection, the ear feels full and the body feels off balance. A ringing in the ear can occur, along with vertigo (dizziness). When Prolotherapy is performed on the head and neck, the posterior sympathetic nervous system begins to function correctly. Conditions such as dizziness, tinnitus, and vertigo (Ménière's disease) can all be eliminated with Prolotherapy, if the symptoms are due to cervicocranial syndrome.

If sympathetic output to the sinus area is low, fluid will also accumulate in this area. Often, immediately after Prolotherapy injections to the posterior head and neck areas, patients with cervicocranial syndrome who have had sinus trouble for years experience clear breathing, which they have not had in years. People using decongestants for years for "chronic allergies" and "chronic sinus infections" are often immediately helped by Prolotherapy injections into the head and neck region.

The other symptoms, such as blurred vision, severe fatigue, dysesthesias (pins-and-needles sensation down the arm), low blood pressure, and low heart rate, are easily understood by a decrease in the output of the sympathetic system of the head, neck, and face areas.

CAUSES AND DIAGNOSIS

Cervicocranial syndrome occurs because of ligament weakness in the neck. Weakness of the neck ligaments commonly occurs because most people spend a good portion of their days looking down at phones and hunched over while working. Their work may consist of typing on a computer or being constantly tethered to their mobile devices for many hours per day, as well as the huge surge in computer gaming. Increasing amounts of patients have suffered from "text neck." All of these tech activities precipitate the head-forward position and put the cervical vertebral ligaments in a stretched position. *(See Figure 5-6.)* Over time, these ligaments weaken and cause pain (creep). The ligament laxity causes an even more head-forward position, as the ligaments can no longer keep the cervical vertebrae in their proper posterior alignment. The paracervical muscles (the neck muscles) tighten to stabilize the joints and head. As the muscles tighten, they create more pain.

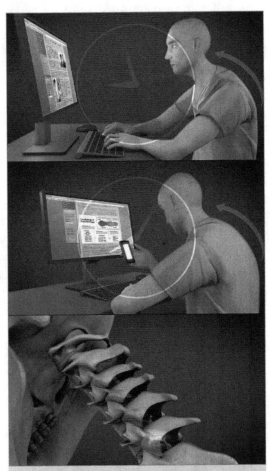

Figure 5-6: Forward head posture from hours of computer work and texting resulting in cervical ligament laxity. Creep, which is a term signifying the slow stretching of ligaments, most commonly occurs by a forward head posture from computer work or looking at a smart phone. Once the ligaments weaken, the muscles contract to give support but this causes chronic neck pain and headaches. Typically, Prolotherapy is required to resolve the pain.

Eventually, the muscles can no longer stabilize the vertebrae and the ligaments are stretched even more. Neck pain increases and the cycle continues to repeat itself. Massage therapy, physical therapy, chiropractic/osteopathic manipulation, and pain medicines all help to temporarily relieve the pain. They do not, however, correct the underlying problem of ligament laxity. Prolotherapy addresses the root cause of neck pain, ligament laxity, and is consequently effective at eliminating the problem.

TREATING CERVICOCRANIAL SYNDROME

The main medicines used to abort severe headache and migraine pain, such as ergotamine, and sumatriptan, constrict the blood vessels. These medicines work, but only temporarily. The medicines act on the symptom of the dysfunction, but not the cause. The correlation is between cervical instability and sympathetic symptoms.[13] Thus, the benefit is only temporary. Prolotherapy to the vertebrae in the neck is the treatment of choice to permanently eliminate cervicocranial syndrome. This occurs because Prolotherapy causes the vertebrae in the neck to move posteriorly (back) and no longer pinch the sympathetic nerves.

Daniel Kayfetz, MD, reported treating 189 patients, from March 1956 through May 1961, who had whiplash injuries to their necks, with Prolotherapy. Fifty-two percent had associated sympathetic nervous system symptoms (as seen in cervicocranial syndrome), 55% of the people had symptoms longer than three months, 81% had symptoms and injuries in other parts of the body, in addition to the neck, and 49% had some kind of legal action because of an auto accident (79% were involved in auto accidents). By all practical purposes these were not simple cases of neck strain, yet Prolotherapy totally eliminated the pain in 60% of the patients, and 86% of the patients considered the end result to be satisfactory (in other words, they had pain relief with the Prolotherapy).[16] Cervicocranial syndrome can also be a late sequela of whiplash injury. C.F. Claussen noted that in Germany in 1992 they had 197,731 cases of whiplash injuries due to traffic accidents. About 80% recovered within a few months. However, about "15-20% developed the so-called late whiplash injury syndrome, with many complaints of the cervico-encephalic syndrome, including headache, vertigo, instability, nausea, tinnitus, hearing loss, etc." It is evident that these symptoms are compatible with cervicocranial syndrome, and this explains why Prolotherapy is so effective in treating whiplash injury and its sequelae.[13]

In our own case series published in the *European Journal of Preventative Medicine*, neck pain, migraines, and other cervicocranial syndrome (Barré-Lieou syndrome) symptoms were resolved following a prescribed series of Prolotherapy injections administered in a pain clinic setting. These patients experienced complete or nearly complete amelioration of pain with relief that lasted months to years after Prolotherapy treatment. **(See Figure 5-7.)** The use of pain medication, chiropractic adjustments, and other therapies were no longer needed by the patients.[14]

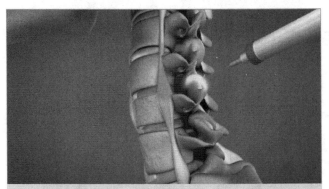

Figure 5-7: Prolotherapy to the cervical facet joints. Prolotherapy is the treatment of choice when cervical instability is the cause of a patient's chronic neck pain, headaches, migraines, vertigo, ringing in the ears and other symptoms of cervicocranial syndrome. By stabilizing the vertebral motion, Prolotherapy resolves the impingement of the cervical sympathetic ganglion and the resultant symptoms.

NECK AND HEADACHE TREATMENTS

Most people say a headache starts at the base of the neck, moves up the neck, behind the eyes, in the temples, and into the head. Migraine sufferers know that pain on one side in the base of the neck may be the beginning of a migraine headache. This is an important clue that the etiology of the headache is in the neck and is producing referred pain. George S. Hackett, MD, the father of Prolotherapy, described the referral patterns of the ligaments of the neck in detail. *(See Figure 5-8.)* These patterns are important to know because the most common cause for pain radiating from the neck to the arm is not a pinched nerve in the neck, but actually a weak ligament in the neck. The most common reason for a pins-and-needles sensation or numbness in the arm is not a pinched nerve, but ligament laxity in the neck.

Dr. Hackett reported good to excellent results in 90% of 82 consecutive patients he treated with neck and/or headache pain.[17,18] Dr. Kayfetz and associates treated 206 patients who had headaches caused from trauma. They found that Prolotherapy was effective in completely relieving the headaches in 79% of patients.[19] John Merriman, MD, of Tulsa, Oklahoma, reported at the 1995 Hackett Foundation Prolotherapy Conference that in treating the necks of 225 patients with Prolotherapy, 80% had good to excellent results.[18] These studies did not differentiate between the different types of headaches. Prolotherapy is effective against migraine, cluster, and tension headaches, if ligament laxity is present.

There are several possible reasons why the cure rate is not even higher. Tension headache, also called muscle-contraction headache, affects at least 80% of the world's population.[20] It is a problem principally of adult life, with women affected three times as often as men. Aching or squeezing discomfort is typically bilateral in the occiput (base of the skull) or the frontotemporal muscle mass (temple area). There is often also an aching in the base of the neck. This typically occurs because of the head position we all subject ourselves to every day. Whether as a computer operator typing at the terminal, a cook cutting up carrots, or a surgeon performing an operation, the head-forward neck-bent posture stretches the cervical ligaments and the posterior neck muscles, including the levator scapulae and trapezeii. *(See Figure 5-6.)*

HACKETT HEAD AND NECK REFERRAL PAIN PATTERNS
LIGAMENT AND TENDON RELAXATION

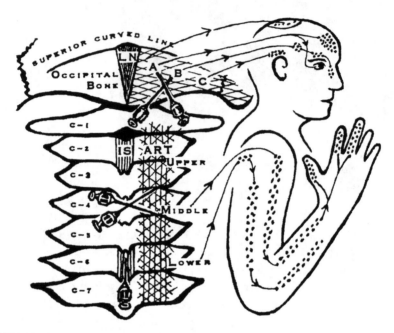

AREA OF WEAKNESS	REFERRAL PATTERN
OCCIPUT AREA A	FOREHEAD AND EYE
OCCIPUT AREA B	TEMPLE, EYEBROW, AND NOSE
OCCIPUT AREA C	ABOVE THE EAR
CERVICAL VERTEBRAE 1-3 (UPPER)	BACK OF NECK AND POSTERIOR SCAPULAR REGION (NOT SHOWN)
CERVICAL VERTEBRAE 4-5 (MIDDLE)	LATERAL ARM AND FOREARM INTO THE THUMB, INDEX FINGER, AND MIDDLE FINGER
CERVICAL VERTEBRAE 6-7 (LOWER)	MEDIAL ARM AND FOREARM INTO THE LATERAL HAND, RING FINGER, AND LITTLE FINGER

Figure 5-8: Head and neck ligament referral pain patterns.

Prolotherapy controls the pain of muscle-contraction headache and neck pain. Prolotherapy, however, will not overcome poor posture or poor dietary and lifestyle habits. If a person is continually sleep-deprived, stressed-out, nutritionally starved (a coffee and doughnut diet), and types on a computer all day, no amount of Prolotherapy will cure that person's neck aches. The cure begins with a proper diet, adequate rest, appropriate stress management, and proper ergonomics at the workstation. If pain persists after the above measures are taken, most assuredly a positive response from Prolotherapy treatment will be experienced.

CERVICAL INSTABILITY DIAGNOSTICS

Often, those who suffer from neck pain due to instability have normal x-rays, MRIs, CT scans, and other radiological studies. This can be frustrating because it does not give any clear indication as to what is causing their pain. Patients are commonly told that the pain is "in their heads" or given refills upon refills of pain medication to help ease their pain.

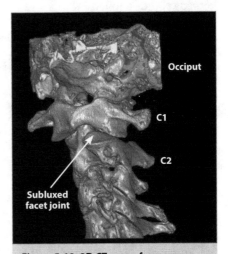

Figure 5-9: Digital Motion X-ray (DMX). In our office, we utilize DMX to document cervical instability and improvement after Prolotherapy.

The diagnosis of cervical instability is often made from a thorough history of the patient's neck pain.[21,22] This is because there is no gold standard diagnostic test for cervical instability or ligament laxity in the cervical spine. That being said, we can use objective methods to document neck instability through specific imaging, such as a Digital Motion X-ray (DMX) or functional MRI or CT. In our office we utilize DMX to essentially take a movie of a patient's cervical spine with motion. *(See Figure 5-9.)*

This is more advantageous than a standard x-ray because it allows the clinician to visualize the bones while moving. Instability or ligament injury is likely to present with a DMX versus a standard x-ray where patient is holding still.[23] In most cases, patients with cervical instability do not have pain at rest but do with motion, so it is easy to understand why a plain radiograph would not show any underlying cause for pain, as the patient is holding still in a position that doesn't hurt. Often, cervical instability patients experience the most symptoms with neck rotation, so rotational views on a DMX are key because they allow the clinician to see what is happening in the spine during that motion (i.e. able to visualize cervical instability with these movements).

Functional MRI and CT scans are useful because they can provide images of the cervical spine in different positions.[24-26] Unlike a DMX, these imaging studies do not present like a "movie," but instead take separate images of the cervical spine

Figure 5-10: 3D CT scan of upper cervical spine. C1-C2 instability can be seen, as 70% of C1 articular facet is subluxed posteriorly (arrow) on C2 facet when the patient rotates his head (turns head to the left then the right). This patient came from Germany because of severe symptoms of cervicocranial syndrome from C1-C2 instability. Prolotherapy to the C1-C2 capsular ligaments tightened this joint and resolved his symptoms, which included severe headaches and neck pain, tinnitus, vertigo, balance trouble and difficulty swallowing.

in different positions. For example, a functional MRI or CT scan will take images while you hold your neck in flexion, extension, or rotation. For this reason, they can offer valuable information about the displacement of cervical vertebrae and ligament injuries that become evident during these motions which can be helpful in the diagnosis of cervical instability.[25] Again, someone may only experience dizziness, blurry vision, or ringing in the ears when the head is rotated. Plain MRIs or CT scans would likely appear normal because the patient is not in a position that causes the symptoms.

Additionally, images from functional CT scans can actually be used to create a 3D image of the patient's neck *(See Figure 5-10.)* and can clearly depict dislocation of facet joints and upper cervical vertebrae.

FACET JOINTS

Some of you may have heard of the term "facet joints" through the mention of "facet joint syndrome." Perhaps you or a loved one has been diagnosed with this condition by your doctor, which essentially just means that the facet joints in your spine are causing pain. Facet joints are the small joints that connect one vertebra to the vertebrae below and above it and have been shown to be a significant generator of neck pain (and thoracic and lumbar

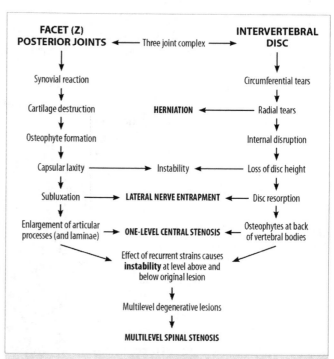

Figure 5-11: The process of facet (Z) joint and disc degeneration and the interrelation between the two.
Adapted from Kirkaldy-Willis WH, et al. *Spine*. 1978;3:319-328.

pain as well).[27,28] If these joints (that connect vertebrae together) suffer injury from trauma, whiplash, or poor posture, it seems reasonable to believe that they will no longer be able to hold the cervical spine in proper position, thus leading to instability. *(See Figure 5-11.)* Unstable and injured facet joints can be very painful[29] and often lead patients to search for a cure for their chronic neck pain. A common treatment for facet joint syndrome involves injections of local anesthetic with or without steroid into the affected facet joint(s) through x-ray guidance. The patient may feel better right away, but these effects often do not last long-term.[29] This is because nothing has stimulated healing to strengthen the ligaments around the facet joint and stabilize the spine. This begins to lead to more instability, and eventually disc herniation, nerve entrapment, and spinal stenosis. Before this happens, it is much easier for a person to regenerate the ligament tissue that allow the proper movement of facet joints, and stability of the spine through Prolotherapy.

ATLANTO-AXIAL INSTABILITY

The cervical spine is divided into two parts – the upper and the lower cervical spine. The upper cervical spine contains C0 (the occiput or base of the skull) and C1 and C2 (the atlas and axis, respectively). Instability of the upper cervical spine is often referred to as "atlanto-axial instability." Ligament injury can happen to any part of the neck, but injury to the upper part of the neck may cause unique symptoms. These include neck pain, headaches, dizziness, vertigo, fatigue, numbness and tingling of the face and tongue, tinnitus, nausea/vomiting, balance difficulties, drop attacks, difficulty swallowing, and migraines. *(See Figure 5-12.)*

Those that have atlanto-axial instability almost always have experienced some sort of trauma to the neck, often involving a car accident or traumatic fall. Again, standard x-rays and MRIs are normal after these types of injuries because instability and ligament injury is usually not evident. Once these imaging studies come back normal, there is often not much else traditional medicine can offer the patient in terms of relieving lingering neck pain and instability. In our experience, Prolotherapy can offer a tremendous amount of hope and relief of symptoms in these cases.[30]

Symptoms for C1-C2 (Atlantoaxial) Instability:

- Balance problems
- Blurred vision
- Continuous pain in the head or neck
- Dizziness
- Fullness in the ear
- Migraine or sub-occipital headaches
- Neck pain with the "head-shaking" motion
- Severe fatigue
- Tinnitus
- Vertigo

Figure 5-12: Upper cervical instability can be the sole cause for any of these symptoms.

POST-CONCUSSION SYNDROME

The diagnosis of post-concussion syndrome (PCS) is often made after suffering a head injury where the patient loses consciousness and develops a myriad of symptoms a year after the injury.[31] These symptoms include headache, neck pain, dizziness, fatigue, irritability, nausea, anxiety, and memory problems. Many of these symptoms overlap with those of atlanto-axial instability, cervicocranial syndrome, and whiplash-associated disorder. *(See Figure 5-13.)* This is not just a coincidence. Typical causes of concussion include blows to the head or falls. If you fall and hit your head on the ground, it is easy to understand that the fall would put a large force on the skull. In addition to that, however, that same force can also be transmitted to the ligaments of the upper cervical spine. A blow to the head or a fall could also cause a hyperextension-hyperflexion type movement of the neck, insinuating that those who suffer concussions also suffer a concurrent whiplash injury. For that

Symptoms	Atlanto-axial instability	Whiplash-associated disorder	Post-concussion disorder	Cervico-cranial syndrome	Vertebrobasilar insufficiency
Neck pain/stiffness	X	X	X	X	X
Headaches	X	X	X	X	X
Dizziness	X	X	X	X	X
Vertigo	X	X	X	X	X
Paresthesias (upper extremities)		X			
Paresthesias (face)	X			X	X
Fatigue	X	X	X	X	
Difficulty sleeping	X	X	X	X	X
Irritability	X	X	X		X
TMJ pain		X			
Tinnitus	X	X	X	X	X
Nausea/vomiting	X		X	X	X
Visual disturbances	X		X	X	X
Cognitive impairment	X	X	X	X	
Anxiety	X	X	X	X	X
Light headedness	X	X	X	X	X
Memory problems	X		X	X	
Ear pain	X			X	
Crepitation	X	X	X	X	
Balance difficulty	X		X	X	X
Drop attacks	X			X	X
Dysphagia	X			X	X
Speech disturbances	X				X
Migraines	X	X	X	X	

Figure 5-13: Overlap in symptomology between atlanto-axial instability, whiplash-associated disorder, post-concussion syndrome, cervicocranial syndrome, and vertebrobasilar insufficiency. Overlap in symptoms exists due to underlying cervical instability found in each of the conditions.

reason, patients who suffer from one or multiple concussion(s) can easily develop upper cervical instability and associated symptoms. Further explanation could be that post-concussion syndrome, which was once thought to be due to residual brain trauma, could be the result of upper cervical instability that develops during the injury. Symptoms of post-concussion syndrome occur long after imaging of the brain appears normal, suggesting that there is another cause for the headaches, dizziness, etc. that develop weeks after the fall/injury. It is likely that this other cause is ligament laxity in the upper cervical spine.

WHIPLASH-ASSOCIATED DISORDER

Whiplash occurs when the neck suffers a "hyperflexion-hyperextension" injury, often after a rear end collision or other car accident. Anyone that has ever been rear-ended knows that a lot of force is placed on your neck when your head moves forward and then backward after the car has been hit. Research shows that when the head is rotated, there is a significant increase in the amount of force placed on the neck during whiplash injuries.[32-34] By simply having your head turned to the side, a significant increase in force is placed on the facet joints in your neck, which can predispose you to more ligament injuries and subsequent symptoms. Common symptoms of whiplash-associated disorder include neck pain, headache, dizziness, vertigo, crepitation in the neck, fatigue, irritability, tinnitus, nausea/vomiting, cognitive impairment, anxiety, lightheadedness, and memory problems. The facet joints in the cervical spine can be easily injured easily with rotational forces, such as the whiplash scenario explained above.

VERTEBROBASILAR INSUFFICIENCY

The vertebral artery supplies 20% of the blood flow to the brain. Vertebrobasilar insufficiency, also known as vertebrobasilar artery insufficiency, occurs when blood flow is disrupted, such as from blood clots or ruptures of the artery. We most commonly see that this condition is due to underlying upper cervical instability. The vertebral arteries travel up through the cervical vertebrae (one on each side) through foramina (or "holes") in a bony prominence called the transverse process. When it gets to the upper cervical spine at C1, the vertebral arteries follow more of a serpentine path up to the brain. It is here that these arteries are at risk of "kinking" and therefore shutting off blood flow to the brain. How does instability cause this? With normal neck rotation (i.e. looking over your shoulder), C1 rotates over the dens of C2. This simple rotation can partially occlude the vertebral arteries (more specifically, the artery on the same side you are looking over) with normal movement. In someone with an unstable cervical spine who suffers from neck hypermobility, this can occur on a more regular basis and cause a plethora of symptoms. One of the most common symptoms in vertebrobasilar insufficiency is drop attacks, which cause the person to suddenly fall to the ground without warning (but remains conscious). It has been proposed that drop attacks may occur from transient loss of blood flow to the brain stem (from the vertebral arteries).[35] Other symptoms include dizziness, fainting, blurred vision, visual and auditory disturbances, flushing, sweating, tearing of the eyes, runny nose, vertigo, numbness and tingling, and difficulty swallowing or talking. It should be noted that instability along any of the entire cervical spine can cause kinking of the vertebral arteries as they travel through each vertebrae, but it is often related to the upper cervical spine.

CERVICAL RADICULOPATHY

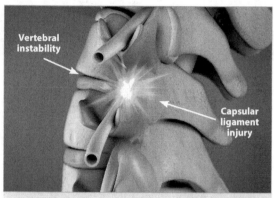

In many cases we see at Caring Medical, people have been diagnosed with radiculopathy, but cannot find permanent help for it. They are prescribed rounds of steroids, nerve blocks, heavy duty pain medications and physical therapy from their general practitioner, but the radiculopathy returns. When someone truly has a pinched nerve, it is one of the worst types of pain a person can experience. They cannot concentrate on anything more than trying to

Figure 5-14: Capsular ligament injury causing cervical radiculopathy. When a person has a ligament injury in the neck, the vertebrae can sublux or move and then encroach on a nerve. This causes pain down the arm with certain neck movements. Prolotherapy resolves this type of cervical radiculopathy by stabilizing the vertebral movement by stimulating ligament repair.

contort themselves into a position that relieves the burning, unrelenting pain. Cervical radiculopathy is a dysfunction of a nerve root in the neck or cervical spine from its exit point at the neuroforamen. *(See Figure 5-14.)* As we've been discussing with cervical vertebrae abnormally pressing on nerves, there is a reason why the bone is now pressing on the nerve. Athletes may experience this type of scenario just by implementing a new technique in their sport. Dr. Hauser is a good example of this.

When concentrating so hard on learning bilateral breathing in swimming, he ended up torquing his cervical ligaments. The continuous over stretching of the cervical ligaments without enough rest between workouts caused instability in the vertebrae and allowed them to pinch one of his cervical nerves, especially when lifting his head. You can see his Digital Motion X-ray in *Figure 5-15.*

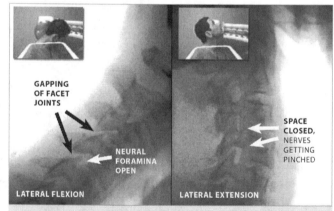

Figure 5-15: Digital Motion X-ray of neck before Prolotherapy. When Dr. Hauser bent his head down and to the side, gapping of the facet joints occurred due to capsular ligament stretching. Extending his head back and to the side caused the facet joints to move, encroaching on the cervical nerves producing excruciating pain down the right arm. This extreme example of cervical instability resulting in cervical radiculopathy was successfully treated with a few Prolotherapy treatments producing complete resolution of the pain and facet joint instability.

The zinging pain shot like a lightning bolt down his arm. He developed cervical instability causing radiculopathy. By now, you understand that the permanent cure for cervical instability is not long-term narcotic medications or steroids, though sometimes a prescription or nerve block is necessary to get a person through the most acute phase. Decreasing the acute pain allows the patient to sleep and rest while the Prolotherapy stimulates the ligaments to tighten and properly restore vertebral alignment. In the fourth issue of the *Journal of Prolotherapy*, we published an article on the non-operative treatment of cervical radiculopathy, along with the physical therapy and chiropractic approach.[36]

TMJ SYNDROME

One reason why a person may not respond adequately to Prolotherapy is that some of the affected areas may not have been treated. A common area forgotten in headache and neck pain is the temporomandibular joint. The temporomandibular joint (TMJ) is the physical connection where the jaw meets the skull. The TMJ is necessary to keep the jaw in proper alignment, especially when talking and eating. A painful and clicking TMJ is called temporomandibular joint syndrome (TMJS). The symptoms of TMJS are essentially the same as cervicocranial syndrome. It is our belief that the symptoms, such as dizziness, vertigo, etc., that physicians ascribe to TMJS, are actually due to cervicocranial syndrome/ Barré–Lieou syndrome.

CAUSES OF TMJ SYNDROME

Typically in TMJS the lower jaw (mandible) is extended forward. A head-forward posture exaggerates the problem.[37,38] This forward mandible aggravates the cervical ligament laxity, which increases the neck pain. Again, an endless cycle of pain and disability is created in the neck, head, and face region. Prolotherapy injections to strengthen both the cervical

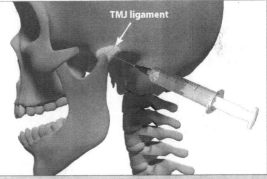

Figure 5-16: Prolotherapy to the TMJ. Prolotherapy is very effective at eliminating the pain and clicking of TMJ syndrome.

vertebrae and the temporomandibular joint will solve this problem. *(See Figure 5-16.)*

Eventually, the mandible moves forward to the extent that it will stretch the lateral TMJ ligament and produce pain. Once the lateral TMJ ligament becomes lax, the joint will click. It is important to note that clicking in any joint is an indication of ligament laxity of that joint. Joint clicking is never normal or a good sign. Joint clicking, whether it is in the TMJ, knee, neck, or lower back is always abnormal. It is a sign that the bones are beginning to rub against each other. The body's compensatory mechanism for such a situation is to tighten muscles and to grow more bone. The end result will be degeneration, arthritis, and stiffness in that joint. Prolotherapy can stop this process. Prolotherapy will stop a joint from clicking and stop the arthritic process from continuing.

Another cause of lax TMJ ligament is the patient's sleeping position. For example, if a patient sleeps with his or her head turned to the right, the TMJ on the left side will be continually stretched throughout the night. Over many decades, continually sleeping in this manner puts the left TMJ at risk for TMJ ligament laxity. The patient with a TMJ problem is advised to sleep with the head turned to the side of the problematic TMJ.

We will never forget Terry who came to Caring Medical with one of the worst cases of TMJS we have ever seen. His jaw popped so loudly that the action of opening his mouth could be heard in the other room. The first Prolotherapy session to his TMJ caused a 60% reduction in the clicking of his jaw. After the second treatment, the clicking was eliminated completely. Terry told us that his dentist was amazed. Most dentists and oral surgeons believe TMJ syndrome is permanent and the best hope is for temporary symptom relief. We can verify in our own practice that TMJ syndrome can be cured with Prolotherapy. By the way, did the dentist call us to find out what we did to finally help Terry find relief? No, they never do.

TREATMENT OF TMJ SYNDROME

Louis Schultz, MD, an oral surgeon, reported in 1956 that after 20 years of experience in treating hypermobile temporomandibular joints with Prolotherapy, the clicking, grating, or popping was controlled in all of the several thousand patients that had been under his care, without any reported complications or deleterious effects.[39,40] Other Prolotherapists have noted similar improvements in their patients.[41-44] In our study, published in *Practical Pain Management*, we reported on 14 patients with TMJ pain. The average number of treatments received was 4.6, and the average pain level decreased from 5.9 to 2.5, on a scale of 1-10.[45]

Prolotherapy solution is injected into and around the temporomandibular joint. The patient is placed on a soft diet until the mouth is able to fully open. The TMJ Prolotherapy injections cause an awkward bite and a tight jaw for a couple of days. The patient should not force the mouth open during this time period.

Options now available for people with head and neck pain are TMJ arthroscopic surgery, TMJ implants, cervical spine surgery (many varieties), botulism toxin injections into muscles,[46] and surgical cauterization, which zaps the bones with a radiofrequency wave, destroying the treated area.[47] This last technique may eliminate a patient's pain because it destroys the fibro-osseous junction, where the pain originates. Why destroy or remove a structure when there is a treatment that will help strengthen and repair it? Prolotherapy causes a permanent strengthening of ligaments and tendons and eliminates the root cause of the pain.

EAR AND MOUTH PAIN

EAGLE SYNDROME AND ERNEST SYNDROME

One of our patients, Jim, told us, "I have been to a hundred doctors and all I get is a hundred different creams. I am drowning in creams, drops, and pills." Some doctors tell him that the problem is in his ear, others say the ear is fine.

Jim, like many others, suffered from terrible ear and mouth pain. Various diagnoses are typically given for such complaints, including *otitis media, otitis externa* (ear infections), trigeminal neuralgia, atypical facial pain, or TMJ syndrome. These diagnoses may be accurate for some; however, chronic unresolved ear, mouth, face, temple, or head pain generally has a ligament laxity etiology. Instead of creams, drops, or pills, Jim needed a physician to press on his stylomandibular ligament. Most likely he would jump off the table in pain. Chronic pain must be reproduced in the doctor's office to properly diagnose the source of the problem, and thereby provide appropriate treatment.

The stylomandibular ligament originates at the styloid process underneath the ear and inserts on the medial side of the mandible (the lower jaw). *(See Figure 5-17.)* Pain from the styloid portion of the ligament is called Eagle syndrome.[48,49] Pain from the mandibular portion is called Ernest syndrome.[50,51]

The following symptoms have been described with both Eagle and Ernest syndromes:[52,53]

• Bloodshot eyes	• Forehead pain	• Shoulder pain
• Cough	• Jaw pain	• Sinusitis
• Difficult jaw opening	• Mouth pain	• Stuffy nose
• Dizziness	• Neck pain	• Throat pain
• Ear pain	• Pain on swallowing	• Tinnitus
• Excessive lacrimation (tearing)	• Pain upon opening the mouth	• TMJ pain
• Eye pain	• Pain upon turning the head	• Tooth pain
• Facial pain		• Vertigo
		• Voice alteration

Most physicians have not heard of these syndromes and do not know where the stylomandibular ligament is located. For this reason, many people with the above complaints do not obtain relief from their pain.

If someone chronically experiences any of these symptoms, the stylomandibular ligament must be palpated. If a positive "jump sign" can be elicited, the culprit for the chronic ear-mouth pain has most likely been located. Prolotherapy injections at the stylomandibular ligament bony attachments will start the repair process. Once the stylomandibular ligament is strengthened, the chronic ear-mouth pain, tinnitus, dizziness, vertigo, and other pain complaints subside.

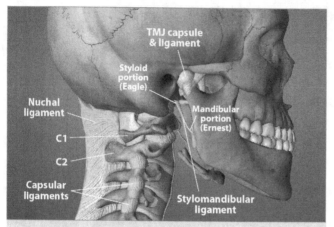

Figure 5-17: Stylomandibular ligament. Weakness of the stylomandibular ligament is responsible for the symptoms of Ernest and Eagle syndromes.

SPASTIC TORTICOLLIS

Joan struggled with spastic torticollis for several years prior to coming to our office. Spastic torticollis is a condition in which the head will twitch or turn uncontrollably and tilt to one side. Joan needed to turn her body to the side in order to see straight ahead. In addition to the social stigma, she experienced debilitating neck pain. Her attempts to relieve her pain with physical therapy, muscle relaxants, and Valium® proved unsuccessful. Spastic torticollis is not due to a Valium® deficiency. Joan had heard about Prolotherapy and wanted to give it a try.

Like all chronic painful conditions, spastic torticollis has a cause, which is typically ligament laxity. Spastic torticollis causes involuntary muscle spasms in the neck.[54] The muscle spasms cause the neck to continually jerk the head to one side. Eventually, because the muscles continue to tighten, it becomes impossible to turn the head to the side.

Upon examining Joan, a positive "jump sign" was elicited when the cervical vertebral ligaments were palpated. Her twitching neck made the treatment difficult, but with persistence it was successfully completed. After the second treatment, Joan reported that she could sleep facing to the left. After five treatments, Joan was a new woman. She was fortunate to have heard about Prolotherapy. She became pain-free, with the ability to turn her head in both directions.

Once a ligament is loose, as occurs in a neck injury, the overlying muscles must tighten to support the structure. If only one side of the neck ligaments loosen, then the muscles on that side of the neck will become spastic. This is how spastic torticollis may form.

If significant shortening of the neck muscles has already occurred, botulism injections may be helpful in conjunction with Prolotherapy. If shortening of the muscles has not occurred, the person with spastic torticollis has an excellent chance of achieving complete neck pain relief with Prolotherapy.

SUMMARY

Some of the most debilitating conditions are those due to cervical instability and ligament laxity. The ligaments that hold the cervical vertebrae in alignment can be damaged via a sudden trauma, such as a whiplash or concussion, or through the slow stretching of ligaments, known as creep. This can be attributed to extended hours of poor posture in front of a computer or smart phone, or other position that slowly stretches the ligaments. Without addressing the ligament laxity, conditions that originate from joint instability can wreak havoc on a patient's life in the form of chronic headaches, migraines, neck pain, TMJ syndrome, ear and mouth pain, to name a few. Prolotherapy strengthens the weakened ligaments and has demonstrated an estimated 80-90% elimination of chronic headaches and neck pain.

There is much overlap in the symptoms caused by cervical instability, and especially upper cervical instability (C0-C2): cervicocranial syndrome, atlanto-axial instability, whiplash, post-concussion syndrome, and vertebrobasilar insufficiency. Prolotherapy permanently strengthens the cervical ligaments and effectively treats the migraine headaches, vertigo, tinnitus, dysthesias, and other symptoms that accompany these syndromes.

Cervical radiculopathy due to a pinched nerve in the neck can cause excruciating, burning pain that radiates into the arms and hands. We know cervical instability causes the facet joints to move too much and this can cause nerves to be pinched, among other symptoms. This movement can clearly be seen by using Digital Motion X-ray (DMX) technology. It allows the practitioner and the patient to observe the vertebrae movement as the patient moves his or her neck through the full range of motion. DMX is an excellent tool for assistance to diagnose the problem as well as for needle guidance during the Prolotherapy treatment.

Ear and mouth pain from Eagle syndrome or Ernest syndrome are also successfully treated with Prolotherapy because it targets the underlying ligament damage associated with these syndromes.

Prolotherapy is an extremely effective treatment for chronic neck, head, TMJ, facial, ear, and mouth pain because it strengthens the structures that are causing the pain. This is why many people are choosing to Prolo their head and neck pain away! ■

CHAPTER

6

PROLO YOUR SHOULDER PAIN AWAY!

Shoulder pain is one of the most common reasons patients give for a physician visit, third only to headache and back pain[1] The incidence of shoulder pain is escalating, especially among office workers with intensive computer use.[2,3]

The shoulder was uniquely designed by God to have tremendous mobility. The shoulder enables a person to scratch

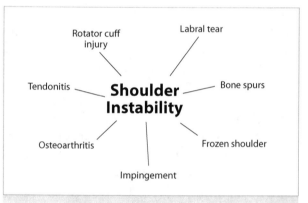

Conditions which commonly cause shoulder pain, instability, and/or joint degeneration.

the head, between the shoulder blades, and even the back without pivoting anything but the shoulder. The lack of big ligamentous structures supporting this joint allow its mobility. The shoulder, when abducted and externally rotated, is more vulnerable to injury due to a lack of bony and ligamentous stability in this position. The primary support for the shoulder involves the rotator cuff muscles, which also move the shoulder. People who frequently abduct and externally rotate their shoulders, especially athletes such as pitchers, gymnasts, tennis players, quarterbacks, swimmers, and volleyball players, are prone to chronic shoulder problems. Any activity done with the hand away from the body involves some sort of shoulder abduction and external rotation.[4] *(See Figures 6-1A & 6-1B.)*

A shoulder that crunches and "pops out of joint" is unstable, and is always a sign of weakness in the joint. *(See Figure 6-2.)* People who suffer from this condition will feel their shoulders coming out of the sockets when they abduct and externally rotate them, because the ligamentous and bony support of the joints is minimal in this position. When this occurs, a person is said to have shoulder subluxation or instability. This diagnosis can be confirmed by abducting and externally rotating the shoulder and pushing the arm forward from the back. In the case of anterior

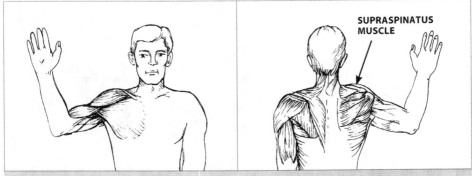

Figure 6-1A: The "Hi" stance. This is the position of shoulder abduction and external rotation.

Figure 6-1B: The "Hi" stance supported by the supraspinatus muscle. This position pulls the shoulder in a compromised position making it more likely to sublux.

shoulder instability, a positive "frighten sign" (the cousin of the infamous positive "jump sign") will be displayed on the patient's face; the patient is afraid his or her shoulder is going to dislocate.

CAUSE AND TREATMENT OF SHOULDER INSTABILITY

Traditional treatment for shoulder instability is rotator cuff strengthening exercises, specifically of the supraspinatus muscle, the primary muscle responsible for the external rotation of the shoulder. The rotator cuff is a group of four muscles: the supraspinatus, infraspinatus, subscapularis, and teres minor. *(See Figure 6-3.)* The rotator cuff muscles help stabilize the shoulder and assist with movement. Rotator cuff strengthening exercises help strengthen shoulder muscles but often do not cure the underlying problem of shoulder instability: joint laxity.

To cure shoulder joint instability, the ligamentous and shoulder capsular structures must be strengthened. The main capsular structure involved in the stability of the shoulder is the glenoid labrum, which holds the humerus bone to the glenoid cavity of the scapula. A shoulder is usually unstable because the structures are torn or stretched. Once these structures are stretched or loosened, no

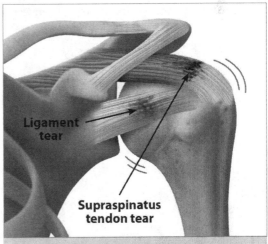

Ligament tear

Supraspinatus tendon tear

Figure 6-2: Shoulder instability increases the force on rotator cuff tendons. The rotator cuff is designed to move the shoulder joint, not stabilize it. This causes the tendons to weaken and degenerate, increasing susceptibility to tearing. Rotator cuff tears are indicative of joint instability and respond great to Prolotherapy.

amount of exercise will strengthen the shoulder joint enough to permanently hold it in place. *(See Figure 6-4.)*

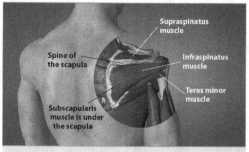

Figure 6-3: Rotator cuff muscles (viewed from back). Rotator cuff muscles support and move the shoulder.

IDENTIFYING GLENOID LABRUM TEARS

The glenoid labrum is one of the most important soft tissue stabilizing structures of the shoulder. Because of this, athletes who depend on powerful shoulders and an excellent range of motion are particularly susceptible to injuries of the glenoid labrum, especially those with hypermobile shoulders. Injuries to the glenoid labrum can be associated with and can cause instability, dislocation, and pain. When the labrum is torn or damaged, the shoulder is susceptible to recurrent dislocations, subluxation, as well as, clicking, catching, and locking secondary to partially attached fragments becoming entrapped between the articular surfaces. Tears are the most common form of glenoid labral injury. There are several different types of tears the labrum can sustain and these types are typically categorized based on the lesion location and/or arthroscopic appearance. In addition, many potential mechanisms of labral injury have been identified. Some of the most commonly reported labral injuries include Superior Labral Anterior to Posterior (SLAP) tear, flap tear, Bankart lesion, and degenerative lesions. Mechanisms of injury can include, but are not limited to compression, avulsion, traction, shear, and chronic degenerative changes.

GLENOID LABRUM ANATOMY AND FUNCTION

The shoulder joint consists of three bones: the scapula (shoulder blade), the clavicle (collar bone), and the humerus (upper arm bone). The head of the humerus comes into contact with a shallow socket in the scapula called the glenoid. The glenoid labrum is a smooth ring of

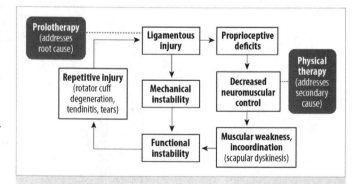

Figure 6-4: Shoulder instability paradigm. Ligament injury is what causes the mechanical instability and proprioceptive deficits that leads to joint mechanical and functional instability (in the shoulder and other joints). Prolotherapy should be started first before rehabilitation because muscles cannot be adequately strengthened and rehabilitated when the joint they move is unstable.

fibrous cartilage that surrounds the glenoid portion of the scapula and stabilizes the glenohumeral (shoulder) joint by allowing the humerus to fit into the glenoid portion of the scapula. The labrum is distinct from both the fibrous shoulder capsule and the hyaline cartilage of the glenoid. Because the head, or ball, of the humerus is much larger than the glenoid socket, the labrum helps to stabilize the shoulder by increasing the socket depth of the glenoid and providing a point of attachment for the glenohumeral ligaments and the tendon of the long head of the biceps. *(See Figure 6-5.)*

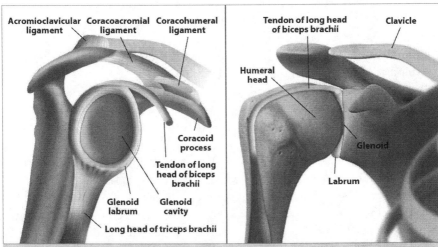

Figure 6-5: The glenoid labrum (a fibro-cartilagenous rim that acts to deepen the glenoid by 50%) is attached to the underlying bony glenoid and is confluent at its area with the long head of the biceps tendon. The labrum has a triangular configuration when viewed in cross section and serves to effectively deepen the glenoid, increasing the stability of the glenohumeral joint.

Adapted from: Nordin M, et al. *Basic Biomechanics of the Musculoskeletal System.* 4th Edition. Lippincott Williams & Wilkins. Baltimore, MD. 2012.

GLENOID LABRUM TEAR SYMPTOMS

The symptoms of a labral tear are very similar to symptoms resulting from injuries to other structures of the shoulder. Patients usually report pain with overhead activity and popping, locking, catching, or grinding with movement. Patients will also commonly report a feeling of instability and/or weakness with decreased range of motion. Glenoid labrum tears are especially significant because they are the most common lesion observed in recurrent shoulder dislocations.

POOR VASCULARITY IN THE LABRUM

An important factor to consider regarding labral pathology is the vascularity of labral tissue. Similar to the meniscal structure of the knee, the vascular supply to the labrum is greater peripherally than centrally. Additionally, the superior and anterosuperior portions of the labrum are less vascular than other portions of the labrum and the vascular density of the entire labrum decreases with age. In short, the blood supply to the glenoid labrum is poor and this is often responsible for glenoid labrum tears not healing.

LESIONS OF GLENOID LABRUM TREATED WITH PROLOTHERAPY

The advantages of using Prolotherapy versus surgery for labral tears:

- Prolotherapy requires no general anesthesia.
- Prolotherapy does not involve big scopes in the joint.
- Prolotherapy does not typically require time out of work.
- Prolotherapy stimulates repair.
- Prolotherapy allows the labrum to retain its flexibility.
- Prolotherapy accelerates the return to athletics.
- Prolotherapy is a fraction of the cost of surgery.
- Prolotherapy risks are minimal.
- Prolotherapy can treat all the injured structures.

Our glenoid labrum lesion study did show that Comprehensive Prolotherapy eliminated 69% of the symptoms in patients with lesions, primarily tears of the glenoid labrum.[5] The patient–reported assessments were taken 16 months after their last Prolotherapy session. Treated patients reported highly significant improvements with respect to pain, stiffness, range of motion, crunching, exercise and need for medication. *(See Figure 6-6.)* Only 1 out of the 33 shoulders treated experienced a worsening of symptoms. Prolotherapy should be the treatment of choice for labral tears. Surgery is needed on rare occasions, and should be a last resort.

TRADITIONAL MEDICINE TREATMENT OF LABRAL TEARS

A typical scenario in our office is a patient who has shoulder instability

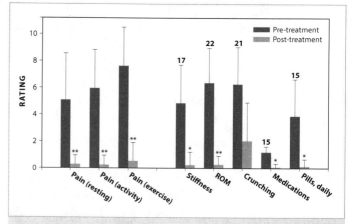

Figure 6-6: Before and after Prolotherapy treatment data on patients who were treated at Caring Medical for glenoid labrum tears.
Patients reported pain, stiffness, range of motion (ROM) and crunching on a 0-10 rating scale. For consumption of medications, the ordinate represents the number of medications used or the number of daily pills taken. For pain reports, n = 33. For stiffness, ROM, crunching and medications, only reports with non-zero baseline values were analyzed, the numbers of which are indicated above the bars. * $p \leq 0.01$, ** $p \leq 0.0001$ by Wilcoxon signed-rank test.

and received corticosteroid injections, which further weakened the cartilage and led to complete shoulder destruction and the eventual need for shoulder replacement. A better option than corticosteroid injections or anti-inflammatory medications is Prolotherapy because it gets at the root cause of the shoulder pain from labral tears which is instability.

When joint instability occurs, the body has three protective mechanisms: engage the muscles, swell the joint, and grow more bone. This is why bone spurs and arthritis are the long-term result of joint instability which was treated only for the symptoms it produced: inflammation and muscle spasms. *(See Figure 6-7.)* Corticosteroid shots and anti-inflammatories address the joint swelling, so the

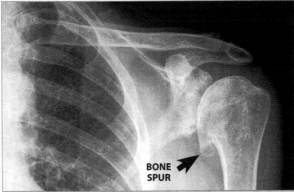

BONE SPUR

Figure 6-7: Shoulder x-ray showing large bone spur.
This young patient (30's) presented with significant pain and limitation of motion. Notice the cartilage is fairly well preserved but the large osteophyte on the humeral neck is present. While Prolotherapy can eliminate much of this person's pain, the restriction of motion may necessitate surgery.

symptoms appear better and people keep taking them, but these do nothing for the joint instability. The joint instability without the "protection" of the joint swelling, which helps brace the joint, puts further pressure on such vital structures in the joint like the articular cartilage. Without resolution of the labral tear, ligament injury, or tendinopathy causing the shoulder instability, the body will eventually overgrow bone to stabilize the joint. This is why long-term labral tears that are not treated lead to shoulder immobility and impingement. So when a patient has waited too long before getting Prolotherapy there are times when even Prolotherapy can only partially resolve the symptoms, and more treatments are typically needed. Thus, it is best to get Prolotherapy as soon as symptoms start.

ROTATOR CUFF TENDONITIS

A supraspinatus tendon problem is manifested by pain with abduction and external rotation of the shoulder, especially when reaching for things above shoulder level, or pain in the shoulder after sleeping due to compression of the supraspinatus tendon. The supraspinatus tendon often refers pain to the back of the shoulder. The supraspinatus tendon is the main abductor and external rotator of the shoulder.

Supraspinatus tendinopathy can be induced by large amounts of swim training, for instance, and is worsened when a swimmer's shoulder is hypermobile. The key muscle group of the shoulder is the rotator cuff, made up of (from anterior to posterior) the subscapularis, supraspinatus, infraspinatus, and teres minor. The primary role of the rotator cuff is to function as the dynamic and functional stabilizer of the glenohumeral joint. Specifically, the supraspinatus muscle helps seat the humeral head (ball) into the glenoid cavity (socket) when the arm is raised from the side. For the serious athlete or those performing a lot of overhead work, this happens thousands of times, so it is no wonder the supraspinatus tendon becomes injured.

Sleeping on the shoulder causes a pinching of the rotator cuff muscles and can lead to rotator cuff weakness. There are cases where the cause of the rotator cuff tendon laxity was due to years of sleeping on the shoulder.

In most cases, traditional therapies such as exercise and physical therapy will resolve rotator cuff tendonitis. It is not uncommon, however, for rotator cuff injuries to linger because blood supply to the rotator cuff tendons is poor.[6] Poor blood supply is a reason the rotator cuff is so commonly injured. In chronic cases of shoulder pain due to rotator cuff weakness, Prolotherapy is the treatment of choice. Prolotherapy will cause the rotator cuff to strengthen and eliminate shoulder pain. If rotator cuff weakness is not corrected, the shoulder's range of motion will deteriorate. Rapid deterioration can occur, especially in people over 60 years of age.

As previously stated, the supraspinatus muscle causes shoulder abduction and external rotation. When this muscle weakens, movement becomes painful. Those who have supraspinatus tendon laxity causing pain will stop moving their arms into the painful position. Although they may not realize it, they are slowly but surely losing shoulder movement. What begins as a simple rotator cuff muscle weakness, easily treated with Prolotherapy, has the potential to become a frozen shoulder because of scar tissue formation inside the shoulder that was left untreated. The scar tissue formation, which causes a decrease in the ability to move the shoulder, is called adhesive capsulitis. Pain means something is wrong.

FROZEN SHOULDER (ADHESIVE CAPSULITIS)

A frozen shoulder is also treatable with Prolotherapy, but healing occurs over a longer period of time. The term adhesive capsulitis refers to scar tissue that forms inside the joint due to lack of movement. If a joint is not moved through its full range of motion every day, scar tissue will form inside the joint. Adhesive capsulitis is especially common in stroke victims who are paralyzed on one side, because they are unable to move their shoulders through a full range of motion.[6]

The first line of treatment for a frozen shoulder is physiotherapy. Physical therapy modalities, such as myofascial release, massage, range-of-motion exercises, and ultrasound, can often release scar tissue. If these do not relieve the problem, then the scar tissue can be broken up within the joint by the physician injecting the shoulder full of a solution made up of sterile water mixed with an anesthetic.

The numb shoulder can then be gently manipulated. Often several sessions of this treatment regimen are needed to achieve the shoulder's original full range of motion.

Since the initial cause of the adhesive capsulitis was supraspinatus (rotator cuff) weakness, Prolotherapy injections to strengthen the rotator cuff are done in conjunction with the above technique. Complete to near-complete resolution can be accomplished using this combined approach.

A misunderstanding of the supraspinatus tendon's referral pattern keeps clinicians from diagnosing the rotator cuff problem. This tendon refers pain to the back and side of the shoulder, leading clinicians to believe their patients have a muscle problem, when in fact they have a tendon problem. A complaint of shoulder pain is almost always a rotator cuff weakness problem. Prolotherapy is extremely effective at strengthening the rotator cuff tendons.

CASE OF AN UNLUCKY YEAR

Kathy missed a step while coming out of a busy San Francisco restaurant and fell directly onto her right shoulder. After the bruising and scrapes healed, she experienced unrelenting pain in her shoulder. She tried icing it, heat pads, taking some pain medication, and rest. Within three months, she had a frozen shoulder. She could not put on a bra or shirt without assistance. She did her best to shower and wash her hair with the other arm, but knew she could not continue to live like this. Her new retail job required her to stock shelves and she needed to keep working. Kathy tried physical therapy, but it was too painful for her to make it through a whole session. Kathy had known about Prolotherapy for years, and decided to fly to our Chicagoland office. Dr. Hauser emphasized that healing her shoulder would be part Prolotherapy and part her dedication to perform the rehabilitation exercises. After only one treatment, she soon started feeling pain relief, enough that she could finally do the recommended exercises that took her the rest of the way to a full recovery.

Nearly a year later, Kathy ran smack into a door, with her left shoulder taking the brunt this time. Again, she tried ice, rest, and massage. But the result was the same as with her right shoulder. She was aware of the pain all the time and getting through work was becoming more difficult. Her shoulder was becoming more painful and less mobile until she could barely lift her arm. Again, she decided it was overdue for her to just get Prolotherapy and stop living that way. With one treatment to her left shoulder, she was able to return to work without pain and her motion was fully restored. We've encouraged her not to wait so long if she has any more bad luck with shoulder injuries! She did just that a few years later when she came in for hip pain, which resolved with only one visit. While the average number of treatments is three to six, some people only need one or two to achieve pain relief!

ACROMIOCLAVICULAR JOINT/CORACOID PROCESS

Another common cause of chronic shoulder pain is a weak attachment of the clavicle to the acromion. This joint is called the acromioclavicular joint and is noted on the surface of the skin at the apex (top) of the shoulder. *(See Figure 6-8.)* This joint is usually injured in a fall or by a hyperextension of the shoulder.[7] When this occurs, the weight of the body is transmitted to the acromioclavicular joint. This joint, like all joints, is held together by ligaments. When these ligaments are injured and become lax, the joint grinds and grates and causes pain. Acromioclavicular ligament laxity causes pain upon lifting or activity involving the hands in front of or across the body. Prolotherapy is extremely effective at strengthening the acromioclavicular ligaments, eliminating the shoulder grinding and chronic shoulder pain from this area.

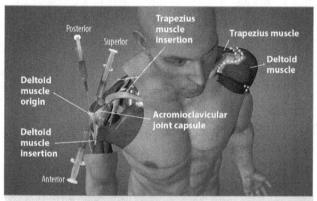

A lesser-known cause of shoulder pain emanates from the coracoid process. From this little nub of bone, stem some very important structures, including the pectoralis minor muscle, coracobrachialis muscle,

Figure 6-8: Prolotherapy of the top of the shoulder. Common sites of tenderness are marked along the scapular spine, clavicle, and deltoid insertion. The approaches to the acromioclavicular joint are demonstrated.

biceps muscle, coracoacromial ligament, coracoclavicular ligament, coracohumeral ligament, and parts of the articular capsule. All attach on a nub of bone no bigger than the tip of the little finger. Although small, this area is "mighty" in regards to importance. This area of the shoulder is palpated during a routine Prolotherapy shoulder examination. Chronic shoulder pain patients are typically very tender in this area and a positive "jump sign" can be elicited upon palpation. Prolotherapy injections are given to strengthen the fibro-osseous junctions of all the above structures at the coracoid process. *(See Figure 6-9.)* This area is routinely treated to relieve chronic shoulder pain.

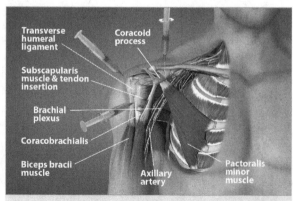

Figure 6-9: Prolotherapy of the shoulder. Frequent sites of injection are demonstrated, including the coracoid process, subscapularis tendon, and the greater tuberosity.

IMPINGEMENT SYNDROME

Approximately 5% of patients with chronic shoulder pain do not find relief from Prolotherapy injections. These people usually have impingement syndrome, caused by the pinching of the supraspinatus tendon between the coracohumeral ligament—from the clavicle above and the humerus below. People often develop a bone spur on the clavicle that decreases the space through which the supraspinatus tendon must travel.[8]

Occasionally, surgery is needed to give the supraspinatus tendon more room to move. The diagnosis can be easily confirmed in the office by observing a grimaced and painful face upon abducting and internally rotating the shoulder, producing a positive "impingement sign." *(See Figure 6-10.)* It should be noted that even with an initial diagnosis of impingement syndrome, the majority of people obtain complete or satisfactory relief of their pain with Prolotherapy alone. For the few patients who have needed surgery for impingement syndrome after Prolotherapy, the response rate of the combined approach has been excellent. The Prolotherapy has strengthened the rotator cuff tendons and surgery has eliminated the impingement of those tendons, leading to complete relief of the chronic shoulder pain.

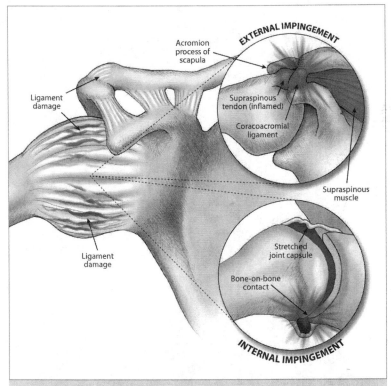

Figure 6-10: Shoulder impingements caused by shoulder instability.
In external impingement, the rotator cuff tendons are compressed by the acromion process. In internal impingement, the structures within the glenohumeral joint themselves are impinged. Both are primarily caused by joint instability.

CHRONIC SHOULDER PAIN TREATED WITH PROLOTHERAPY

We investigated the outcomes of patients undergoing Hackett-Hemwall dextrose Prolotherapy treatment for unresolved shoulder pain at a charity clinic in rural Illinois.[9] We studied a sample of 94 patients with an average of 53 months of unresolved shoulder pain that were treated quarterly with Prolotherapy. An average of 20 months following their last Prolotherapy session, patients were contacted and asked numerous questions in regard to their levels of pain and a variety of physical and psychological symptoms, as well as activities of daily living, before and after their last Prolotherapy treatment. The results of this study showed that patients had a statistically significant decline in their level of pain, stiffness, and crunching sensations (crepitation), after Prolotherapy. This also included 39% of patients in a sub-group who were told by their medical doctors that there were no other treatment options for their pain and 21% who were told that surgery was their only option.

Over 82% of all patients experienced improvements in sleep, exercise ability, anxiety, depression, and overall disability with Prolotherapy. Ninety-seven percent of patients received pain relief with Prolotherapy. *(See Figure 6-11.)*

UNRELIABILITY OF MRI FOR DIAGNOSIS OF LIGAMENT INJURY

MRI of the shoulder is notoriously misleading. It is why we do not order them frequently. Numerous studies done on asymptomatic patients regularly show abnormalities on MRI, including glenoid labrum abnormalities, supraspinatus tendinopathy, and rotator cuff tears.[10-15] It is scary to think about the thousands of surgeries based primarily on MRI readings without a correlating physical exam.

Prolotherapy Shoulder Study Results

Demographics	All Shoulder Patients	No Other Treatment Option	Surgery Only Option
Total number of shoulders	94	37	20
Avg. years of pain	4.6	5.2	3.9
# of pain meds used before Prolotherapy	1.2	1.3	1.5
# of pain meds used after Prolotherapy	0.3	0.4	0.4
Pain level before Prolotherapy	7.1	7.1	7.0
Pain level after Prolotherapy	2.3	2.2	2.6
Stiffness level before Prolotherapy	5.4	5.8	5.1
Stiffness level after Prolotherapy	2.0	2.0	2.3
Greater than 50% pain relief	87%	81%	90%
Athletic ability > 30 minutes of exercise before Prolotherapy	29%	17%	15%
Athletic ability > 30 minutes of exercise after Prolotherapy	78%	46%	80%
Prolotherapy changed life for the better	97%	97%	95%

Figure 6-11: Summary of results of Hackett-Hemwall dextrose Prolotherapy shoulder study.

But it happens all the time that patients are signed up for surgery and say the doctor barely touched them. Remember, these studies were conducted on people who did not have any symptoms of shoulder pain. It is imperative that an evaluation be done by a Prolotherapist because diagnostic tests can often lead a clinician astray.

Even in cases where the MRI reading notes a "complete tear" of the rotator cuff, a consultation for Prolotherapy is a good idea. Upon physical exam, we have found that the tear truly is not a "complete" tear, making Prolotherapy an ideal option in place of surgery. After several sessions of Prolotherapy, the patient's shoulder was symptom-free. There is no substitute for a listening ear and a strong thumb. If physicians cannot reproduce their patient's pain in the office, they probably cannot get rid of it either. A Prolotherapist can reproduce a patient's pain using his or her own MRI (My Reproducibility Instrument, the thumb) and can eliminate the pain. Reproduction of pain by a good physical examination *(See Figure 6-12.)*, combined with elimination of the pain by Prolotherapy, is far more effective in diagnosing the cause of chronic shoulder pain than an MRI scan.

SUMMARY

Chronic shoulder pain is due to joint instability which may involve weakness in the rotator cuff, specifically in the supraspinatus tendon, because the tendon has poor blood supply. If left untreated, this supraspinatus tendon laxity leads to adhesive capsulitis, or frozen shoulder. Other common reasons for shoulder joint instability involve

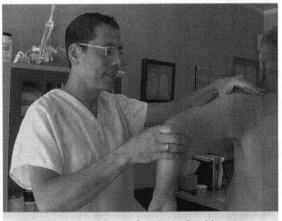

Figure 6-12: Dr. Hauser performing a shoulder exam.

acromioclavicular ligament laxity, a weakened glenohumeral ligament or glenoid labrum tear, and weakness of the structures that attach to the coracoid process.

MRI scans of the shoulder are often abnormal in individuals without any shoulder symptoms whatsoever. The best diagnostic procedure for chronic shoulder pain is palpation of the structure, causing a positive "jump sign," and relief of the pain immediately after the structure is treated with Prolotherapy. Prolotherapy is the treatment of choice for chronic shoulder pain because it corrects the underlying weakness causing the pain. This is why many people are choosing to Prolo their shoulder pain away! ∎

CHAPTER

7

PROLO YOUR KNEE PAIN AWAY!

It is dangerous to have knee pain and walk into an orthopedic surgeon's office. Arthroscopic surgery is the favorite pastime of orthopedic surgeons. When patients are asked the reasons for their surgery, the typical response is "to shave cartilage" or "I don't know." The best treatment, as long as it is a partial tear, is to help the body repair the injured area.

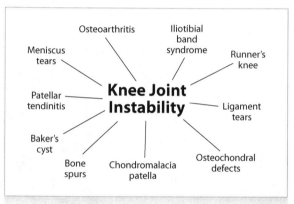

Conditions caused by knee joint instability.

Remember, removing any tissue that God has put in the body will have a consequence. That consequence is often joint instability, the primary cause of chronic pain and degenerative arthritis of the knee. The tissues most commonly removed during arthroscopic surgery in the knee are parts of the meniscus and the articular cartilage. Both of these structures are needed by the body to help the femur bone glide smoothly over the tibia. *(See Figure 7-1.)* When either structure is removed, the bones do not glide properly. Eventually, whatever meniscus or articular cartilage is left after the arthroscopic surgery is worn away. Once this occurs, bone begins rubbing against bone and proliferative arthritis begins. After a course of cortisone shots, nonsteroidal anti-inflammatory drugs, and several trials of physical therapy, the patient is again under the knife, this time for a knee replacement. Once an arthroscope touches the knee, the chance of developing arthritis in the knee tremendously increases. This is because surgery, especially when any tissue is removed, increases joint instability.

Before letting an arthroscope touch you, it is imperative to have an evaluation by a physician familiar with Prolotherapy. Prolotherapy will begin collagen formation both outside and inside the knee joint depending on the structure(s) that are injected.[1] Prolotherapy stimulates the body to repair itself, specifically the ligaments

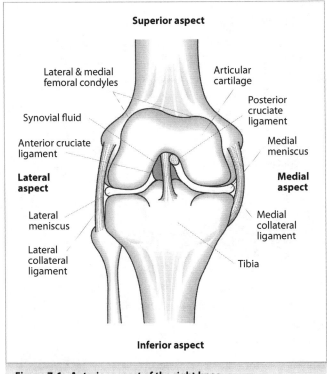

Figure 7-1: Anterior aspect of the right knee.

that stabilize knee motion. Surgery in the knee is appropriate when a ligament is completely torn, such as would occur from a high-velocity injury. Prolotherapy is only helpful to regrow ligaments if both ends of the ligament remain attached to bone. Remember, 98% of ligament injuries are partial tears for which Prolotherapy would be helpful.

Numerous studies have shown Prolotherapy is an effective treatment for a variety of knee pain, including osteoarthritis, ligament tears, meniscal injuries, and more.[2-13] Every year the list of studies gets longer. It is no longer acceptable for a physician who treats chronic pain to say that he or she has not heard of Prolotherapy or that there is not evidence for its effectiveness!

In our own study of 119 knees, Prolotherapy showed statistically significant improvement in pain levels (VAS 1-10), stiffness, crunching sensation, and range of motion.[14] More than 82% of patients also showed improvement in walking ability, medication usage, athletic ability, depression, and overall disability due to Prolotherapy treatment. The average patient reported pain for an average of 5 years prior to Prolotherapy. Additionally, 2 out of 5 patients were taking at least one pharmaceutical pain medication. The population represented chronic, and often hopeless, cases who had exhausted the traditional medicine system. This reinforced what we see everyday in our clinic: quality of life can be drastically improved with Prolotherapy! *(See Figure 7-2.)*

DIAGNOSIS OF KNEE CONDITIONS

The primary cause of knee pain is knee joint instability. This can be due to a number of ligaments and tendons attachments becoming torn or degenerated, as well as damaged or removed cartilage and meniscal tissue.

It is also important to understand the referral patterns of knee ligaments that can trigger pain sensations further down the leg and into the foot. The medial collateral ligament refers pain down the leg to the big toe and the lateral collateral ligament refers pain to the lateral foot.

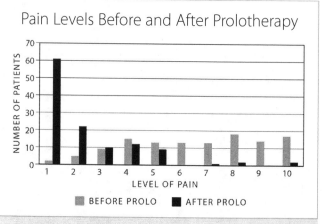

Pain Levels Before and After Prolotherapy

Figure 7-2: Starting and ending pain levels before and after receiving Hackett-Hemwall dextrose Prolotherapy in 80 patients (119 knees) with unresolved knee pain.

The ligaments inside the knee are called the anterior and posterior cruciate ligaments. These ligaments help stabilize the knee, preventing excessive forward and backward movement. If these ligaments are loose, even in a young person, degenerative arthritis begins to form.[15] Prolotherapy causes a stabilization of the knee after these ligaments are treated.[1]

The feeling of a loose knee is reason enough to suspect a cruciate ligament injury. The cruciate ligaments are the power horses that stabilize the knee. They refer pain to the back of the knee. Posterior knee pain may be an indication of cruciate ligament injury.

A common cause of chronic knee pain is weakness in the pes anserinus tendons. Below the knee cap, on the inside of the knee, are the attachments of three tendons: semimembranous, semitendinosus, and gracilis. Together, these tendons create the pes anserinus area. **(See Figure 7-3.)** When left untreated, may contribute to developing arthritis. Even in cases of significant arthritis, crippling knee pain is often due to pes anserinus tendonitis or bursitis. This condition is easily treated with Prolotherapy, eliminating the chronic knee pain.

The pes anserinus tendons are also known as the inside hamstring muscles. Most of us have very weak hamstring muscles that are short because we sit for a large portion of our day.

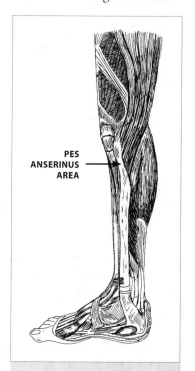

PES ANSERINUS AREA

Figure 7-3: Muscles and tendons of the inside leg.
The pes anserinus area is a common site of chronic pain.

The pes anserinus tendons flex the knee and stabilize the inside of the knee. Patients with fallen arches are prone to strains in these muscles. The tibia tends to rotate outward to compensate for the fallen arch. Running, hiking, pregnancy, and aging may predispose a patient to develop a fallen arch. This outward rotation of the tibia places additional stress on the pes anserinus tendons. Eventually, these tendons become lax and are no longer able to control the tibial movement, adding to the chronic knee pain. Addressing the fallen arches of the foot may also be required to fully alleviate the knee pain. Prolotherapy injections strengthen the tendon attachments of the pes anserinus, resolving the chronic knee pain.

CHONDROMALACIA PATELLA

Another common source of knee pain is known as chondromalacia patella. (*Chondro* means cartilage, *malacia* means breakdown, and *patella* means knee cap.) Thus, chondromalacia patella refers to cartilage breakdown underneath the knee cap. This condition is also called patellofemoral dysfunction or patellar-tracking dysfunction, and is common among runners and also athletes where the sport involves a lot of running (soccer, tennis, etc.) A more accurate description is that chondromalacia patella begins as a patellar-tracking problem. This means that the knee cap scrapes the bones underneath when the knee is moved. Typical conventional treatments for this condition include taping the knee, exercising to strengthen the thigh muscles, and stretching exercises. These treatments may be effective but are usually not curative. Prolotherapy, on the other hand, can help patellar tracking and relieve chondromalacia pain.[17] **(See Figure 7-4.)**

MENISCUS INJURIES

Articular cartilage has a huge job within the knee. Many factors work against it, as it has the high pressure job of handling hundred of pounds of weight with each step the body takes, all the while receiving very little nourishment from the synovial fluid. Fortunately, the super strong menisci are present to help "lighten the load." Unfortunately, however, the menisci are

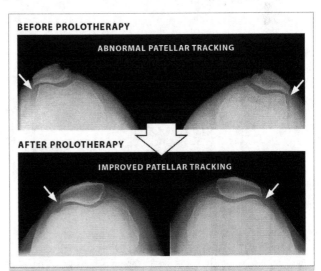

Figure 7-4: Sunrise views of knees before and after Prolotherapy. The alignment in this patient's knees after Prolotherapy is much improved. She suffered from chondromalacia patella and patellofemoral pain syndrome. Prolotherapy helped her get back to running pain free.

often injured, representing one of the most common knee injuries that patients seek care for.

The menisci (plural of meniscus) are a pair of C-shaped fibrocartilages which lie between the femur and tibia in each knee, extending peripherally along each medial and lateral aspect of the knee. *(See Figure 7-1.)* The anatomy of both menisci is essentially the same, with the only exception being that the medial meniscus is slightly more circular than its hemispherical lateral counterpart. Each meniscus has a flat underside to match the smooth top of the tibial surface, and a concave superior shape to provide congruency with the convex femoral condyle. Anterior and posterior horns from each meniscus then attach to the tibia to hold them in place. The meniscus is comprised of approximately 70% water and 30% organic matter. This organic matter is primarily a fibrous collagen matrix consisting of type I collagen, fibrochondrocytes, proteoglycans, and a small amount of dry noncollagenous matter.[18,19]

The mighty menisci are responsible for load transmission, shock absorption, lubrication, and improvement of stability of the knees. Most studies indicate that the menisci transmit about 50% of the load at the knee, while the remaining 50% is borne directly by the articular cartilage and surfaces.[20,21] The menisci, therefore, protect the articular cartilage from high concentrations of stress by increasing the contact area on the femur and tibia bones.

Tears are the most common form of meniscal injury, and are generally classified by appearance into four categories: longitudinal tears (also referred to as bucket handle tears), radial tears, horizontal tears, and oblique tears.[22] *(See Figure 7-5.)* Research indicates that radial or horizontal tears are more likely to occur

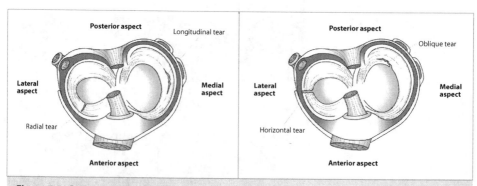

Figure 7-5: Common types of meniscal tears.

Longitudinal (bucket handle) tears - vertical tear around the long axis of the meniscus often with displacement of the inner margin (bucket handle).

Radial tears - extend from the medial rim toward the lateral rim of the meniscus.

Horizontal tears - tears that are in the same horizontal axis as the meniscus tissue.

Oblique tears - full thickness tears running obliquely from the inner edge of the meniscus out into the body of the meniscus.

Complex tears - more than one of the above patterns.

in the elderly population while younger patients have a higher incidence of longitudal tears.[22-25] Each can be further described as partial thickness tears or complete thickness tears, depending on the vertical depth of the tear.

Essentially every study shows that articular cartilage pressures escalate when the menisci are removed. Ahmed and Burke showed a 40% increase in the contact stress while Baratz and associates found a 235% increase in articular cartilage contact force following total meniscectomy.[26,27] *(See Figure 7-6.)* If that is not bad

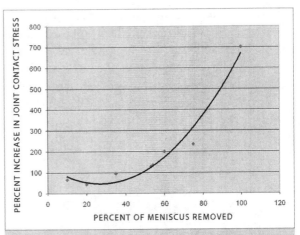

Figure 7-6: Increase in joint contact stress versus percent of meniscus removed. As the percentage of meniscus removed during surgery increases, joint contract stress increases exponentially. Thus arthroscopic meniscectomy dramatically increases the incidence of future degenerative knee arthritis.

Source: 1. Baratz ME, et al. Meniscal tears: the effect of meniscectomy and of repair on intraarticular contact areas and stress in the human knee. A preliminary report. *Am J Sports Med.* 1986;14:270-275. 2. Lee SJ, et al. Tibiofemoral contact mechanics after serial medial meniscectomies in the human cadaveric knee. *Am J Sports Med.* 2006;34(8):1334-1344.

enough, other researchers found 450-700% increases in articular cartilage pressure. A reasonable average estimate taken from the available literature indicates that total meniscectomy results in a two- to three-fold (200-300%) increase in contact stresses.[28-30]

Removal of the menisci will produce knee instability and hasten arthritic changes. Following partial or total meniscectomy, articular degenerative changes have been described, including the formation of osteophytic ridges, generalized flattening of the femoral articular surface, and narrowing of the joint space. *(See Figure 7-7.)* Roughening and degeneration of the articular cartilage is seen and seems to be proportional to the size of the segment removed. Degenerative changes appear first in the tibiofemoral contact areas, with those areas formerly covered by the meniscus involved later.[28,31]

Once the menisci are removed, aggressive proliferative arthritis is inevitable. It occurs early in 40% of individuals, but is essentially guaranteed long-term.[31-33] This sad fact needs

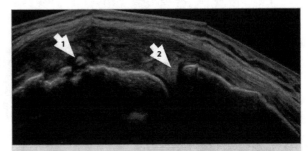

Figure 7-7: Ultrasound of knee showing medial meniscus defect. This ultrasound not only shows this patient's post-traumatic calcifications (1), but also a medial meniscus tear (2).

serious consideration when an arthroscopy is proposed. Arthroscopic partial meniscectomy is an extremely common procedure. Besides the proliferative arthritis that results, a concomitant decrease in the ability to function follows. Let no one, especially someone in a white coat with an arthroscope, do anything to your menisci. The health of your articular cartilage depends upon it!

Meniscal removal leads to increased forces on the articular cartilage. This may produce articular cartilage breakdown, which leads to thinning of the articular cartilage. As a result of this, increased pressure on the underlying tibia bone is observed, which leads to more pressure on the ligaments. Ligament tears, worsened instability, and chronic pain often result, which further weaken the joint. In response to this weakness, the joint overgrows bone, which is called arthritis.

RESULTS OF PROLOTHERAPY FOR MENISCAL TEARS

In 2010, our team published a study on the Hackett-Hemwall technique of dextrose Prolotherapy for 28 knees (in 24 patients) with MRI documented meniscal pathology, including tears and degeneration. Patients were interviewed an average of 18 months after their last Prolotherapy treatment. This retrospective pilot study documented multiple areas of improvements in the patients' quality of life. *(See Figure 7-8.)* Most patients reported statistically significantly less pain and stiffness and major improvements in

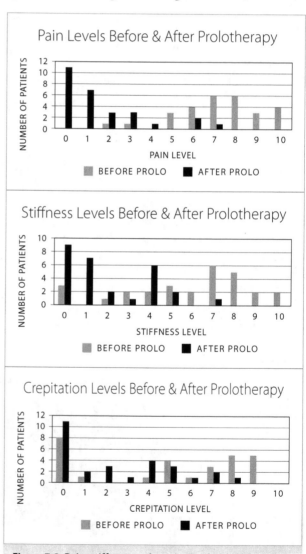

Figure 7-8: Pain, stiffness, and crepitation levels before and after Hackett-Hemwall Prolotherapy in 28 patients with unresolved knee pain due to meniscal injuries.

range of motion, crepitation of the knee, medication usage, walking ability, and exercise ability. The improvements with Prolotherapy met the expectations of the patients in over 96% of the knees to the point where surgery was not needed. Prolotherapy improved knee pain and function regardless of the type or location of the meniscal tear or degeneration. The improvements were so overwhelmingly positive that Hackett-Hemwall Prolotherapy should be considered as a first-line treatment for pain and disability caused by meniscal tears and degeneration.[34]

KNEE LIGAMENT INJURIES (ACL, PCL, MCL AND LCL)

The knee condyles (medial=middle; lateral=outside) are bony structures that sit in the bottom of the thigh bone in the knee joint that assist in keeping the knee from hyperextending. The medial condyle is larger bone structure because it bears more weight. As we age, these bones wear, and their degeneration has been clearly associated with meniscus degeneration.

As we stated earlier, the meniscus is the cartilage padding that acts as a shock absorber. When damaged the protective cartilage that covers the thigh and shin bones is now stressed. This is the beginning of bone-on-bone knees.

Knee stability is maintained by the scope of the condyles and menisci. Instability occurs when these structures suffer degenerative changes, tears, or OA.

The four major ligaments of the knee are the anterior cruciate (ACL), the posterior cruciate (PCL), the medial collateral ligament (MCL), and the lateral collateral ligament (LCL). The medial collateral ligament and posterior cruciate ligament are attached to the medial condyle; the lateral collateral ligament is attached to the lateral condyles. Instability in these ligaments can start the degenerative cascade of the condyles and the menisci. Wear and tear, impact injuries, and anything that might occur in the knee affects the ligaments and the ligaments affect every structure in the knee. When these bony attachments begin degenerating, the attached ligaments lose their tautness and even become looser.

When patients experience an MCL injury, they typically also injure the other knee ligaments such as the ACL, PCL, and LCL. Traditional medicine likes to treat these types of injuries with surgery. Surgery, however, means cutting and removing. Cutting through important knee structures will eventually lead to more instability and degeneration of the knee joint. *(See Chapter 19 on Surgery.)*

Prolotherapy, conversely, is a non-surgical regenerative option that strengthens the attachments, thus eliminating the ligament laxity and stabilizing the knee joint. At Caring Medical we inject all of the ligament attachments in the knee versus just placing one injection into the knee joint. If we do not tighten the loose supporting structures, the knee remains unstable, and will continue to cause pain and injury. Comprehensive Prolotherapy addresses all of the ligament attachments and ensures that the treated knee will be strong and stable. *(See Figures 7-9 & 7-10.)*

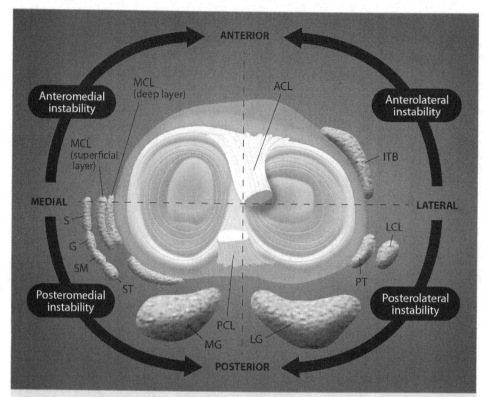

Figure 7-9: Instabilities about the knee. ACL = anterior cruciate ligament; ITB = iliotibial band; LCL = lateral collateral ligament; PT = popliteal tendon; LG = lateral gastrocnemius; PCL = posterior cruciate ligament; MG = medial gastrocnemius; ST = semitendinosus; SM = semimembranosus; G = gracilis; S = satorius; MCL = medial collateral ligament.

Modified from Magee DJ. Orthopedic Physical Assessment. 6th Edition. St Louis, 2014, Elsevier Saunders, p. 811.

BAKER'S CYSTS

As we have discussed, when a joint is unstable, it can swell. In the case of a Baker's cyst, the accumulation of fluid occurs in a sac behind the knee, causing discomfort and difficulty bending the knee. *(See Figure 7-11.)* Often, patients get these cysts drained only to have them fill right back up again. Why does that happen? Draining a cyst does not address the joint instability that caused the cyst to form in the first place. Address the instability by receiving Prolotherapy to tighten the loose ligaments and the joint will stop swelling! We have excellent results using Prolotherapy to help patients with Baker's cysts resolve the pain and keep the cyst from returning!

PROLOTHERAPY IS THE IDEAL TREATMENT FOR KNEE ARTHRITIS

Arthritis in the knee is one of the most common complaints that patients present to us at Caring Medical. More often than not, they have experienced years of traditional care for knee pain, from regularly taking NSAIDs to cortisone injections, and even a surgery to "clean out" the joint as they tell us. By the time they arrive in our office, the possibility of a future knee replacement has already been discussed with their local orthopedic surgeon as the progression of arthritis appears unstoppable. No doubt, continuing with most of the traditional pain management methods, a person will end up with a knee replacement. Preferring to not take that route, Prolotherapy, and often Stem Cell Prolotherapy, is an excellent alternative to surgery because it addresses the root cause of what started the arthritic progression in addition to the ongoing damage. The underlying cause of the arthritis is

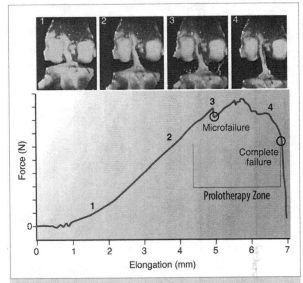

Figure 7-10: Load-elongation curve of cadaver human anterior cruciate ligament. As the ligament is stretched at a physiologic strain rate, damage begins at 5mm of elongation (stretch) and completely tears at 7mm. The Prolotherapy zone (areas 2 and 3) is the point where Prolotherapy is able to repair the ligament damage so that complete joint stabilization results. If complete failure of the ligament occurs, surgery is typically required.

Used with permission from: Nordin M, et al. *Basic Biomechanics of the Musculoskeletal System.* 4th Edition. Lippincott Williams & Wilkins. Baltimore, MD. 2012.

actually due to structural damage that leads to degenerative changes in the knee. **(See Figure 7-12.)** Meniscus tears or injuries to the supporting knee ligamentous system will eventually lead to degenerative arthritis. Determine the underlying cause of the weakness and instability; stop the degenerative process with regenerative injection treatments such as Prolotherapy and/or Cellular Prolotherapy; halt the progression of arthritis. It is as simple as that! **(See Chapters 13 and 19 for more on Arthritis and Surgery.)**

SUMMARY

Knee pain can start from a traumatic event, such as a fall or football tackle. Or it can become more apparent over time, with increasingly stiff and swollen knees. The underlying cause of knee pain is joint instability due to weakness

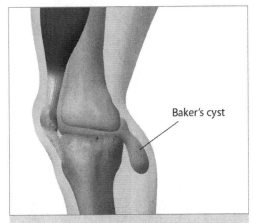

Figure 7-11: Schematic diagram of Baker's cyst. A Baker's cyst is joint fluid which has leaked into the back of the knee.

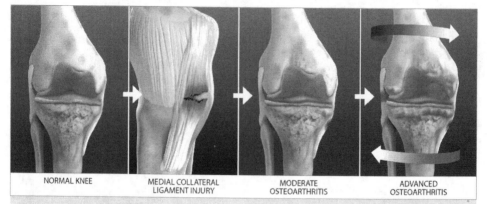

| NORMAL KNEE | MEDIAL COLLATERAL LIGAMENT INJURY | MODERATE OSTEOARTHRITIS | ADVANCED OSTEOARTHRITIS |

Figure 7-12: The progression of knee osteoarthritis. When a simple ligament injury (medial collateral ligament depicted here) is not resolved, the resultant joint instability can progress to the complete breakdown of the articular cartilage and the joint.

in the ligaments and tendons surrounding the knee joint. Knee joint instability can also result in the knee cap tracking abnormally, causing pain and the cartilage under the knee cap to wear down. Surgical intervention to remove tissues, including the meniscus or cartilage, puts increased pressure on the other areas of the knee and worsens knee instability. Over time, this worsened joint instability leads to severe cartilage defects, osteoarthritis, and additional surgeries that will eventually include joint replacement. Prolotherapy is an excellent first-line treatment that can stabilize the knee joint, regenerate cartilage, and stop the accelerated degenerative cascade. Because of these facts, many people are choosing to Prolo their knee pain away! ■

CHAPTER

PROLO YOUR HIP PAIN AWAY!

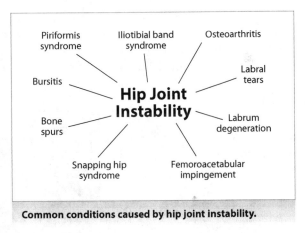

Piriformis syndrome

Iliotibial band syndrome

Osteoarthritis

Bursitis

Labral tears

Hip Joint Instability

Bone spurs

Labrum degeneration

Snapping hip syndrome

Femoroacetabular impingement

Common conditions caused by hip joint instability.

The hip joint joins the leg to the pelvis. Unfortunately for most people, both legs are not exactly the same. They may look the same, but from a biomechanical standpoint, they are not the same. One leg may be rotated either in or out, or one leg may be shorter than the other. The latter is especially common if one leg was broken during childhood. Because the hip joint connects the leg to the pelvis, the hip joint will sustain the brunt of any biomechanical abnormality that may occur. If one leg is shorter than the other, the hip joints will be stressed because the leg-length discrepancy causes an abnormal gait. The gait cycle is most efficient when the iliac crests are level. Unequal leg lengths cause the pelvis to move abnormally. This is evidenced by the waddling gait of someone with a hip problem. This waddling gait helps remove pressure on the painful hip.

With leg-length discrepancy, either hip joint can cause pain and usually both hip joints hurt to some degree.[1] To propel the leg forward, the hip joint must be raised which strains the gluteus medius muscle and the posterior hip ligaments. Leg-length problems are also associated with recurrent lower back problems because they cause the pelvis to be asymmetric.[2] Prolotherapy to the sacroiliac and hip joints will correct the asymmetries in the majority of cases. The leg-length discrepancy disappears as a result of the leveling of the pelvis. If asymmetry remains after treatment, a shoe insert or heel lift will generally correct the problem.

HIP INSTABILITY AS A CAUSE OF REFERRED PAIN

A problem in the hip may commonly manifest itself as groin or inguinal pain. Someone suffering from groin pain should be examined at the pubic symphysis, sacroiliac joint, iliolumbar ligaments, and hip joint. Pain from the hip joint may also be felt locally, directly above the hip joint in the back. When the hip joint becomes lax, the muscles over the joint compensate for the laxity by tensing. As is the case with any joint of the body, lax ligaments initiate muscle tension in an attempt to stabilize the joint. This compensatory mechanism to stabilize the hip joint eventually causes the gluteus medius, piriformis muscle, and iliotibial band/ tensor fascia lata muscles to tighten because of chronic contraction in an attempt to compensate for a loose hip joint. The contracted gluteus medius can eventually irritate the trochanteric bursa, causing a trochanteric bursitis. A bursa is a fluid-filled sac which helps muscles glide over bony prominences. Patients with chronic hip problems often have had cortisone injected into this bursa, which generally brings temporary relief. But this treatment does not provide permanent relief because the underlying ligament laxity is not being corrected. Prolotherapy injections to strengthen the hip joint and iliocapsular ligaments will provide definitive relief in such a case.

It is interesting to note that trochanteric bursitis, piriformis syndrome, and weakness in the iliotibial band also cause "sciatica."[3,4] We find that patients suffering from so-called sciatica often have weakness in the sacroiliac joint, hip joint, sacrotuberous and sacrospinous ligaments, trochanteric bursa, and iliotibial band/tensor fascia lata. *(See Figure 8-1.)* The sciatic nerve runs between the two heads of the piriformis muscle. When the piriformis muscle is spastic, the sciatic

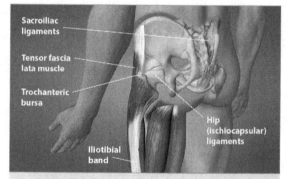

Figure 8-1: Pelvic and hip ligament anatomy.
The tensor fascia lata muscle overlays the hip joint which is supported by the hip ligaments.

nerve may be pinched. Lumbosacral and hip joint weaknesses are two main causes of piriformis muscle spasm. Stretches and physical therapy directed at the piriformis muscle to reduce spasm help temporarily, but do not alleviate the real problem. Prolotherapy to the hip and lower back strengthens those joints, thus eliminating the piriformis muscle spasms.

The iliotibial band/tensor fascia lata extends from the pelvis over the hip joint to the lateral knee. Its job is to help abduct the leg, especially during walking so the legs do not cross when walking. When this band/muscle is tight, it puts a great strain on the sacroiliac and lumbosacral ligaments.[3] Stretching this muscle is beneficial to many people with chronic hip/back problems. Stretching and massage feels good to people with chronically "tight IT bands." Take this one step further though to understand why the bands/muscles become tight in the first place, which is joint instability generally in the hip or the knee. This instability needs to be properly identified and treated for the chronic tightness to be eliminated, along with the need to regularly stretch or massage the area in order to feel relief. Once the joint becomes stable, the continual tightness subsides.

HIP REPLACEMENT SURGERY EPIDEMIC

The top reason why patients with hip pain are referred to our office is to avoid a hip replacement surgery. Many of these patients received years of traditional care that include numerous cortisone injections and prescriptions for NSAIDs, which, as discussed in **Chapter 2**, can quickly degenerate articular cartilage. Clearly modern medicine and especially orthopedic surgeons have not determined how to stop degenerative arthritis from occurring in hip joints. The mention of a hip replacement often sends patients looking for referrals outside the surgical arena. Comparing the effects of Prolotherapy and cortisone gives patients a good reason to reconsider before scheduling hip replacement surgery. **(See Figure 8-2.)**

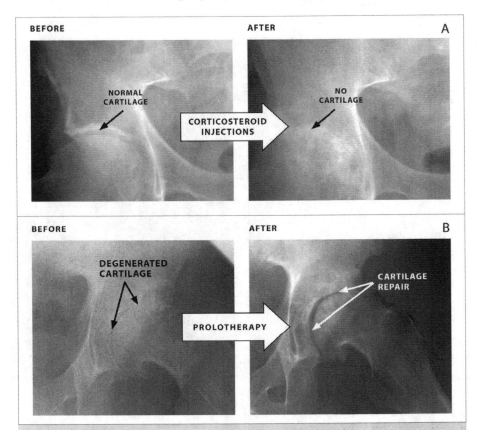

Figure 8-2: A. X-ray of a normal hip compared to a steroid-injected degenerated hip. Right hip degeneration was accelerated in a patient following multiple steroid injections. **B. Prolotherapy regeneration of hip cartilage.** Before and after hip X-rays of a patient treated with Prolotherapy.

In 1994, the National Institutes of Health gathered 27 experts in hip replacement and component parts to evaluate hip replacements. In their report, they noted that 120,000 artificial hip joints are implanted annually in the United States. They further stated, "Candidates for elective total hip replacement should have radiographic evidence of joint damage and moderate to severe persistent pain or disability, or both, that is not substantially relieved by an extended course of nonsurgical management."[5]

Hip replacement surgeries are out of control! According to the U.S. government's own records, hip replacement surgeries have gone from 120,000 in 1994 to 336,000 in 2003 to about 450,000 in 2010 when we include total hip replacements, partial hip replacements, and revisions. If this is not insane enough, then consider that by 2030 that number will climb past 1 million with 50,000 occurring in people under age 45! These replacement parts come with their own risks that include corrosion, metal poisoning, loosening and malalignment, infection, postoperative fracture, pulmonary embolism, malunion, leg length discrepancy, trochanteric bursitis, peroneal or sciatic nerve palsy, among others.[6-9] *(See Figure 8-3.)* Fortunately there is Prolotherapy to help stop this epidemic from continuing! Specifically, Stem Cell Prolotherapy is often the treatment of choice in more advanced cases where a replacement is already a possible option.

DEGENERATIVE ARTHRITIS OF THE HIP

It is much easier to prevent a hip problem than solve it once it has developed. Consider a patient who came for an initial visit to Caring Medical. He suffered a severe trauma several years prior to seeing us. On physical examination, his left hip had almost no motion, so we sent him for an x-ray. *(See Figure 8-4.)*

As you can see, one hip is totally destroyed while the other one has only mild hip osteoarthritis. Hip replacement surgery was recommended for the severely degenerated hip. Yes, there are occasionally times where it is required. We treated his other hip when it became symptomatic

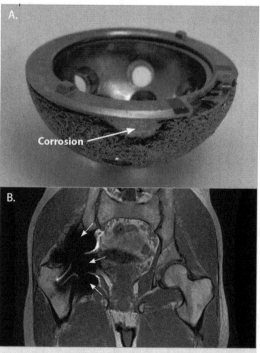

Figure 8-3: Examples of the risks of hip replacement surgery. A. Corrosion in acetabular component of hip replacement. This necessitated a revision surgery with placement of a new prosthesis. **B.** Metallosis of right hip. The depositition and build-up of metal debris (arrows) in the soft tissue can be easily seen on MRI.

which was very successful and kept him from requiring another hip replacement surgery.

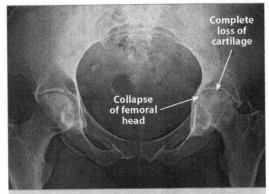

Figure 8-4: X-ray of our patient with hip pain. One hip is mildly arthritic and the other is completely degenerated. The patient also exhibits pubic symphysis diastasis.

Many patients that we see at Caring Medical report a history of trauma and have undergone some type of hip procedure prior to seeing us. Most surgeries attempt to reshape the hip and supposedly "repair" the labrum. What the patient does not realize is the procedure itself stretches out all of the hip ligaments! During arthroscopy the hip joint must be expanded with water under pressure, so the large arthroscopes, at least two of them, are put inside the joint. Realize sometimes this lasts for two hours! The net result can be ligament laxity and joint instability, not joint stabilization!

Numerous structural risk factors for the development of hip arthritis exist including labrum tear, labrum degeneration, femoroacetabular impingement, hip dysplasia, slipped capital femoral epiphysis, degenerative arthritis on the opposite hip, as well as joint instability.[10-14] From an orthopedic surgeon's point of view, if for instance femoroacetabular impingement and labrum tears are risk factors for later development of hip osteoarthritis and current operations are not halting the development of the hip osteoarthritis, then what is needed are newer operations. Thus every year new operations are developed. Conservative methods, including Prolotherapy, should be exhausted prior to receiving surgery for these types of instability-based conditions.

PROLOTHERAPY RESULTS FOR CHRONIC HIP PAIN

We performed a study on patients who were treated with Prolotherapy at a charity clinic where we analyzed a sub-group of patients who had been told by other providers that no other treatment was available for their conditions, as well as a sub-group who were told surgery was their only option.[15] It is interesting to note that 100% of patients felt that Prolotherapy changed their lives for the better. *(See Figure 8-5.)* Improvements were seen across the board in pain and stiffness levels, as well as an increased ability to exercise and a decreased need for pain medication.

FEMOROACETABULAR IMPINGEMENT SYNDROME

Sometimes the hip has an acetabular deformity that can get complicated. The femoral head may have an odd shape. For example, it may have a non-spherical head or the orientation of the acetabulum may be off (i.e. retroverted) or have some

Demographics	All Hip Patients	No Other Treatment Option	Surgery Only Option
Total number of patients	61	20	8
Months of pain	59	69	44
# of pain meds used before Prolotherapy	1.1	1.5	1.8
# of pain meds used after Prolotherapy	0.3	0.5	0.2
Pain level before Prolotherapy	7.2	5.0	7.1
Pain level after Prolotherapy	2.6	3.0	2.4
Stiffness level before Prolotherapy	4.4	6.0	4.0
Stiffness level after Prolotherapy	2.1	2.7	2.0
Greater than 50% pain relief	89%	80%	100%
Athletic ability > 30 minutes of exercise before Prolotherapy	40%	35%	0%
Athletic ability > 30 minutes of exercise after Prolotherapy	83%	88%	74%
Prolotherapy changed life for the better	100%	100%	100%

Figure 8-5: Summary of results of Hackett-Hemwall dextrose Prolotherapy hip study.

other "weird angle" compared to the femur bone.

Some patients have conditions that predispose them to less range of motion. A person may present with 50% of normal motion in his right hip with regard to external rotation compared to his left hip, but not have any pain in the right hip. He may be able to run and continue sports with no problem, as the range of motion deficiency does not necessarily hinder sports performance or feel painful. *(See Figure 8-6.)*

DO CONGENITAL HIP ABNORMALITIES REQUIRE SURGERY?

Many patients ask us if a congenital (genetic) hip problem requires surgical correction. The answer is – sometimes. Sometimes pelvic osteotomy, femoral osteotomy, or joint replacement surgeries are needed. If someone has avascular necrosis of the hip, sometimes surgery is needed. If the patient has some reasonable range of motion remaining, ie 50% or greater normal range of motion, then Prolotherapy works great at helping with the pain and exercises like cycling and swimming will slowly allow the patient to regain some of the lost range of motion.

Sometimes the patient will only achieve pain relief, which, of course, the patient is excited about. However, some sports like martial arts require not only improved pain levels, but also improved range of motion. So sometimes, even though the patient is a good Prolotherapy candidate for decreasing pain levels, the patient may still need arthroscopy or some other surgical procedure to help with range of motion. It is surprising, however, the high number of patients we have seen over the years who do not really get much improved range of motion with surgical procedures! For those who are inquiring about a surgical procedure for premature osteoarthritis of the hip, have a frank discussion not just with your Prolotherapy doctor, but also with your orthopedic surgeon. If you end up choosing surgery, you can always get Prolotherapy after the surgical procedure. Better yet, if Prolotherapy does not fully meet your expectations, you can always then choose surgery. Our philosophy is always to go the least invasive, most potentially successful route first.

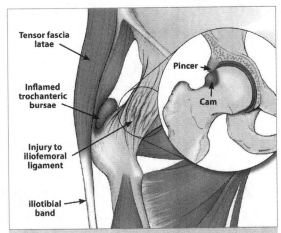

Figure 8-6: Femoroacetabular impingement of hip. Hip instability caused by injury to the labrum or any of the hip ligaments (illustrated as iliofemoral ligament injury), is typically the cause of the two main types of femoroacetabular impingement (pincher and cam types). Prolotherapy is often an effective treatment for femoroacetabular impingement because it addresses the cause of the condition.

FEMOROACETABULAR IMPINGEMENT (FAI) TREATMENT WITH PROLOTHERAPY

Many patients ask if a structure is impinged, doesn't someone have to un-impinge it? Again, the answer is sometimes. Let's say, for instance, a patient has FAI and his main symptom is groin pain. The patient is a cyclist and is experiencing pain with cycling. In seeing this particular patient, we would try and determine if he truly has FAI on physical examination, looking for a positive impingement sign and then determine the cause of it. If the cause is some tremendous structural problem with the hip like a dysmorphic problem or orientation problem of the femur, then surgical correction may be needed. However, remember, the most common cause of FAI and other premature osteoarthritic conditions is simply some type of soft tissue injury such as a ligament injury, so thus Prolotherapy is the best treatment! Injury to the iliofemoral or ischiofemoral ligaments, as well as a torn hip labrum, can cause hip joint instability. Given enough time this can cause premature osteoarthritis and eventually FAI.

TWO DIFFERENT TYPES OF FAI

Potential patients will email us frequently about the two different types of FAI: the "cam-type" FAI, where the femoral head-neck junction is abnormal; and the "pincher-type" FAI, where the acetabulum shape or its configuration within the pelvis is abnormal. Some people have both types of FAI. Both types of femoroacetabular impingement cause injuries to the labral area because of repetitive impingement stress. They either cause labrum degeneration or labrum tears.

HOW TO TELL THE DIFFERENCE AND DOES IT MAKE A DIFFERENCE?

In pincher femoroacetabular impingement when the hip is in full flexion, the femoral head-neck junction hits or abuts the anterosuperior aspect of the acetabulum. It is commonly caused by too deep of an acetabular socket as in coxa profunda or protrusion acetabuli. One can easily imagine that if the socket portion of the hip is too deep that when the patient flexes the femur bone (thigh), it will pinch structures like the labrum between the acetabulum and the femur neck, so it pinches the labrum. In cam femoroacetabular impingement, abnormal contact between the head and socket of the hip occurs because of a loss of roundness of the femoral head. Cam comes from the Dutch word meaning "cog" because the femoral head is not round. This loss of roundness causes an abnormal contact between the head and the socket of the hip. In cam FAI, the impingement typically occurs when the hip is flexed, but also internally rotated. As already mentioned, patients often have "mixed" FAI, meaning they have a combination of both.

Both types of FAI can cause premature osteoarthritis of the hip because both types progress to hip labral and cartilage damage. For the person who desires a more conservative approach, we recommend Prolotherapy inside the joint, as well as around the structures of the joint causing some or all of the pain. What most patients may not realize is the cartilage has no nerve endings, so pain in a joint originates from some other structure(s) than cartilage. This is another reason that just getting injections inside the joint does not make much sense. Hackett-Hemwall dextrose Prolotherapy, along with other proliferants, addresses all the pain-producing structures. It typically works well with FAI, along with the other conditions causing premature hip osteoarthritis. Again, this is used along with an exercise program geared at stimulating joint health. Like other causes of premature hip osteoarthritis, sometimes surgical procedures are needed. The operative procedures are designed to address the adverse mechanical effects of impingement and hopefully address the reasons for it. Sometimes a combination of Prolotherapy and surgery is required.

SNAPPING HIP SYNDROME

Snapping hip syndrome is a condition characterized by a snapping sensation, and often an audible popping noise, when the hip is flexed and extended. The syndrome occurs most often among individuals 15 to 40 years-old, and affects females slightly more often than males. In one clinic, the rate of some form of snapping hip syndrome among female ballet dancers with hip complaints was close to 50%, and approximately 30% noted pain with this condition.

HOW DOES SNAPPING HIP SYNDROME DEVELOP?

Snapping hip syndrome has three primary causes. The most common cause involves the iliotibial band, or IT band, which is a thick, wide tendon that runs over the outside of the hip joint. Snapping hip syndrome occurs when the iliotibial band snaps over the bony prominence over the outside of the hip joint. Patients with this type of snapping hip syndrome may also develop trochanteric bursitis from the irritation of the bursa in this region. The second cause for snapping hip syndrome is the iliopsoas tendon, which can catch on a bony prominence of the pelvis and cause a snap when the hip is flexed. When the iliopsoas tendon is the cause of snapping hip syndrome, patients typically experience no problems other than the annoying snapping. Finally, the third and least likely cause of snapping hip syndrome involves a tear in the hip cartilage or labral tear in the hip joint. This type of snapping hip usually causes pain and may be disabling. In addition, a loose piece of cartilage can cause the hip to catch or lock up. *(See Figures 8-7.)*

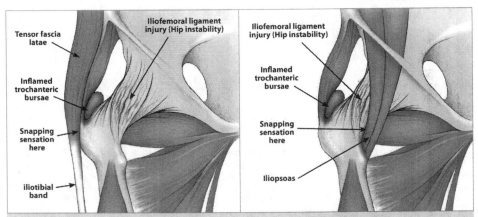

Figure 8-7: Snapping hip syndrome. The tensor fascia latae or iliopsoas muscle snapping sensation is actually from the muscle tightening to help stabilize the hip because of an underlying hip instability issue from either a ligament or labrum injury (laxity or tear). Trochanteric bursitis can also occur because of the hip instability.

PROLOTHERAPY STICKS IT TO SNAPPING HIP SYNDROME

A better approach than the traditional steroid shot, RICE, and endless rounds of physical therapy is to strengthen the hip ligaments with Prolotherapy. Prolotherapy to the posterior hip capsule and ischiofemoral ligaments generally resolves the problem if the condition involves snapping of the iliotibial band or gluteal muscles, because posterior hip laxity is involved in these conditions. Prolotherapy to the anterior hip ligaments, namely the iliofemoral ligament, will tighten the joint and stop the anterior protrusion of the hip. Prolotherapy helps resolve snapping hip syndrome because the underlying etiology of the problem is most often hip ligament laxity, and not tight muscles or tendons.

HIP LABRUM TEARS

In a retrospective study we performed at Caring Medical on hip labrum lesions treated by Prolotherapy, all patients reported improvements in pain relief and functionality. Patients reported complete relief of 54% of recorded symptoms.[16]

(See Figure 8-8.) Prolotherapy is a highly successful non-surgical option for hip labrum tears. Our opinion is that Prolotherapy should be the treatment of choice before surgery is even considered.

Hip instability is the major cause of hip osteoarthritis and subsequently the need for hip replacement surgery. The hip labrum along with the capsular ligaments iliofemoral, pubofemoral, ischiofemoral and articularis, as well as internal ligaments, ligamentous teres and transverse ligament; and the normal deep-socket configuration of the hip joint provide most of the stability of the hip. The labrum specifically deepens the socket by 20% and increases the acetabular contact area by 25%.[17]

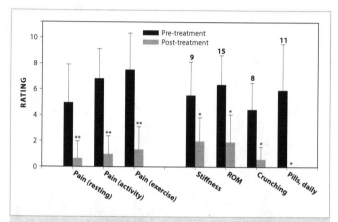

Traditional allopathic physicians offer either debridement or titanium sutures for hip labral tears. While short-term results are promising, the verdict is out on long-term

Figure 8-8: Before and after Prolotherapy treatment data on patients who were treated at Caring Medical for acetabular labrum tears. Patients reported pain, stiffness, range of motion (ROM) and crunching on a 0 – 10 rating scale. For consumption of medications, the ordinate represents the number of daily pills taken. For pain reports, n = 21 hips (19 patients). For stiffness, ROM, crunching and medications, only reports with non-zero baseline values were analyzed, the numbers of which are indicated above the bars. * $p \leq 0.01$, ** $p \leq 0.0001$ by Wilcoxon signed-rank test.

results. It is our opinion to only use surgery as a last resort because removing the labrum will definitely make the joint more unstable and will limit labrum pliability by stapling part of it down, only making it more prone to tears and degeneration. The blood flow to this area is already compromised, so what will happen with a metal object sticking through it? You can be the judge of that!

We have treated hip labrum tears with Prolotherapy for many years at Caring Medical. Cellular Prolotherapy solutions such as Platelet Rich Plasma or stem cell injections are sometimes required, especially in active people with hip labral tears. Generally 3-6 treatments at 4-8 week intervals are required.

A myriad of conditions lead to chronic hip pain, including trochanteric tendinitis or bursitis, pelvic floor dysfunction, ischiofemoral impingement, iliopsoas bursitis, myofascial pain syndrome of the tensor fascia lata, gluteal muscle tears and strain, as well as ligament sprains of the hip. When traditional treatments such as physiotherapy, medications, electrical stimulation, manipulation, exercise, rest, or massage do not work, then consider that you may have a labral tear. If you externally rotate your hip while lying on the ground and keep your foot off of the ground and then run it next to your opposing leg from the groin down to the foot and this increases your pain and you feel a clicking, grinding or popping sound, this correlates highly with the diagnosis of a hip labral tear. If this is the case, then consider receiving Prolotherapy.

SUMMARY

Most painful hip conditions begin with damage to the surrounding ligaments and progress into degenerative conditions that include hip osteoarthritis, labral degeneration, snapping hip syndrome, bone spurs, femoroacetabular impingement and more. Cortisone injections are routinely used in traditional medicine to cover up the pain temporarily and have degenerative effects that lead to early onset of osteoarthritis. Traditional treatments are not targeted to resolve the source of hip pain, which therefore leads to accelerated degeneration and the eventual need for hip replacement. However, hip replacement surgery is fraught with problems from the need for revision and resurfacing to metal poisoning and many others. Staples or other attempts to secure tissue can leave it less pliable and at risk for further long-term damage. While there are times that surgery is needed for more advanced cases that have lost most range of hip motion and have extensive destruction of the joint integrity, Prolotherapy may be an option afterward for post-surgical pain relief and soft tissue repair. Even better is seeking a Prolotherapy evaluation for painful hip conditions before the joint destruction is out of control!

Prolotherapy offers a successful and much-needed alternative to hip surgery by stimulating the body to repair the supportive ligaments around the joint, as well as promoting cartilage regeneration. In our studies, we found Prolotherapy is an excellent option for alleviating chronic hip pain and the need for most hip surgeries. Cellular Prolotherapy is also an excellent option for more advanced hip arthritis and labral tears. ■

CHAPTER

PROLO YOUR PELVIC AND GROIN PAIN AWAY!

The pelvic ring is important for proper load bearing required for all activities. It requires significant ligament strength to provide stability in order to transfer loads through the trunk of the body and between the upper and lower extremities. *(See Figure 9-1.)* If any of the supporting structures, such as the pubic symphysis or the surrounding

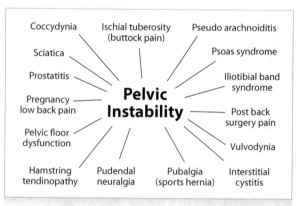

Coccydynia · Ischial tuberosity (buttock pain) · Pseudo arachnoiditis · Sciatica · Psoas syndrome · Prostatitis · Iliotibial band syndrome · Pregnancy low back pain · Pelvic floor dysfunction · Post back surgery pain · Vulvodynia · Hamstring tendinopathy · Pudendal neuralgia · Pubalgia (sports hernia) · Interstitial cystitis

Pelvic Instability

Chronic pelvic conditions caused by pelvic instability.

ligaments become weakened, it can cause disabling groin pain.

The pubic symphysis is actually a disc. It is a fibrocartilaginous disc that, like any other disc in the body, can be disrupted. It is supported on top by the superior pubic ligaments. Typically, people with groin pain are assumed to have a groin strain. This refers to a strain of the adductor muscles that attach to the pubic bone. Chronic pain that does not respond to exercise, massage, or manipulation is most likely a ligament problem. In the case of pain reproduced by palpating the pubic symphysis, the cause of the pain is pubic symphysis diathesis. This means a loose pubic symphysis area. Unfortunately, mild laxity in the joints can only be diagnosed by palpation. There is no x-ray study that can be done to confirm it. This is also why many physicians do not diagnose it. The diagnosis of ligament laxity can generally only be made by a listening ear and a strong thumb.

The pubic symphysis joint is stressed when the leg is pulled out from under-neath, such as a slip and fall accident. In sports, pubic symphysis injuries are relatively frequent. Swimmers who do the breast stroke often suffer groin pain from a pubic symphysis injury. Prolotherapy for pubic symphysis diathesis entails injections into the fibro-osseous junction of the superior pubic symphysis ligament and injections in the pubic symphysis itself. Prolotherapy is extremely effective in strengthening the pubic symphysis and relieving chronic groin pain in this area.[1,2]

CASES OF GROIN PAIN

A patient brought his son, highly touted baseball prospect, into the office. His baseball career was abruptly halted when he was told his chronic groin pain was a sports hernia. He followed the doctor's advice and had surgery for it, which didn't help. The next diagnosis was

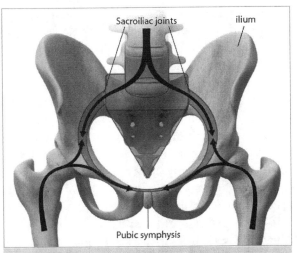

Figure 9-1: The components of the pelvic ring. The arrows show the direction of body weight force as it is transferred between the pelvic ring, trunk, and femurs. The keystone of the pelvic ring is the sacrum, which is wedged between the two ilia and secured bilaterally by the sacroiliac joints.

Adapted from: Magee D. *Orthopedic Physical Assessment.* 6th Edition. St. Louis, MO: Saunders; 2014. From Neumann DA. *Kinesiology of the musculoskeletal system.* Ed 2. St. Louis, 2010, CV Mosby, p. 360. Redrawn after Kapandji IA. *The physiology of joints.* Vol 3. New York, 1974, Churchhill Livingstone.

an iliopsoas muscle strain, so he worked with various therapies to relieve the muscle strain. Those did not help either. His back was finally x-rayed, where they found some degenerative disc changes. At this time, the team doctor began talking surgery.

That's when he came to see us at Caring Medical. On physical exam, the son had significant tenderness over the pubic symphysis, which was expected, tender iliopsoas muscle, and some degenerative changes in the lower lumbar spine on MRI. Palpation of the hip joint did not produce pain, but a positive jump sign was elicited at the iliolumbar ligaments, lumbosacral ligaments, and the sacroiliac ligaments. Dr. Hauser injected him in these areas and saved this young 18 year-old from a needless surgery.

This case illustrates a point that we will continue to emphasize: Prior to any surgical procedure for pain, it is important to have an evaluation by a physician familiar with Prolotherapy. The main cause of unresolved chronic pain is weakness in a ligament. Surgery does not cause ligaments to regrow but Prolotherapy does. Chronic groin pain is easily treated with Prolotherapy because there are multiple ligament laxities that cause groin pain. Iliolumbar ligament laxity should be explored as a diagnosis for any patient with unresolved groin pain.

In another case, a young woman came to see Dr. Hauser at Caring Medical. She had been suffering for more than 10 years with terrible groin pain. She had stepped into an animal trap, which wrapped around her leg. This caused the trap to engage and, before she knew it, she found herself hanging upside down from a tree limb with the rope lassoed around her ankle. Alone in the forest, she hung there for what seemed like eternity until she was finally rescued. As a result of this incident, she was left with chronic groin and back pain. As a health food store owner, she turned to numerous healing techniques. She also sought relief from many doctors who diagnosed her as having, among other things, a groin sprain, a disc problem, and a tendon strain. Nothing permanently relieved her pain.

Her medical history clearly indicated one thing that could have caused the problem. Dr. Hauser compressed the pubic symphysis (the pubic joint ligament) with his thumb on the side of the leg that had been caught in the rope. Wow! That caused a whole-body "jump sign." He treated that area with Prolotherapy. For the first time in a decade, she walked without pain.

Only once has a patient said that a physician had examined the pubic symphysis. The pubic symphysis is the front joint of the pelvic bone. The back joint of the pelvic bone is the sacroiliac joint. If the sacroiliac joint is lax, there is a good chance that the pubic symphysis will also be lax. Regarding the treatment of chronic pain with Prolotherapy, it is advisable to treat both sides of a joint to ensure its strength. Someone suffering from low back pain should not only have the sacroiliac joints examined, but the pubic symphysis as well. Likewise, patients with groin pain should have the sacroiliac joints palpated. Sacroiliac ligament laxity can also refer pain to the groin.[3]

ISCHIAL TUBEROSITY PAIN: SIMPLY, A PAIN IN THE BUTT!

Let's be honest, most of us sit all day! We probably don't realize all of the pains that are simply caused by excessive sitting. *(See Figure 9-2.)* The bones we sit on are the ischial tuberosities. Human beings were meant to be standing and moving. If you have a job that involves a lot of sitting, we emphatically urge you to stand more and if you need to sit, make sure you have a rocker bottom chair or sit on a Swiss ball, something that makes you engage your core muscles while sitting. If your core is not contracted while you work, you are putting incredible stresses on various joints in your neck, back, hip and, of course, on your ischial tuberosities. When you contract your core the lordotic curve in your lower back is maintained and this significantly lowers lower back disc pressures. However, prolonged static sitting without contracting the core is one of the

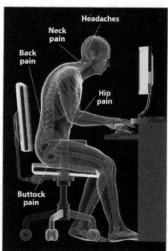

Figure 9-2: X-ray analysis of human body while sitting. Human beings were not meant to sit for long periods of time. The negative effects of sitting are the cause for a lot of the chronic neck, headaches, and back pain people suffer from. That is why standing while doing computer work is much better for a person than sitting.

risk factors not only for developing buttock pain, but low back pain! When the core is contracted, one of the beneficial effects is reduced pressure on the ischial tuberosities![4,5] Consider those of you who have careers or lifestyles that involve a lot of driving. In these cases, not only are excessive pressures exerted on your buttocks because of the hours sitting while driving every day, but your right hamstring must undergo an eccentric contraction (elongation) to use the gas pedal. If you drive a truck or a stick shift car, your left hamstring muscle undergoes the same type of stressors using the clutch. When studied, the optimal seat while driving would have an adjustable seat back that includes a 100 degrees from horizontal, a changeable depth of seat back to front edge of seat bottom, horizontally and vertically adjustable lumbar support, adjustable bilateral arm rests, adjustable head restraint with lordosis pad, seat shock absorbers to dampen frequencies in the 1 to 20 Hz range, and linear front-back travel of the seat enabling drivers of all sizes to reach the pedals, and believe it or not, there are several more recommendations. But you get the point![4-6] Sitting is bad for the body, especially the low back and the ischial tuberosity attachments, as is driving for long periods of time because of the way car seats and pedals are designed.

Several structures attach to the ischial tuberosity including the sacrotuberous ligament, hamstring muscles (biceps femoris, semitendinosus, semimembranosus) and adductor magnus muscle. When a person has severe buttock pain along with tenderness on the ischial tuberosity, often the diagnosis of ischial tuberosity pain syndrome or ischial bursitis is made. Bursitis can be ruled out when the area is not significantly red and swollen. When MRIs are performed of this area, occasionally they show tendinosis or degenerated tendon (it is actually the hamstring muscle origin) but more often than not, the MRI is negative. Why is this? *MRIs can never show weakness in a tissue.* When you can stand and your butt no longer hurts, but then it significantly irritates you the more you sit, then clearly the structures you are sitting on do not have the strength to withstand the pressure of sitting! You can buy cushions for your seat or car, but again that does nothing to strengthen the weak area. *(See Figure 9-3.)*

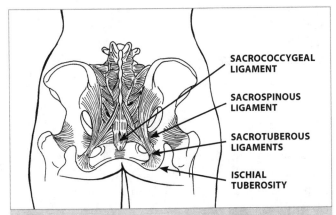

SACROCOCCYGEAL LIGAMENT

SACROSPINOUS LIGAMENT

SACROTUBEROUS LIGAMENTS

ISCHIAL TUBEROSITY

Figure 9-3: Ischial tuberosity and its relationship to the pelvic bones and ligaments. Important structures attach to the ischial tuberosity, including the sacrotuberous ligaments and the hamstring muscles.

ISCHIAL BURSITIS

The most common cause of pain at the cheek line in the buttock area is weakness in the structures that attach to the ischial tuberosity. The condition that is manifested by buttock pain and tenderness over the ischial tuberosity is known in traditional medical lingo as ischial bursitis. A bursa is a fluid-filled sac that allows tendons and muscles to glide over the bones. Bursitis means inflammation of the bursa. True bursitis pain is so painful that any pressure to the bursa would elicit a positive "hit the ceiling" sign. True bursitis is extremely rare. If a physician diagnoses bursitis and recommends a cortisone shot to relieve the inflammation, a fast exit out the door is strongly suggested. Remember, chronic pain is not due to a cortisone deficiency and is rarely due to bursitis.

Prolotherapy injections for buttock pain are given all along the ischial tuberosity, where the hamstring muscles and sacrotuberous ligaments attach. Prolotherapy will strengthen this area. After four sessions of Prolotherapy, the buttock pain is usually eliminated. Unfortunately, the ischial tuberosity is an area that is rarely examined by traditional physicians.

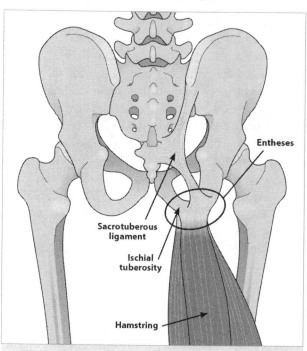

Figure 9-4: Entheses (plural) is the point at which a structure attaches to the bone. One of the enthesis of the hamstring muscles and sacrotuberous ligament is the ischial tuberosity.

ISCHIAL TUBEROSITY ENTHESOPATHY

Entheses (plural) is the point at which a structure attaches to the bone. One of the enthesis of the hamstring muscles and sacrotuberous ligament is the ischial tuberosity. **(See Figure 9-4.)** Disease, degeneration, or weakness of an attachment of a muscle, ligament, or tendon to the bone is called an enthesopathy. If you think about it, this whole book is about enthesopathies. Ligaments and tendons typically first become weakened, degenerated, and injured at their fibro-osseous junctions. *Fibro* signifies connective tissue and *-osseous* stands for bone, so the fibro-osseous junction is the enthesis. Thus, buttock pain from weakness at the ischial tuberosity muscle and ligament attachments should really be called ischial tuberosity enthesopathy.

What should the person do with ischial tuberosity enthesopathy? The same thing someone would do if the MRI showed an injury to the hamstring muscles: get Prolotherapy to the area. For runners and cyclists and others whose activities put a lot of strain on the hamstrings, Prolotherapy to the degenerated or torn areas will stimulate repair. Prolotherapy works great for this condition.

BUTTOCK PAIN IS DUE TO JOINT INSTABILITY

Throughout this book we emphasize the fact that it is important to consider if a condition could result from joint instability. The ischial tuberosity is part of the innominate bone and it attaches to the other side of the innominate bone via the pubic symphysis and its ligaments; and in the back attaches to the sacrum via the sacroiliac ligaments and the lower lumbar vertebrae by way of the iliolumbar ligaments. These areas need to be evaluated, as injuries to these structures would put additional strain on the structures of the ischial tuberosity and would also need to be treated to obtain long-term pain relief. The person who had complete relief of his/her buttock pain with Prolotherapy to the ischial tuberosity only to have it recur, should make sure to eliminate excessive static sitting and consider whether or not joint instability in the lower back or pubic area is associated with the condition.

RECTAL, VAGINAL AND TESTICULAR PAIN

Some of the most heartbreaking chronic pain cases involve pelvic and groin pain. Patients who deal with this pain are brave. Many tell us of the difficulty of going from doctor to doctor explaining problems that involve their most intimate bodily functions from painful orgasms to frequent urination to difficult bowel movements, and being given numerous prescription pills that chase the symptoms, until finally, they are called "crazy" or "depressed" and counseling is recommended. Chronic pain that extends to the pelvic floor and rectum, vagina, testes, and tailbone can be devastating. It can disrupt work, sports, marriages, childbearing, household duties with a constant awareness of pain or pressure that begins to rule a person's life. Just finding a comfortable position can be difficult as any adjustment may put pressure on different areas and cause a different type of pain. Ah ha! So again, we see that pain is positional and is caused upon joint movement.

It is interesting to hear the diagnoses people have been given for their conditions. One particularly memorable patient was very happy that someone had finally given her a diagnosis for her pain: vulvodynia. She was crushed when she was told that this meant nothing more than vaginal pain. *Vulva* means vaginal and *dynia* means pain. All the doctor did was tell her something she already knew. She had vaginal pain. Diagnoses like lumbago or lumbalgia (back pain), cervicalgia (neck pain), fibromyalgia (body pain), or proctalgia (rectal pain) are not diagnoses. They are terms for the symptoms. *(See Figure 9-5.)*

Roughly 15% of the population at one time or another will experience rectal pain, which is commonly diagnosed as proctalgia or proctalgia fugax.[7] It is characterized by episodic sharp pain in the rectal region, lasting for several seconds to several minutes. Traditional treatments include pain medications, steroid injections, counseling, or biofeedback.[8] Since no standard medical treatment is very effective, both the physician and the patient are easily frustrated. Often the patient is labeled as having irritable bowel syndrome, again a fancy diagnosis which just labels the symptoms.

Rectal, vaginal, or testicular pain, like pain anywhere else in the body, has a cause. Generally, these pains can be reproduced when the ligaments around the pelvis are palpated. The most commonly affected areas are the ligaments around the sacrococcygeal junction, which includes the sacrococcygeal ligament, sacrotuberous, and sacrospinous ligaments. Since these ligaments are near the rectum, it makes sense that rectal or groin pains originate

Diagnoses Associated with Pelvic Floor Dysfunction

- Chronic pelvic pain syndrome
- Chronic prostatitis
- Coccydynia
- Dyspareunia
- Interstitial cystitis
- Irritable bowel
- Levator ani syndrome
- Overactive bladder
- Painful bladder syndrome
- Pelvic congestion
- Prostatodynia
- Pudendal neuralgia
- Urinary incontinence
- Vaginismus
- Vulvar vestibulitis
- Vulvodynia

Figure 9-5: Various symptoms or associated diagnoses of pelvic floor dysfunction.

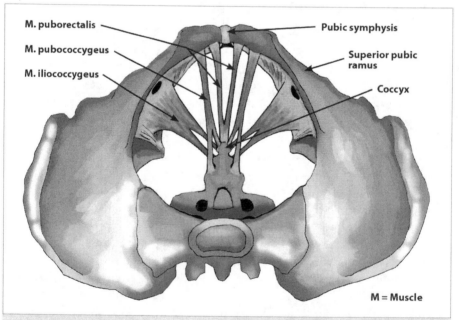

Figure 9-6: Female pelvis, superior view showing muscular attachments on the coccyx.
As can be seen from this illustration, the muscles that make up the levator ani (puborectalis, pubococcygeus, ilococcygeus) attach to the coccyx and pubis. Injury to the pelvic ligaments, including the pubic symphysis, superior pubic ligaments, sacrococcygeus ligaments or sacroiliac ligaments) could cause spasm to the levator ani muscle causing incontinence and/or severe pain. Prolotherapy, by tightening up the "loose" or stretched out ligaments, resolves the pelvic instability and pelvic floor dysfunction syndrome.

from these structures. When Prolotherapy has strengthened these ligaments, chronic rectal pain dissipates. *(See Figure 9-6.)* Another common cause of chronic groin, testicular, or vaginal pain is iliolumbar ligament weakness, because this ligament refers pain from the lower back to these areas. Prolotherapy of the iliolumbar ligament can be curative for chronic groin, testicular, vaginal pain, and symptoms associated with pelvic floor dysfunction. *(See Figure 9-7.)*

TAILBONE PAIN

Shelly, a 46 year–old woman came to Caring Medical with a

Symptoms Associated with Pelvic Floor Dysfunction

· Abdominal pain/fullness
· Constipation
· Difficulty initiating bowel movements
· Difficulty initiating the urine stream
· Frequent urination
· Increased discomfort when sitting for long intervals
· Pain with orgasm
· Pain with vaginal penetration
· Pelvic pressure or pain
· Post-ejaculatory pain
· Sensation of incomplete bladder emptying
· Sensation of needing to urinate immediately after urinating
· Severe fatigue
· Severe pain or burning with urination or defecation
· Sexual dysfunction
· Straining with urination
· Testicular or penis pain
· Vaginal pain

Figure 9-7: Symptoms associated with pelvic floor dysfunction syndrome.

history of constant tailbone pain for almost six years. The area above the tailbone was tender and swollen. Shelly suspected that the injury stemmed from a fall on ice where her tailbone hit the corner of a concrete step. The pain was unbelievable at the time, so she subsequently went to the emergency room where x-rays did not reveal any damage. Shelly stated that she was to the point of not wanting to go on, having been to numerous doctors without any solutions.

The tailbone, or coccyx, attaches to the sacrum via the sacrococcygeal ligaments. When ligaments are injured, as in the case of this woman who fell, the joints they support sustained excessive movement, which put additional strains on the injured ligaments. A swollen joint after trauma typically indicates ligament injury. Ligament injuries do not show up on x-ray. Shelly received a series of four Prolotherapy treatments and was completely healed of her pain. She is one happy lady thanks to Prolotherapy! She only wishes she found out about it sooner!

Chronic rectal or tailbone pain can be horribly disabling as this case illustrates. After extensive testing, patients are often given dubious diagnoses such as proctalgia fugax, anorectal neuralgia, levator ani syndrome, coccygodynia, or spastic pelvic floor syndrome.[7-10] Typical conservative traditional treatments include pain medicines, sitz baths (sitting in a warm tub), local anesthetic creams, massage, muscle relaxants, electrical stimulation gizmos, or the end-all pain treatment, an anti-depressant medication. Such treatments generally have unsatisfactory results because they do not correct the underlying cause of the chronic rectal pain.

SUMMARY

Chronic pain that does not respond to exercise, massage, or manipulation is most likely a ligament problem. As in other parts of the body, the most important evaluation in analyzing chronic pain is palpation of the area. When a positive "jump sign" is elicited over the painful ligament, both the patient and the doctor know that the cause of the pain is a weakened ligament.

In cases of pain in groin, rectal, vaginal, testicular, pelvic floor, and pubic symphysis areas, generally these pains can be reproduced when the ligaments around the pelvis are palpated. The most commonly affected areas are the ligaments around the sacrococcygeal junction, which includes the sacrococcygeal ligament, sacrotuberous, and sacrospinous ligaments. Patients with pain should have the sacroiliac joints palpated because sacroiliac ligament laxity can also refer pain to the groin. Another common cause of chronic groin, testicular, or vaginal pain is iliolumbar ligament weakness, because this ligament refers pain from the lower back to these areas. In the case of pain reproduced by palpating the pubic symphysis, the cause of the pain is pubic symphysis diathesis. This means a loose pubic symphysis area.

Prolotherapy treatments to the weakened ligaments help these areas heal and return to normal strength. Once the ligaments are strong again, the chronic pain abates. In cases of pelvic floor dysfunction, the additional symptoms such as difficulty with urination and bowel movements, as well as sexual dysfunction and abdominal pressure, can be eliminated as well. Athletes with chronic groin pain find that return to sports after Prolotherapy is generally quick and provides the desired long-term stability. This is why many people with chronic rectal, tailbone, groin, testicular, and vaginal pains are choosing to Prolo their pain away! ∎

CHAPTER

10

PROLO YOUR ANKLE AND FOOT PAIN AWAY!

When we watch an MMA fight, we are amazed to see the pounding those fighters take! What's even more remarkable is that they choose to do it. Even that pounding is minor compared to the pounding our feet take every day. The average person takes 3,000 to 10,000 steps per day. The foot's job during the process of walking is to traject the body weight up one inch with each step. For example, if a woman weighing 125 pounds takes 5,000 steps in a day, her feet have lifted 625,000 pounds during that day. If a 150-pound person walks one mile, 60 tons of force is exerted through the small area that encompasses the ankle and feet. Is it any wonder feet are sore by the end of the day?[1]

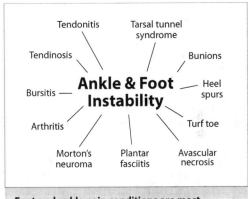

Foot and ankle pain conditions are most commonly a result of joint instability.

FOOT BIOMECHANICS

Poor foot biomechanics may be responsible for a myriad of chronic complaints, including pain in the feet, knees, lower back, and neck.[2] The feet act as a spring, propelling the body forward with each step. If the spring is not working, the propelling force must come from the knees, hip, or lower back. Because these areas are not designed to function in this manner, they eventually deteriorate and the chronic pain cycle begins.

The most important factor in evaluating a person's gait (walking cycle) is to observe the stability of the arch and the ability of the foot to spring the body forward. The most important arch in the foot is the medial arch. *(See Figure 10-1.)* It is abnormal for the arch to collapse during the gait cycle or while at rest. This

collapsing of the arch is known as
flat feet, or pes planus. A collapsed
arch indicates tissue breakdown.
Supporting tissue is no longer able
to elevate the inside of the foot.
The plantar fascia is the first tissue
to be affected. Pain resulting from
this weakened tissue is called plantar
fasciitis. If the condition continues,
a terrible thing will occur. The
person will pay a visit to a podiatrist
and receive a cortisone shot for
the inflamed fascia. Cortisone will

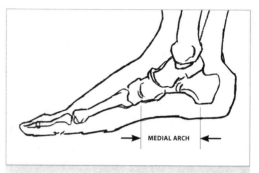

Figure 10-1: Side view of the foot showing the medial arch. Collapsing of the medial arch is known as pes planus (flat feet).

eventually weaken the fascia. If the fascia is not strengthened, a painful heel spur
will result. Prolotherapy to strengthen the fascia is a superior treatment option.

The next affected structures are the ligaments that support the inside of the foot,
especially the calcaneonavicular ligament. *(See Figure 10-2.)* When this ligament is
weakened, the arch pain will increase. Eventually, the posterior tibialis tendon in
the knee must help support the arch. This tendon eventually weakens, resulting in
knee pain added to the original foot pain, as the arch continues to collapse. Because
the arch and the knee can no longer elevate the foot, the entire limb must be raised

during a step, putting additional
strain on the hip. The spring in the
foot and the efficiency of the gait
are drastically reduced due to the
collapsed arch. This requires more
energy from the foot, resulting in
further deterioration of the medial
arch. The more severe the collapse
of the arch, the greater the likelihood
of pain. The deterioration cycle will
continue until something is done
to support the arch. Contrary to
popular belief, cortisone shots will
not accomplish this! Arch pain in
the foot is not a cortisone deficiency!
(See Figure 10-3.)

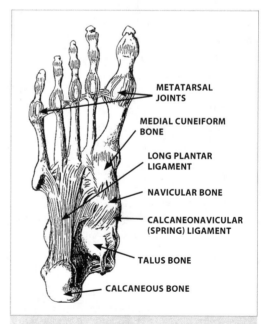

METATARSAL JOINTS

MEDIAL CUNEIFORM BONE

LONG PLANTAR LIGAMENT

NAVICULAR BONE

CALCANEONAVICULAR (SPRING) LIGAMENT

TALUS BONE

CALCANEOUS BONE

Figure 10-2: Bone and ligament anatomy of the bottom of the foot. The plantar fascia has been removed to show the spring ligament and other bones of the foot.

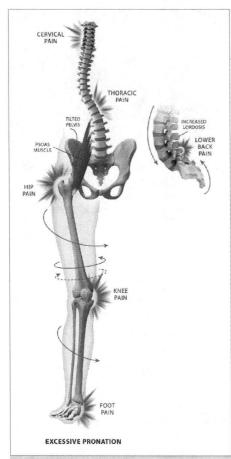

CERVICAL PAIN

THORACIC PAIN

TILTED PELVIS

INCREASED LORDOSIS

PSOAS MUSCLE

LOWER BACK PAIN

HIP PAIN

KNEE PAIN

FOOT PAIN

EXCESSIVE PRONATION

Figure 10-3: The kinetic chain-joint instability connection. The shin bone is connected to the thigh bone and explains why the collapse of the foot works it's way up the kinetic chain to affect the knee, hip, and eventually the lower back.

Adapted from: Foot instability causes skeletal instability poster. Somathotics Inc.

FALLEN ARCHES

The medial arch is supported by fascia and ligaments. As previously explained, ligaments maintain proper bone alignment. Loose ligaments allow the bones to shift, resulting in chronic pain. The main supporting structure is the plantar fascia, also known as the plantar aponeurosis. The plantar fascia is essentially a strong, superficially placed ligament that extends in the middle part of the foot from the calcaneus to the toes. Another important structure is the plantar calcaneonavicular ligament which passes from the lower surface of the calcaneus to the lower surface of the navicular bone. *(See Figure 10-4.)* This ligament resists the downward movement of the head of the talus, supporting the highest part of the arch, and is responsible for some of the elasticity of the arch. This ligament is also known as the spring ligament.

An arch support insert is the typical treatment for a fallen arch. Many people experience dramatic pain relief, while others continue to suffer from chronic achy feet.

Prolotherapy is the treatment that makes the most sense for a fallen arch due to weak ligaments. Prolotherapy injections into the fibro-osseous junctions of the plantar fascia and calcaneonavicular ligament, which supports the arch, will strengthen this area. If the condition is diagnosed early on, the ligaments can be strengthened to support the arch. If the process has gone on for years, an arch support may be needed in addition to Prolotherapy. But even in the latter case, Prolotherapy can eliminate the chronic arch pain.

HEEL SPURS AND PLANTAR FASCIITIS

Many patients with foot pain come to Caring Medical saying they have been diagnosed with "heel spurs." Others were told they had "plantar fasciitis." Patients have anxiety night and day because they have "heel spurs" and "plantar fasciitis." (It does sound kind of scary, doesn't it?) Such a diagnosis resulted from an x-ray that revealed some extra bone where the plantar fascia attaches to the calcaneus.[3] This extra bone is called a "spur." *(See Figure 10-4.)* Because it involves the heel, it is ingeniously named a "heel spur." It is located where the plantar fascia attaches to the heel, hence plantar fasciitis.

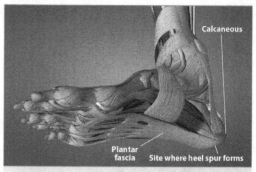

Figure 10-4: Heel spur formation. Weakness in the plantar fascia (called plantar fasciitis) causes inflammation to occur at the calcaneal attachment, causing a heel spur.

Treatments such as the dreaded cortisone shot or, even worse, surgery to remove the spur, have claimed many victims. These treatments do not correct the underlying defect. The plantar fascia supports the navicular, talus, and medial cuneiform bones. When the plantar fascia must also attempt to support the arch, excess pressure is placed on the calcaneus bone. The calcaneal spur forms because the plantar fascia cannot adequately support the arch. The plantar fascia is "holding on for dear life" to its attachment at the calcaneus. This "holding on for dear life" causes the body to grow more bone in that area in an attempt to reduce the pressure on the ligament, resulting in a heel spur. The same kind of pressure would occur if you were hanging from a ledge of a tall building by the tips of your fingers. You can bet when you were finally rescued that the ledge might have some marks in it where your fingers were located.

Cortisone may temporarily relieve the pain in some cases, but it will always weaken tissue long-term. Prolotherapy to the fibro-osseous junction of the plantar fascia will cause a permanent strengthening of that structure. Once the plantar fascia returns to normal strength, the chronic heel pain will be eliminated. "But what about the heel spur?" people complain. Remember, the heel spur is just an x-ray finding. Many people have heel spurs without any pain. Prolotherapy will not remove the heel spur, but it will eliminate the chronic pain by eliminating the cause. So relax and enjoy a foot without pain.

BIG TOE AND BUNION PAIN

The most common foot condition is pain in the first metatarsophalangeal joint. This is the joint that handles the most amount of force in the foot with walking and running. Instability of this joint, not only causes significant big toe pain, but if left untreated results in a bunion.

Bunions are another problem that excite the surgeons. Nothing makes a foot surgeon happier than an elderly patient with bunions. Bunions are an overgrowth of bone at the first metatarsophalangeal joint. *(See Figure 10-5.)*

What causes an overgrowth of bone? You're learning...ligament weakness. When ligaments weaken, the bones move. This is visually evident because bunions are a result of a gross displacement of the bone. Bone movement due to ligament laxity causes the bones to hit each other. This hitting causes an overgrowth of bone, as an attempt to stabilize the joint. Thus, a bunion is the body's response at the great toe to compensate for a weak ligament.

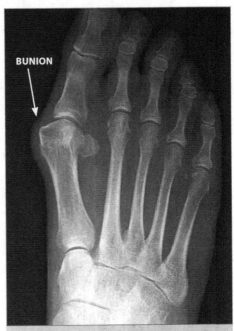

Figure 10-5: X-ray image of a bunion of the big toe. Weakness of the ligaments leads to a crooked big toe and subsequent bunion.

In our study published in the *Foot and Ankle Online Journal*, 12 of our patients were treated for pain and deformity of the first metatarsophalangeal, commonly referred to as a bunion.[4] Patients received traditional dextrose Prolotherapy with added Human Growth Hormone (HGH), as we have found this Prolotherapy solution helpful in arthritic conditions for the big toe and other joints. Upon completion of three to six Prolotherapy sessions, 11 of 12 patients had a favorable outcome—the relief of symptoms, which included pain levels during activity, stiffness levels, and numbness. *(See Figure 10-6.)* The average patient required four treatments, for those suffering from toe pain and stiffness due to bunions.

PROLOTHERAPY RESULTS FOR FOOT PAIN

The foot is similar to the wrist. It consists of several bones in a sea of ligaments. Stretching of any of these ligaments can be a source of chronic pain. John Merriman, MD, in a 1995 study, obtained good to excellent results in 79% of the 204 patients with foot pain who were treated utilizing Prolotherapy as the only modality.[5]

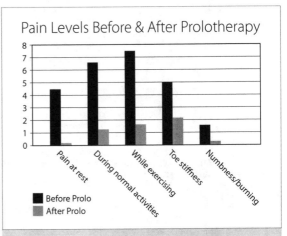

Figure 10-6: Survey responses before and after Prolotherapy on levels of big toe pain with various activities.

In our study on unresolved foot and toe pain, published in the *Journal of Prolotherapy*, 19 patients who had been in pain an average of 54 months were treated quarterly with Hackett-Hemwall dextrose Prolotherapy.[6] This included a subset of eight patients who were told by their medical doctor(s) that there were no other

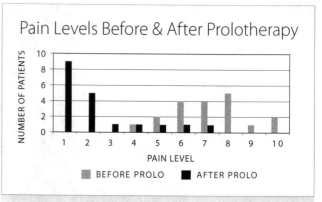

Figure 10-7: Pain levels before and after receiving Hackett-Hemwall dextrose Prolotherapy in patients with unresolved foot pain.

treatment options for their pain. Patients were contacted an average of 18 months following their last Prolotherapy session and asked questions regarding their levels of pain, physical and psychological symptoms, as well as activities of daily living, before and after their last Prolotherapy treatment. In these 19 patients, 100% exhibited improvements in their pain. *(See Figure 10-7.)* Eighty-four percent experienced 50% or more pain relief. Dextrose Prolotherapy helped the patients make large improvements in walking and exercise ability, as well as produced decreased levels of anxiety and depression. *(See Figure 10-8.)*

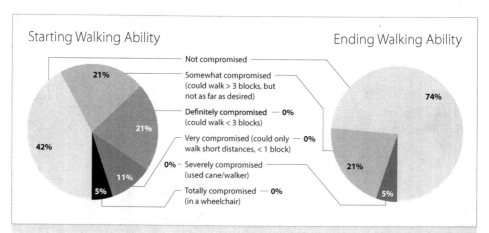

Figure 10-8: Walking ability before and after Hackett-Hemwall dextrose Prolotherapy in 19 patients with unresolved foot pain.

MORTON'S NEUROMA AND TARSAL TUNNEL SYNDROME

CHRONIC FOOT PAIN AND/OR NUMBNESS

It is quite common for people with the diagnosis of a neuroma, or nerve entrapment, to undergo multiple surgeries attempting to alleviate the entrapment. One individual came to us with a history of 15 surgeries! This occurs primarily because most physicians incorrectly believe numbness is equated with a pinched nerve. Ligament and tendon weakness in the limb also cause chronic numbness in an extremity.

Morton's neuroma is often diagnosed from the symptom of burning pain in a toe or toes. This is a neuroma involving the nerves located between the toes. These nerves allow sensation to be felt on the skin of the toes. A neuroma is a nervous tissue tumor. Despite years of experimental research and clinical investigation, the painful neuroma has remained difficult to prevent or to treat successfully when it occurs. More than 150 physical and chemical methods for treating neuromas have been utilized, including suturing, covering with silicone caps, injecting muscle or bone with chemicals such as alcohol, and many others.[7]

Surgical treatment has been problematic with poor results and complications. In one study, 47% of the patients continued to have symptoms of foot pain after surgery.[8] The reason for continued symptoms after surgery or chemical injections may be that the chronic foot pain or numbness is due to ligament weakness and not only a pinched nerve.

In our study on 19 feet with pain diagnosed as having Morton's neuroma, in 17 patients, we found that dextrose Prolotherapy was extremely effective at improving a number of pain factors: pain at rest; pain with normal activities; pain with exercise; pain while walking barefoot.[9] Patients' subjective experience of pain offers the best measure for statistical accuracy, and all patients in our study reported pain as a symptom. Patients were additionally asked about numbness levels and stiffness.

This prospective, non-controlled study demonstrated that Hackett-Hemwall dextrose Prolotherapy decreases pain and improves the quality of life for patients with Morton's neuroma, which was unresolved by previous therapies, medications, and interventions. Prolotherapy provided relief of at least 74% for 14 out of 17 of the patients at least six months after their last treatment. Two out of three patients who were told they needed surgery prior to Prolotherapy, felt sufficient pain relief with Prolotherapy and were able to avoid surgery. After the study period, patients experienced overall improvement in range of motion, ability to walk and exercise, as well as relief of stiffness and numbness/burning. *(See Figure 10-9.)*

REFERRAL PAIN PATTERNS OF THE FOOT

As we all know, the foot bone is connected to the leg bone, is connected to the hip bone, is connected to the back bone. The hip and back also need to be poked on if someone suffers from foot pain and/or numbness. Hip joint weakness and ligament laxity can refer symptoms to the big toes. *(See Figure 10-10.)* The sacroiliac

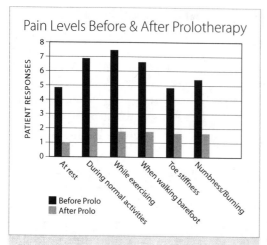

Pain Levels Before & After Prolotherapy

Figure 10-9: Survey responses before and after Prolotherapy on levels of pain from Morton's Neuroma with various activities.

joint commonly refers pain to the lateral foot area. The sacrospinous and sacrotuberous ligaments in the pelvis refer pain and/or numbness to the heel area. So all these areas must be examined to see if they are contributing to a person's symptoms.

It is quite common for a doctor to limit an examination of a patient with foot pain to just the foot. This is a mistake, as foot pain is often a reflection of a knee or back problem. Treatment directed at the foot in such cases may have unsatisfactory results.

Most chronic foot pain and numbness are not primarily due to a nerve being pinched but due to weakness in the ligaments and soft tissue structures that support the ball of the foot and the arch. Prolotherapy injections start these areas to grow new and stronger tissue. Once this tissue gains normal strength the pain, numbness, and disability normally stop. If it does not, the nerve entrapment can be "unpinched" quickly and non-surgically with Nerve Release Injection Therapy (NRIT). We will discuss this issue in greater detail in **Chapter 16**. In our office, we frequently combine dextrose Prolotherapy with Nerve Release Injection Therapy (NRIT) and/or Lyftogt Perineural Injection Therapy for nerve-related pain. This combined approach works well to correct the underlying joint instability, as well as free up and nourish the entrapped nerve.

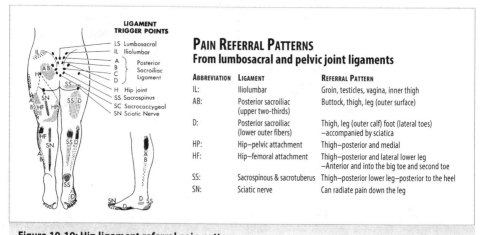

Pain Referral Patterns
From lumbosacral and pelvic joint ligaments

Abbreviation	Ligament	Referral Pattern
IL:	Iliolumbar	Groin, testicles, vagina, inner thigh
AB:	Posterior sacroiliac (upper two-thirds)	Buttock, thigh, leg (outer surface)
D:	Posterior sacroiliac (lower outer fibers)	Thigh, leg (outer calf) foot (lateral toes) –accompanied by sciatica
HP:	Hip–pelvic attachment	Thigh–posterior and medial
HF:	Hip–femoral attachment	Thigh–posterior and lateral lower leg –Anterior and into the big toe and second toe
SS:	Sacrospinous & sacrotuberus	Thigh–posterior lower leg–posterior to the heel
SN:	Sciatic nerve	Can radiate pain down the leg

Figure 10-10: Hip ligament referral pain pattern.
Hip instability from ligament injury can refer pain into the foot from the big toe.

Many people, despite surgery, still have pain in their feet from so-called Morton's neuroma or tarsal tunnel syndrome. Tarsal tunnel syndrome is very similar to carpal tunnel syndrome of the hand *(See Chapter 11.)* except it involves the foot. The tibial nerve runs in a canal on the inside of the foot called the tarsal tunnel. When the tibial nerve gets pinched here, it is called tarsal tunnel syndrome. The symptoms described for this syndrome include pain in the ankle, arch, toes, or heel.[10] Chronic burning arch, toe, or heel pain is most often due to ligament weakness in the foot and/or ankle or soft tissue weakness in the arch of the foot, which has allowed the pinching or entrapment of a nerve.

The ball of the foot is called the metatarsal joints and supports half the body weight during walking.[11] Since these structures bear the bulk of the body weight when a person stands, walks, or runs, it is no wonder that these are generally the first structures to weaken. Metatarsal ligament weakness is manifested by pain at the ball of the feet which often radiates into the toes. This is called metatarsalgia. Both the instability of the foot and peripheral nerve entrapments can be alleviated with a combination of Prolotherapy and NRIT. NRIT provides instant nerve pain-relieving results for the patient while Prolotherapy stimulates the long-term repair of the supportive ligament structures. The success of this combination significantly decreases the need for surgery for most cases.

ANKLE PAIN

An ankle sprain is one of the most common ligament injuries in the body. It is estimated that 26,000 people sprain their ankles every day. Unfortunately, ankle sprains are not always simple injuries and can result in residual symptoms in 30-40% of patients.[12] The most common ankle sprain is an inversion injury,

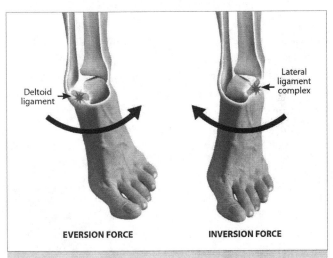

EVERSION FORCE   **INVERSION FORCE**

Figure 10-11: Ankle instability. Inversion forces stress the lateral ligament complex; whereas eversion forces stress the deltoid ligament.

turning the ankle inward, injuring the ligaments on the lateral side of the ankle, usually the anterior talofibular and the tibiofibular ligaments. *(See Figure 10-11.)* The most common symptom of this type of injury, besides lateral ankle pain, is a propensity for the ankle to continually turn inward. Many of our young patients with hypermobility, which we discuss in more detail in *Chapter 17*, have problems with continuous ankle subluxations due to weakened, overstretched ligaments. This can become a viscous cycle as the ankle can sublux with every step, worsening the joint instability and accelerating the wear and tear to the joint structures. Patients become frustrated trying to walk, run, dance, and play sports and constantly being afraid of another ankle sprain or feeling that the ankle will give way at any moment.

Exercises designed to strengthen the muscles that support the lateral ankle are beneficial, but rarely solve the problem. Taping ankles, as many trainers and athletes do, only provides temporary benefit. Ankle joint instability is a common finding during an exam of the lateral ankle. *(See Figure 10-12.)* The best long-term solution is to stimulate the body to tighten the ligaments around the ankle. Prolotherapy injections to

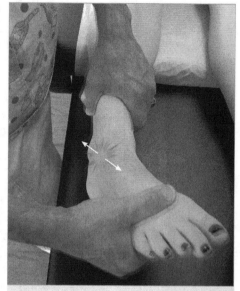

Figure 10-12: Examination of lateral ankle. Excessive movement or soft end feel compared to non-painful side while inverting ankle is a sign of lateral ankle instability.

strengthen the ligaments supporting the lateral ankle provide definitive results, and can eliminate chronic ankle sprains and subluxations.

The inside of the ankle is held together by the deltoid ligament. This ligament is injured from turning the foot outward, as can happen when falling down stairs or mis-stepping. Again, Prolotherapy injections at the fibro-osseous junction of the deltoid ligament eliminate the chronic ankle pain and instability in this area.

If ankle pain and subluxation continues, the tissue continues to degenerate, eventually leading to ankle arthritis or other conditions that demonstrate a cellular deficiency in the area. For more advanced cases like this, Cellular Prolotherapy provides a stronger proliferant to stimulate tissue repair. *(See Figure 10-13.)* For patients at risk of ankle replacement or ankle fusion surgery, Cellular Prolotherapy provides a preferable modality to get long-term pain relief.

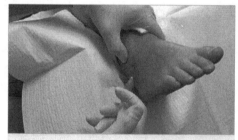

Figure 10-13: Direct bone marrow injection to the ankle.

PROLOTHERAPY RESULTS IN PATIENTS WITH CHRONIC ANKLE PAIN

In the 2010 January/February issue of *Practical Pain Management*, we published data obtained on 19 ankle patients who suffered from chronic ankle pain and were treated with Prolotherapy.[13] Of these, 63% (12) were female and 37% (7) were male. The average age of the patients was 52 years-old. Patients reported an average of 3.3 years (40 months) of pain and on average saw 3.3 MDs before receiving Prolotherapy. The average patient was taking 1.0 pain medication. Sixty-three percent (12) stated that the consensus of their medical doctor(s) was that there were no other treatment options for their chronic pain. Eleven percent (2) stated that the only other treatment option for their chronic ankle pain was surgery.

TREATMENT OUTCOMES

Patients received an average of 4.4 Prolotherapy treatments per ankle. The average time of follow-up after their last Prolotherapy session was 21 months. Patients were asked to rate their pain and stiffness levels on a scale of 1 to 10 on a visual analog scale (VAS) with 1 being no pain/stiffness and 10 being severe crippling pain/stiffness. The 19 ankles had an average starting pain level of 7.9 and stiffness of 5.4. Ending pain and stiffness levels were 1.6 and 1.5 respectively *(See Figure 10-14.)* Ninety-five percent reported a starting pain level of 6 or greater, while none had a starting pain level of four or less. After Prolotherapy none had a pain level of 6 or greater, and 90% of patients reported at least a 50% reduction in pain. One-hundred percent of patients stated their pain and stiffness was better after Prolotherapy. Over 78% reported that pain and stiffness since their last session had not returned.

In regard to quality of life issues prior to receiving Prolotherapy, 74% noted problems with walking, but only 37% experienced compromised walking after. In regard to exercise ability before Prolotherapy, only 47% could exercise longer than 30 minutes, but after Prolotherapy this increased to 90%. To a simple yes or no question, "Has Prolotherapy changed your life for the better," all of the patients treated answered "yes." This question was included in many of our studies, because when it comes down to the point of any medical treatment, we feel this is the point. It's not "Is my x-ray better?" but rather, how has your life changed for the better.

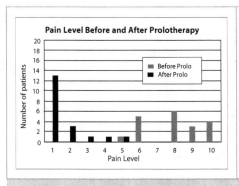
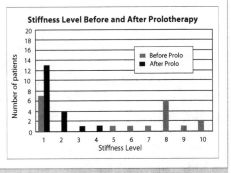

Figure 10-14. Pain and stiffness levels before and after receiving Hackett-Hemwall Prolotherapy in patients with unresolved ankle pain.

ACHILLES TENDINOPATHY

The Achilles is the largest tendon in the body. It is a commonly injured tendon typically due to overuse and running sports injuries. Tendon injuries often start after a demanding workout and initially causes a tendinitis, where the body is trying to repair the weakened tendon. When the tendon doesn't heal on its own and as more time passes, the tendon begins to show signs of cellular damage and collagen degeneration, or tendinosis. Tendinosis makes the Achilles tendon more prone to tearing. *(See Figure 10-15.)* Degenerated tissue needs regeneration, which is why Prolotherapy is such an effective treatment for Achilles tendon pain. For a torn or degenerated Achilles tendon, Cellular Prolotherapy is preferred to bring concentrated growth factors directly to the site of the injury to accelerate repair. Remember, RICE, NSAIDs, and cortisone injections promote degeneration which is not conducive to healing. Cellular Prolotherapy, by stimulating the growth and repair of the Achilles tendon, improves its strength, giving long-term pain relief.

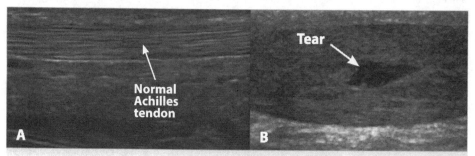

Figure 10-15: Ultrasound demonstrating a normal Achilles tendon (a) and one with a tear (b).

SUMMARY

In summary, chronic ankle and foot pain is relatively common and almost expected, as the feet bear tons of force every day just from the process of walking. Often, chronic foot pain begins from a collapse of the medial arch. This occurs because the spring ligaments and plantar fascia can no longer support the arch. Treatments, such as arch supports, may provide temporary benefit. Prolotherapy injections to strengthen the arch provide permanent results.

Heel spurs are due to weakened ligamentous support of the plantar fascia. Prolotherapy to strengthen the plantar fascia will eliminate chronic heel pain. There is generally not a need for heel spurs to be surgically removed after the supportive ligaments and plantar fascia have been repaired. Big toe pain, including bunion pain, is due to weakness of the metatarsal ligaments. Prolotherapy is superior at eliminating the pain of bunions, but does not correct the deformity.

The most common ligament injury is the ankle sprain. Taping and exercising for this condition often have only temporary results. Prolotherapy can permanently strengthen the ligaments of the ankle, eliminating chronic ankle sprains and subluxations. Because Prolotherapy stimulates the repair of the soft tissue injuries and subsequent instability that are associated with bunions, heel spurs, plantar fasciitis, ankle sprains, fallen arches, and Achilles tendinopathy, chronic pain from these conditions is eliminated. For advanced degenerative conditions, Cellular Prolotherapy is often utilized for accelerated recovery. In conditions, such as tarsal tunnel syndrome and Morton's neuroma, in addition to Prolotherapy to repair the underlying joint instability, Nerve Release Injection Therapy provides instant relief for entrapped nerves.

Cortisone injections, NSAIDs, and surgery work against a patient's best long-term interest because they are degenerative by nature. Patients with chronic ankle and foot pain need regenerative options to stop the degenerative process. This is also true for athletes with acute foot and ankle problems, as well as anyone who wishes to stay active without taking extended time off for surgical recovery. It is for this reason that many people are choosing to Prolo their ankle and foot pain away! ■

CHAPTER

11

PROLO YOUR ELBOW, WRIST, AND HAND PAIN AWAY!

Typically, people who perform repetitive tasks with their hands are the patients with chronic elbow, wrist, and hand pain.[1] This includes mail handlers, assembly line workers, carpenters, computer operators, secretaries, and the thousands of other jobs that keep people in one space doing the same thing day after day. Is it any wonder that after repeating a movement 10 billion times that a part of the body breaks down?

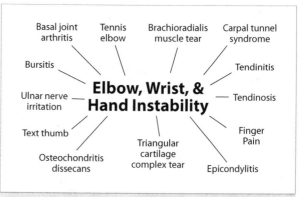

Conditions which commonly cause elbow, wrist, and hand pain and are due to, or cause instability and joint degeneration.

After a long hard day of work or strenuous exercise, it is quite normal for muscles to hurt for a short period of time. This is often a "good hurt." You put your body through strenuous activities that caused the normal soreness. The muscles ache after a good workout because muscle cells were actually injured during exercise. Yes, you read that correctly. Exercise and repetitive work does cause injury to muscle cells. But such injury is good for the muscles because they have a tremendous blood supply, and this "temporary injury" stimulates muscle cells to multiply and grow.

God made muscles with the ability to be ready for a fight. It is a necessary defense mechanism that, at a moment's notice, the blood supply to our muscles can increase tenfold. If you wake up to find that your house is on fire, the blood supply to the muscles can increase to give them the strength to rescue you. Exercise is necessary for good health and keeps the muscles strong.

This "good hurt" with exercise should not last more than an hour or two.

If the muscles hurt longer than this time period, you are either exercising too much or need to take more breaks during work.

Muscle injuries usually heal with plain and simple rest. To speed up recovery from muscle injuries, it is beneficial to stretch the muscles after exercising.[2] Nutritional supplements also help muscle injuries heal.[3]

Chronic pain that is not relieved by rest is likely due to a ligament injury. Pain with repetitive motion may be an indication of tendon injury. Ligaments attach bone to bone. While the ligaments stabilize the bones, the tendons and muscles enable the bones to move. This is why ligaments often hurt when the body is at rest and tendons often hurt from activity.

ELBOW PAIN

ANNULAR LIGAMENT WEAKNESS

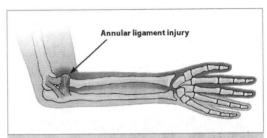

Eighty percent of chronic elbow pain is due to a sprain of the annular ligament. *(See Figure 11-1.)* This ligament is rarely examined by a family physician or an orthopedic surgeon. Nearly all of our patients with chronic elbow pain tell us their doctors told them they have tennis elbow. Tennis elbow is also known as lateral epicondylitis. The latest treatment

Figure 11-1: Annular ligament injury. Injuries to the annular ligament at the lateral elbow can refer pain and/or numbness and tingling down to the wrist and fingers. Often, these injuries can present with symptoms similar to those of carpal tunnel syndrome. Palpation of the annular ligament on physical exam can elicit moderate to severe tenderness and/or reproduction of symptoms.

for this condition is the dreaded cortisone shot! Cortisone weakens tissue, whereas Prolotherapy strengthens tissue. Cortisone has temporary effects in regard to pain control whereas Prolotherapy has permanent effects. However, cortisone does have one permanent effect: continual use will permanently weaken tissue. Anyone receiving long-term prednisone or cortisone shots will confirm this fact.

The annular ligament is located approximately three quarters of an inch distal to the lateral epicondyle. Its job is to attach the radius bone to the ulnar bone. It is this ligament that enables the hand to rotate, as in turning a key or a screwdriver. Because of the tremendous demands placed on the fingers and hands to perform repetitive tasks, the annular ligament is stressed every day. Eventually, this ligament becomes lax and a source of chronic pain.

The lateral epicondyle of the humerus bone is very superficial, so it is much more inviting to the dreaded cortisone-filled needle of an orthopedist than the deeper annular ligament. Typically, people with chronic elbow pain are tender over the lateral epicondyle but do not elicit a positive "jump sign" in that area. Only palpation over the annular ligament elicits the positive "jump sign." The annular ligament also has a distinct referral pain pattern. It refers pain to the thumb, index, and middle fingers.

CARPAL TUNNEL SYNDROME - A LIGAMENT PROBLEM

Unfortunately, many patients with elbow and hand pain have been misdiagnosed with carpal tunnel syndrome. Carpal tunnel syndrome refers to the entrapment of the median nerve as it travels through the wrist into the hand. The nerve supplies sensation to the skin over the thumb, index, and middle fingers. A typical carpal tunnel syndrome patient will experience pain and numbness in this distribution in the hand. Because most physicians do not know the referral pain patterns of ligaments, they do not realize that the fourth and fifth cervical vertebrae and the annular ligament can refer pain to the thumb, index, and middle fingers. Ligament laxity can also cause numbness, as already discussed. Cervical and annular ligament laxity should always be evaluated prior to making the diagnosis of carpal tunnel syndrome.

Surgery for carpal tunnel syndrome should not be done until an evaluation is performed by a physician who understands the referral patterns of ligaments and is experienced in Prolotherapy.

True carpal tunnel syndrome	Pseudo carpal tunnel syndrome
• Atrophy of thenar eminence	• No atrophy of hand muscles
• Positive EMG/NCV	• Negative EMG/NCV
• Positive Phalen's test	• Negative Phalen's test
• Positive Tinel's sign	• Negative Tinel's sign
• Thumb weakness	• Thumb strength normal
• True numbness in thumb, index, and middle finger	• Numbness
	• Tenderness over annular ligament in elbow

Figure 11-2: Signs and symptoms of "true" versus "pseudo" carpal tunnel syndrome. Patients with true carpal tunnel syndrome (constriction of the median nerve) may present with different symptoms that those with pseudo carpal tunnel syndrome, which involves pain referral from another source (often the elbow).

Seldom do patients find relief from the "carpal tunnel" complaints of pain in the hand and elbow with physical therapy and surgery because the diagnosis is wrong. *(See Figure 11-2.)* The most common reason for pain in the elbow that refers pain to the hand is weakness in the annular ligament, not carpal tunnel syndrome. Several sessions of Prolotherapy will easily strengthen the annular ligament and relieve chronic elbow pain.

In addition to Prolotherapy to the elbow, a technique called Nerve Release Injection Therapy (NRIT) can be used for an instant release of an entrapped nerve in cases of carpal tunnel syndrome.

NRIT uses a 5% dextrose solution (or other solution) which is injected under ultrasound around a nerve to free it up from the underlying tissue. *(See Figure 11-3.)* In our office, it is often done along with other types of

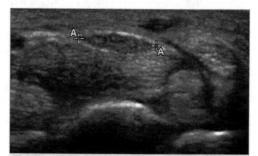

Figure 11-3: Measurement of carpal tunnel dimensions with ultrasound. Ultrasound can be used to document swollen nerves that are being compressed.

Prolotherapy to help stabilize the surrounding joint and alleviate nerve pain. The awesome part for the patient is the significant reduction in symptoms immediately after the treatment.

ULNAR COLLATERAL LIGAMENT WEAKNESS

Another common cause of chronic elbow pain is an ulnar collateral ligament sprain. *(See Figure 11-4.)* This ligament supports the inside of the elbow. It is responsible for holding the ulnar bone to the distal end of the humerus. This enables the arm to flex, pivoting at the elbow. A patient's complaint of pain on the inside of the elbow will cause a physician to examine the medial epicondyle. For example, the diagnosis of golfer's elbow is often made without examining the ulnar collateral ligament.

The ulnar collateral ligament is approximately three-quarters of an inch distal to the medial epicondyle. The ulnar collateral ligament refers pain to the little finger and ring finger. This same pain and numbness distribution is seen with aggravating the ulnar nerve. The ulnar nerve lies behind the elbow and is the reason why hitting your funny bone causes pain. Because most physicians are not familiar with the referral pattern of ligaments, patients with elbow pain and/or numbness into the little finger and ring finger are diagnosed with an ulnar nerve problem, cubital tunnel syndrome. A more common reason is ligament laxity in the sixth and seventh cervical vertebrae or in the ulnar collateral ligament—not a pinched ulnar nerve.

As stated, a patient given the opinion that surgery on the ulnar nerve is needed for a pain complaint should obtain a second opinion from a doctor who is competent in the treatment of Prolotherapy. Surgery should be performed only after all conservative options, including Prolotherapy, have been attempted. Prolotherapy to the ulnar collateral ligament is the most successful way to eliminate medial elbow pain.

If medial epicondylitis (golfer's elbow) or lateral epicondylitis (tennis elbow) is causing elbow pain, the muscles that attach to these areas are attempting to repair themselves, causing inflammation. The treatment should not be to "anti-inflame," as is the case with cortisone or with anti-

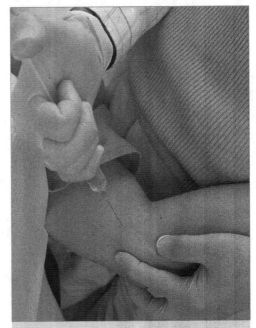

Figure 11-4: Prolotherapy treatment for ulnar collateral ligament weakness.

inflammatories like ibuprofen. The correct treatment is to strengthen the muscle attachments that are inflamed due to the body's attempt to strengthen the area. The muscles that extend the wrist attach at the lateral epicondyle and the muscles that flex the wrist attach at the medial epicondyle. Prolotherapy to strengthen these muscle attachments is very effective in eliminating chronic elbow pain.

UNTREATED TENDONITIS BECOMES TENDINOSIS

Anyone with a nagging elbow injury has probably heard the term "tendonitis," especially in sports circles. What is casually referred to as "tendonitis" is more often chronic "tendinosis," as the condition continues over a period of time. Tendonitis can happen as an acute flare up of pain and inflammation after sports or overuse. The muscles in the area recover quickly because they have a great blood supply. However, tendons, which attach muscle to bone, have a poor blood supply. If the inflamed tendon does not heal and the person continues to exercise or stress the joint, the tendon begins to degenerate and the condition is known as tendinosis. Both painful conditions are indicative of a weakened tendon that needs repair or strengthening in order to continue handling the stress put upon it. The treatment of choice for repairing tendon tissue is Prolotherapy. Most cases of tendinosis and tendonitis are coupled with joint instability from ligament injury as well. **(See Figure 11-5.)** Cellular Prolotherapy, as discussed more in **Chapter 3**, plays a big role in treating degenerative conditions like tendinosis because they tend to lack enough cells to repair on their own. Prolotherapy with Platelet Rich Plasma (PRP) is a favorite of Caring Medical for speeding up the tendon repair process, especially for sports injuries of the elbow!

ELBOW PAIN STUDY RESULTS WITH PROLOTHERAPY

In the October 2009 issue of *Practical Pain Management* we presented a study on 36 patients with unresolved elbow pain who were treated with dextrose Prolotherapy at a quarterly clinic, which included a sub-group of 15 patients who were told by another practitioner that there was no other option for their pain.[4] The patients' average age was 53 years-old. They reported an average of four years and one month of pain and saw 2.4 MDs before receiving Prolotherapy.

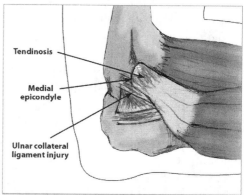

Figure 11-5: Medial view of elbow illustrating tendinosis. A chronically degenerated tendon (tendinosis) occurs when the underlying joint is unstable. In this example, the origin of wrist flexors is degenerated (tendinosis) from medial elbow instability caused by ulnar collateral ligament injury. Prolotherapy to the tendonotic area will be helpful, but to resolve the problem both the tendinosis and the underlying ligament injury have to be treated.

Patients received an average of 4.3 Prolotherapy treatments per elbow. The average time of follow-up after their last Prolotherapy session was 31 months. Patients were asked to rate their pain and stiffness levels on a scale of 1 to 10, with 1 being no pain/stiffness and 10 being severe crippling pain/stiffness. The 36 patients had an average starting pain level of 5.1 and stiffness of 3.9. Their ending pain and stiffness levels were 1.6 and 1.4 respectively. Sixty-one percent had a starting pain level of 6 or greater, while only 11% had a starting pain level of three or less whereas, after Prolotherapy, only 5% had a pain level of 6 or greater and 94% had a pain level of three or less. One hundred percent of patients stated that the pain and stiffness in their elbows was better after Prolotherapy. Over 78% said the improvements in their pain and stiffness since their last Prolotherapy session have continued 100%. *(See Figure 11-6.)*

Demographics	All Elbow Patients	No Other Treatment Options
Total number of patients	36	15
Average months of pain	49	59
Average pain level before Prolotherapy	5.1	6.9
Average pain level after Prolotherapy	1.6	2.2
Paired t ratio	14.43	8.367
P value	$P < .000000$	$p < .000001$
Average stiffness level before Prolotherapy	3.9	4.7
Average stiffness level after Prolotherapy	1.4	1.9
Paired t ratio	6.285	14.992
P value	$p < .000000$	$p < .000001$
Exercise ability > 30 minutes of exercise before Prolotherapy	33%	33%
Exercise ability > 30 minutes of exercise after Prolotherapy	86%	80%
Paired t ratio	-8.371	-6.205
P value	$p < .000000$	$p < .000023$
Greater than 50% pain relief	94%	93%

Figure 11-6: Summary of results of Hackett-Hemwall dextrose Prolotherapy elbow study.

WRIST PAIN

Weakened ligaments commonly cause chronic wrist pain. The weakened ligaments allow one of the eight wrist bones to become unstable and shift positions, leading to wrist instability. *(See Figure 11-7.)* The wrist is actually eight oddly shaped bones in a sea of ligaments.[5] The most common wrist bones that become unstable because of loose ligaments are the capitate, scaphoid, and lunate.[6,7] Thus, the most common ligaments treated with Prolotherapy for chronic wrist pain are the dorsal capitate-trapezoid, hamate-capitate, scaphoid-triquetral, and scapholunate ligaments. Again, the diagnosis is easily made by direct palpation of these ligaments, as the wrist bones are very superficial to the skin. The weakened ligament can be palpated and a positive "jump sign" elicited. Several Prolotherapy sessions in this area resolves the problem.

Our chronic wrist pain study looked at 31 patients who received an average of 3.6 dextrose Prolotherapy treatments.[8] The average time of follow-up after their last Prolotherapy session was 22 months. Patients were asked to rate their pain and stiffness levels on a scale of 1 to 10 with 1 being no pain/stiffness and 10 being severe crippling pain/stiffness. Starting pain level averaged 5.5 and stiffness 3.7. Ending pain and stiffness levels were both 1.4 after Prolotherapy. Seventy-four percent exhibited a starting pain level of 5 or greater, while only 13% had a starting pain level of 2 or less; whereas after

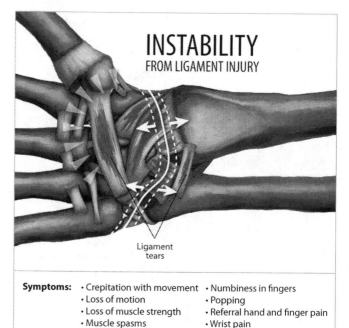

INSTABILITY
FROM LIGAMENT INJURY

Ligament tears

Symptoms:
- Crepitation with movement
- Loss of motion
- Loss of muscle strength
- Muscle spasms
- Numbiness in fingers
- Popping
- Referral hand and finger pain
- Wrist pain

Figure 11-7: Wrist instability. Arrows signify excessive joint motion.

Prolotherapy zero patients reported a pain level of 5 or greater, while 90% had achieved a pain level of two or less. *(See Figure 11-8.)*

Ninety percent of patients stated Prolotherapy relieved them of at least 50% of their pain. Sixty-one percent received greater than 75% pain relief. Ninety-seven percent of patients achieved at least 25% pain relief with Prolotherapy. Eighteen patients (58%) reported wrists with incomplete range of motion before Prolotherapy. After Prolotherapy, only six (19%) patients reported incomplete range of motion in their wrists. *(See Figure 11-9.)*

SUB-GROUPS OF WRIST STUDY POPULATION

Prior to Prolotherapy, 14 (45%) patients were told no other treatment options were available

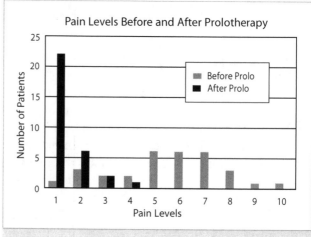

Figure 11-8: Pain levels before and after receiving Hackett-Hemwall dextrose Prolotherapy in 31 patients with unresolved wrist pain.

for their wrist pain. As a group, they suffered with pain an average of 66 months. Analysis of these patients revealed a starting average pain level of 6.2 and a post-Prolotherapy pain level of 1.5. Wrist stiffness averaged 4.0 prior to Prolotherapy treatments and improved to 1.5 after completing the treatments. Eleven out of fourteen (78%) achieved 50% or greater pain relief. Prior to Prolotherapy only 36% of the patients could

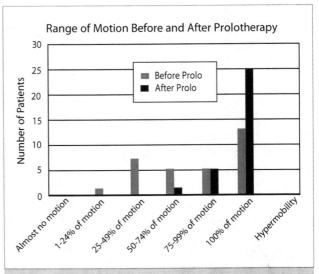

Figure 11-9: Range of motion levels before and after receiving Hackett-Hemwall dextrose Prolotherapy in 31 patients with unresolved wrist pain.

exercise longer than 30 minutes, but this increased to 78% after Prolotherapy.

Five patients (16%) were told that surgery was the only option available to eliminate their wrist pain. Their average pain duration prior to Prolotherapy was 39 months. Their starting average pain level was 4.8 before Prolotherapy, which declined to 1.2 after Prolotherapy. Reported wrist stiffness was 1.8 prior to Prolotherapy and 1.0 after. All five patients (100%) exhibited 50% or greater pain relief. One out of five of the patients could exercise longer than 30 minutes prior to Prolotherapy, but this number increased to four out of five after Prolotherapy. **(See Figure 11-10.)**

TRIANGULAR FIBROCARTILAGE COMPLEX (TFCC)

A common injury from falling on an outstretched hand, or in athletes who put a lot of pressure on their wrists, such as gymnasts, is a tear of the triangular fibrocartilage complex. This small piece of cartilage and ligaments on the ulnar side of the wrist (same side as the little finger) acts as a cushion for the joint. Ligament injury in the front, back, and ulnar side of the wrist causes wrist instability. This is the most common cause of pain and cartilage degeneration in this area. Most patients with wrist instability and damage to the TFCC have a characteristic clicking sound in the wrist. Many have also been diagnosed via x-ray or MRI.

The treatment of TFCC injuries includes splinting or casting, ice, rest, and anti-inflammatory medications. In some cases, surgery to remove the cartilage may be recommended. As we have discussed, these do nothing to actually promote healing, in fact, they have a higher potential of doing further damage to the joint, let alone an athletic career. Prolotherapy works nicely in cases of TFCC tears, and is an excellent alternative to surgically removing the cartilage. In the case of athletes, poor technique can lead to more falls and worse injuries and should be addressed as part of a comprehensive rehabilitation program.

HAND PAIN

When it comes to hand pain, the most common problem involves the thumb because of its unique role in the hand's function. Whenever a doorknob is turned, a screwdriver is used, or something is held, the thumb is part of the action. When typing, what part of the hand must continually hit the

Demographics	All Wrist Patients	No Other Treatment Options	Surgery Only Option Given
Total number of patients	31	14	5
Average months of pain	52	66	39
Average pain level before Prolotherapy	5.5	6.2	4.8
Average pain level after Prolotherapy	1.4	1.5	1.2
Paired t ratio	13.463	9.099	4.811
P value	0.000000	0.000001	0.008579
Average stiffness level before Prolotherapy	3.7	4.0	1.8
Average stiffness level after Prolotherapy	1.4	1.5	1
Paired t ratio	5.014	3.381	1
P value	0.000022	0.004919	0.373901
Exercise ability > 30 minutes before Prolo.	36%	36%	20%
Exercise ability > 30 minutes after Prolo.	87%	78%	80%
Paired t ratio	-8.478	-5.259	-2.138
P value	0.000000	0.000154	0.099311
Greater than 50% pain relief	90%	78%	100%

Figure 11-10: Summary of results for retrospective study of patients with wrist pain treated with dextrose Prolotherapy.

space bar? The thumb. Because thumbs have to work so much harder than fingers, it is usually the first to elicit pain. The thumb ligament that joins the wrist to the base of the thumb is called the radial collateral ligament, the same name as the ligament inside the elbow. The thumb ligament that joins the base of the thumb (the first metacarpal) to the succeeding joint (proximal phalanx) is the collateral ligament. *(See Figure 11-11.)*

These two joints of the thumb, called the carpometacarpal (CMC) and metacarpophalangeal (MCP), are usually the first areas where pain is experienced. If the ligaments in these joints are not strengthened, arthritis will eventually occur. Arthritis starts the day a joint becomes loose. The looser the joint, the greater the chance it has of becoming arthritic. Arthritis in the thumb, as well as other phalangeal joints in the hand, are a major cause of disability, especially among the elderly.[9,10] The progression of osteoarthritis stops the day the ligaments become strong and are able to stabilize the joint.

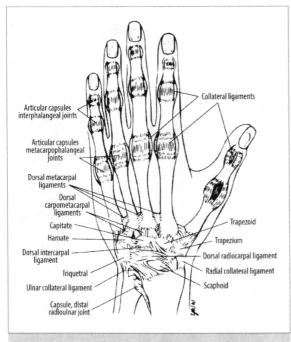

Articular capsules interphalangeal joints
Articular capsules metacarpophalangeal joints
Dorsal metacarpal ligaments
Dorsal carpometacarpal ligaments
Capitate
Hamate
Dorsal intercarpal ligament
Triquetral
Ulnar collateral ligament
Capsule, distal radioulnar joint
Collateral ligaments
Trapezoid
Trapezium
Dorsal radiocarpal ligament
Radial collateral ligament
Scaphoid

Figure 11-11: Ligaments of the hand, thumb, and fingers. Note that all the joints of the hand, thumb, and fingers are primarily supported by ligaments.

Our retrospective, observational study showed that Prolotherapy helps decrease pain and stiffness in patients with previously unresolved hand/finger pain. Forty patients, who had been in pain an average of 55 months (4.6 years), were treated quarterly with Hackett-Hemwall dextrose Prolotherapy.[11] Patients were contacted an average of 18 months following their last Prolotherapy session and asked questions regarding their levels of pain and stiffness before and after their last Prolotherapy treatment. In these 40 patients, 98% had improvements in their pain. Eighty-two percent had 50% or more pain relief. Dextrose Prolotherapy caused a statistically significant decline in patients' pain and stiffness.

Prolotherapy helped all but one patient reduce the amount of pain medication needed. All 40 patients have recommended Prolotherapy to someone. *(See Figure 11-12.)*

Prolotherapy is the treatment of choice for patients suffering from stiff, sore hands or thumbs. Once the ligaments are strengthened, the pain and stiffness in the thumbs and fingers subside. Again, four Prolotherapy treatment sessions are usually all that is needed.

Prolotherapy Hand Study Results	
Total number of patients	40
Average months of pain	55
Average pain level before Prolotherapy	5.9
Average pain level after Prolotherapy	2.6
Paired t ratio	15.534
P value	p < .000001
Average stiffness level before Prolotherapy	5.6
Average stiffness level after Prolotherapy	2.7
Paired t ratio	13.477
P value	p < .000001
Greater than 50% pain relief	82%

Figure 11-12: Summary of results of Hackett-Hemwall dextrose Prolotherapy hand study.

THUMB PAIN

The thumb, unlike the other fingers, is opposable. This allows us to grasp objects with our hands because we are able to oppose or turn back against the other four fingers; thus we develop fine motor skills and are able to use a wide variety of hand tools. Because of the thumb's heavy use, the base of the thumb often receives the brunt of the force in the hand and is frequently the first hand joint to break down. Most thumb, and for that matter, hand and finger pains, begin with basal thumb osteoarthritis. Traditional medicine offers these patients the options of anti-inflammatory medications, corticosteroid shots, splinting of the joint, joint replacement and/or tendon repair surgery. A much better option is Prolotherapy.

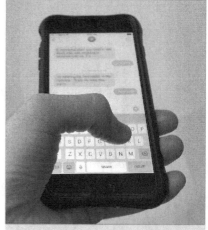

Figure 11-13: Smart Phone Syndrome. The excessive use of smart phones is causing ligament injury and thumb joint instability, also known as text thumb. Fortunately, Prolotherapy is available to help!

We have treated many thumbs with Prolotherapy throughout our years in practice and we are seeing a rise in thumb pain. Why, you ask? *Smart phone syndrome.* **(See Figure 11-13.)** Smart phones are causing increasing levels of thumb and hand pain, and for that matter, neck and back pain as well. People who frequently use their smart phones better wise up and realize the damage they are causing to the carpometacarpal (CMC) joint. The end result is articular cartilage breakdown in the joint which is diagnosed as either basal thumb arthritis or trapeziometacarpal arthritis. Computer work is also putting additional strains on the joint and thumb pain incidence is increasing and becoming a major problem for many people. Fortunately there is a major solution: Prolotherapy!

In our published thumb pain study, Prolotherapy produced significant improvements in pain, range of motion and ability to perform activities such as sports.[12] Prolotherapy is performed around the whole joint. **(See Figure 11-14.)**

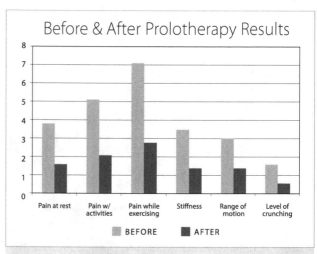

Before & After Prolotherapy Results

BEFORE · AFTER

Pain at rest · Pain w/ activities · Pain while exercising · Stiffness · Range of motion · Level of crunching

Figure 11-14: Visual Analog Scale (VAS) results for 13 patients with CMC joint osteoarthritis in 17 of their thumbs treated with Prolotherapy.

Prolotherapy works great for base of thumb sprains, injuries and osteoarthritis because it gets at the root cause of chronic thumb pain: joint instability. *(See Figure 11-15.)* Research is produced every year confirming that the osteoarthritic process begins with ligament pathology, causing increased pressure on the articular cartilage because of abnormal and excessive motion.[13,14] This is true for the thumb basal joint as well.[15] Most people wait too long before seeking appropriate care. It is best not to wait to receive Prolotherapy until the hand surgeon says, "We need to replace the joint." Remember pain in the base of the thumb means tissues are being damaged. They need repair, strengthening, and healing. Prolotherapy inside the joint and around the stabilizing ligaments causes these structures to heal. Most patients thumb pain resolves to a 0 or 1 level of pain. Sometimes, due to lifestyle factors such as smart phone syndrome, it is impossible to achieve a 0 level of pain. Would Dr. Hauser's thumb pain resolve to 0 if he continued to perform 1000 to 2000 injections every day while receiving Prolotherapy? What about those people who perform tens of thousands of key strokes or text 100s of times per day? You get the point!

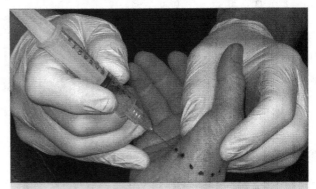

Figure 11-15: Prolotherapy for basal joint arthritis of the thumb.

SUMMARY

Chronic pain in the arms, elbows, wrists, and hands is primarily due to the type of work people perform in a modern high-tech society. Pain is often aggravated by specific sports and workouts when the joint is not strong enough to handle the force. Additionally, smart phone syndrome and thumb pain have become increasingly common pain complaints. The repetitive motions of the upper extremities eventually wear out the ligamentous support of the elbows, wrists, and thumbs. The end result is loose joints that cause pain and stiffness.

Sudden injuries, such as to the triangular fibrocartilage complex (TFCC), can also result in joint instability. Acute injuries are at high risk of becoming chronic conditions if traditional treatments like cortisone is applied when regenerative options would be a better choice. Prolotherapy injections start the healing process to cause the growth of ligaments that stabilize these joints. Once the ligaments return to normal strength, the chronic pain is eliminated, as well as the degenerative cascade that leads to arthritis. In more severe cases of tendon, ligament, and cartilage degeneration, Platelet Rich Plasma Prolotherapy is an excellent option, as are other forms of Cellular Prolotherapy. When nerve entrapment is evident as is the case of carpal tunnel syndrome, Nerve Release Injection Therapy is often the treatment of choice. Patients who want effective, non-surgical treatment options for chronic elbow, wrist, and hand pain are choosing to Prolo their pain away! ■

CHAPTER

12

PROLO YOUR CHEST AND RIB PAIN AWAY!

The rib cage and chest area may not be the most common area to have pain, but it can present tricky symptoms that can mislead both patients and practitioners who are not familiar with pain referral patterns. Just like with other joints of the body, instability in one area can shoot pain to another, and as one joint becomes loose, it begins to

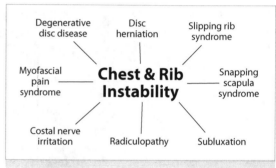

Chronic chest and rib conditions caused by chest or rib instability.

affect the function of adjacent joints. It is common for patients to experience chronic subluxations in these areas that become more extreme with time. Since these joints are almost always in motion, due to breathing and assisting in upper extremity movement and posture, the person is almost constantly aware of the pain.

SLIPPING RIB SYNDROME

Dawn, a 35 year-old, was rushed to the hospital for the fourth time in less than a year complaining of severe chest pain, fearing a heart attack. After EKGs, blood tests, x-rays, and a stay in the intensive care unit, the cause of her pain was still unknown. Everyone began to wonder if she was a little crazy.

As Dr. Hauser examined her, Dawn initially explained that she was not currently having severe chest pain but did feel a dull ache in her chest. She needed one more diagnostic test, the trusty MRI—My Reproducibility Instrument. In a second, the diagnosis was made. Dr. Hauser pressed on her left fourth thoracic rib attachment onto the sternum and Dawn's severe crushing chest pain immediately returned. Had she ever been examined in this fashion? She said she had not. Dawn's pain was caused by slipping rib syndrome.

An extremely important point illustrated by Dawn's case is that even if an x-ray, blood sample, or EKG do not reveal a cause, they do not eliminate the presence of a physical condition as the source of chest pain. It is much more likely that the chronic chest pain is due to weakened soft tissue, such as a ligament or tendon. If heart and lung tests prove normal, yet the patient claims to still be experiencing pain, the patient is often given a psychiatric diagnosis.

Depression, anxiety, and being a little crazy are not the etiological bases for most chronic pain. They can be associated factors involved in the problem, but they are normally not the cause. If depressed people complain of shoulder pain, most likely they have shoulder pain. Chronic pain should be assumed to be originating from a weakened soft tissue, such as a ligament or tendon. A weak tendon, like the rotator cuff, or ligament, such as the coracoacromial ligament, may be the cause.

Slipping rib syndrome, also known as Tietze's syndrome, was first described in 1921 by Alexander Tietze, MD, as chest pain over the sternoclavicular and costochondral junctions.[1] Other names include xiphoidalgia, costochondritis, or anterior chest-wall syndrome. But the most descriptive and accurate name for the actual etiological basis of the condition is slipping rib syndrome.[2] It is interesting to note that just one year after Dr. Tietze's description, slipping rib syndrome was described in medical literature.[3]

In Dawn's case, a rib was slipping out of place because the ligaments that hold the ribs to the sternum, the sternocostal ligaments, were weak. Without muscles to hold the ribs in place, loose ligaments allow slipping of the rib which causes further stretching of the ligament, manifesting itself by producing severe pain. The loose ribs can also pinch intercostal nerves, sending excruciating pains around the chest into the back. Sternocostal and costochondral ligaments refer pain from the front of the chest to the mid back. Likewise, costovertebral ligament sprains refer pain from the back of the rib segment to the sternum where the rib attaches. **(See Figures 12-1.)**

Traditional medicine believes the condition is caused by inflammation in the costochondral junction, causing costochondritis. The treatment of choice in traditional medical circles is, you guessed it, an NSAID, a nonsteroidal anti-inflammatory drug. Chronic pain, no matter what the cause, is not due to an NSAID deficiency. Slipping rib syndrome is caused by weakness of

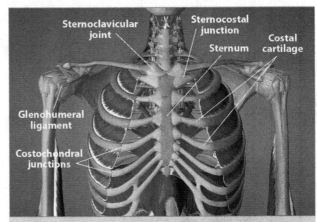

Figure 12-1: Anterior view of chest wall and shoulder joints. Injury to either the costochondral or sternocostal junctions will give rise to slipping rib syndrome.

the sternocostal, costochondral, or costovertebral ligaments. Prolotherapy will strengthen these ligament junctions in all the areas where the ribs are hypermobile.

Slipping rib syndrome may be caused by hypermobility of the anterior end of the costal cartilage, located at the rib-cartilage interface, called the costochondral junction. Most often, the tenth rib is the source because, unlike ribs one through seven which attach to the sternum, the eighth, ninth, and tenth ribs are attached anteriorly to each other by loose, fibrous tissue.[4] This provides increased mobility, but a greater susceptibility to trauma. Slipping rib cartilage may cause no pain or only intermittent pain.[5]

Slipping rib syndrome is also more likely to occur in the lower ribs because of the poor blood supply to the cartilaginous tissue and ligaments. Injury to the cartilage tissue in the lower ribs or the sternocostal ligaments in the upper ribs seldom completely heals naturally. The sternocostal, rib-sternum, and costochondral joints undergo stress when the rib cage expands or contracts abnormally or when excessive pressure is applied on the ribs themselves.

In order for the rib cage to expand and contract with each breath, the costochondral and the sternocostal junctions are naturally loose. Humans breathe 12 times per minute, 720 times per hour, 19,280 times per day, which stresses these ligamentous-rib junctions. Additional stressors include any condition that makes breathing more difficult. A simple coughing attack due to a cold may cause the development of slipping rib syndrome. Conditions such as bronchitis, emphysema, allergies, and asthma cause additional stress to the sternocostal and costochondral junctions. Another cause of slipping rib syndrome is the result of surgery to the lungs, chest, heart, or breast, with resection of the lymph nodes, which puts a tremendous stress on the rib attachments because the surgeon must separate the ribs to remove the injured tissue. Unresolved chest or upper back pain following a thoracotomy, chest operation, or CPR is most likely due to ligament laxity in the rib-sternum or the rib-vertebral junction.

The ribs are attached in the front as well as in the back of the body. A loose rib in the front is likely also loose in the back. The rib-vertebral junction is known as the costovertebral junction, and is secured by the costotransverse ligaments. Unexplained upper back pain, between the shoulder blades and costovertebral, (rib-vertebrae pain) is likely due to joint laxity and/or weakness in the costotransverse ligaments.

Chronic chest pain, especially in young people, is often due to weakness in the sternocostal and costochondral junctions. Chronic mid-upper back pain is due to weakness at the costovertebral junction. Both conditions may lead to slipping rib syndrome, where the rib intermittently slips out of place, causing a stretching of the ligamentous support of the rib in the front and back. The result is periodic episodes of severe pain and underlying chronic chest and/or upper back pain. Prolotherapy, by strengthening these areas, provides definitive results in the relief of the chronic chest pain or chronic upper-back pain from slipping rib syndrome.

THORACIC OUTLET SYNDROME

"I have thoracic outlet syndrome." "No you don't." "Yes, I do!" "No, you don't!" Such is the typical conversations we have with patients when they come in with this diagnosis.

The thoracic outlet consists of the space between the inferior border of the clavicle and the upper border of the first rib. *(See Figure 12-2.)* The subclavian artery, subclavian vein, and brachial plexus nerves (the nerves to the arm) exit the neck region and go into the arm via this space. In thoracic outlet syndrome (TOS), the space is, presumably, narrowed, causing a compression of these structures. The symptoms of TOS include: pain in the neck, shoulder, and arm; coldness in the hand; and numbness in the arm and hand. However, in severe cases of compression of the subclavian vessels, Raynaud's phenomenon, claudication, thrombosis, and edema can occur in the involved extremity.[6] **TOS is a legitimate condition and does occur but its prevalence is extremely rare! Most people who come to Caring Medical with the diagnosis of TOS leave with other diagnoses such as glenohumeral ligament sprain, rotator cuff tendinopathy, cervical ligament sprain, or slipping rib syndrome.** All of the pain and numbness symptoms of TOS can occur from these later four conditions, all of which respond beautifully to Prolotherapy.

The reason it makes sense that Prolotherapy would be a cure for the symptoms of so-called "TOS" is the fact that the condition almost exclusively occurs in women with long necks and low-set droopy shoulders.[7] Activities that involve abduction of the shoulders, such as combing the hair, painting walls, and hanging pictures, cause worsening of the symptoms. Passively abducting the arm (having someone do it for the person) relieves the symptoms. In other words, when the shoulder is actively raised over the head (the person does it themselves) the symptoms of pain and/or numbness down the arms occur, however, when the exact same movement is done passively (by another person) the symptoms do not occur. This type of symptomatology is a perfect description of ligament and tendon weakness (laxity). The injured ligament and tendon give localized and referral pain when doing strenuous movements, but when someone else takes the brunt of the force, no such symptoms occur.

The people with so-called TOS almost unanimously have normal reflexes and nerve conduction studies.

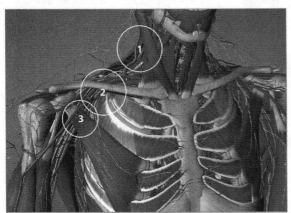

Figure 12-2: Thoracic outlet syndrome (TOS) locations.
TOS can occur at the level of the scalene muscles (1), ribs (2), or at the shoulder joint (3).

This gives further indication that a nerve is not getting pinched. Furthermore, surgically slicing structures to give the nerve more room will not eliminate the symptoms the person is having and could, quite possibly, cause more problems. Instead, Prolotherapy to the neck ligaments, shoulder ligaments and tendons, or to a rib that is slipping is all that is needed to cure the symptoms of so-called TOS.

SNAPPING SCAPULA SYNDROME

Snapping syndromes in the body, including the scapula, are due to underlying joint instability. The scapula lies over the ribs and helps make up the shoulder joint. *(See Figure 12-3.)* In snapping scapula syndrome, the snapping occurs as the muscles that move the shoulder joint contract against an unstable base and allow the scapula to rub against the ribs. The problem is not due to muscle weakness, rather, instability. This joint instability can occur where the ribs that attach to the thoracic spine, causing a rib to stick out too far. Or the instability can occur in the shoulder joint, such as from a labral tear or overstretched glenohumeral ligaments. For those with snapping scapula syndrome, the great news is that once the instability is identified, Prolotherapy is an excellent curative treatment for this condition.

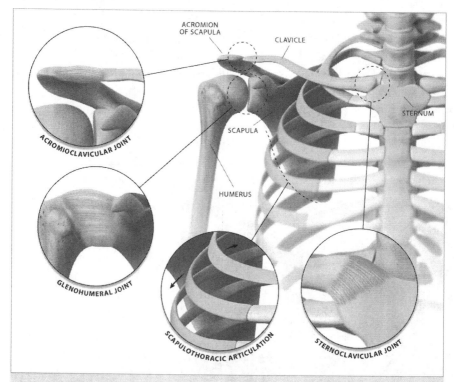

Figure 12-3: The bony structures of the shoulder and their four articulations. The circular insets show three synovial joints—sternoclavicular, acromioclavicular, and glenohumeral—and one bone-muscle-bone articulation—the scapulothoracic joint.

Adapted from: De Palma AF. Biomechanics of the shoulder. *In Surgery of the Shoulder*, 3rd edition. Philadelphia: JB Lippincott Co. 1983;65-85.

STERNOCLAVICULAR JOINT SUBLUXATION

The sternoclavicular joint (SCJ) attaches the clavicle, or collarbone, to the sternum. *(See Figure 12-4.)* It is an underappreciated joint that allows us more upper extremity movement. We frequently see weightlifters, wrestlers, or other athletes who have chronic subluxation and weakness of this joint. They complain of a constant "pop, pop, pop" sound every time they do upper body work. In others, they can physically see and feel the joint subluxing. Again, we see how joint instability, even in this smaller joint, causes a good deal of pain and weakness during and after workouts. Often when an athlete hears the word "weakness" he or she thinks they just need to work out harder. Let us assure you that is not the case with SCJ injuries. As we have been discussing throughout this book, muscles are not typically the problem. If you have been doing physical therapy, exercising the surrounding muscles, massage, and the popping is still happening, you have to consider that the joint instability is not being addressed. While some athletes do have to take more care to use good form during their workouts, most SCJ problems are best dealt with using Prolotherapy. The ligament attachments of the SCJ typically need a few Prolotherapy treatments, and once the SCJ is more stable, an athlete gets back to the gym without restriction. Ultimately, this is what our patients are after.

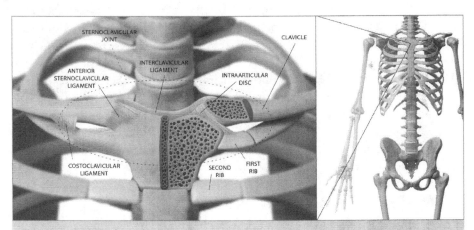

Figure 12-4: Sternoclavicular joint.
Adapted from Oatis CA. *Kinesiology: The Mechanics and Pathomechanics of Human Movement.* 2008. Baltimore, MD. Lippincott Williams & Wilkins, 128.

SUMMARY

Just like any other joint in the body, patients can have instability of joints through the chest, ribs, and thoracic area. These instabilities can cause chest pain, popping, loss of breath, catching sensations, weakness, and other painful subluxation symptoms. Prolotherapy is very effective at eliminating the chronic pain caused in conditions including slipping rib syndrome and thoracic outlet syndrome, as well as chronic subluxations of the sternoclavicular joint and the ribs. ■

CHAPTER

13

PROLO YOUR ARTHRITIS PAIN AWAY!

It is important to first note what arthritis is not. It is not a consequence of old age. There is always a reason for the pain. The most common reason for chronic pain—regardless of age—is joint instability due to ligament laxity. This includes the formation of osteoarthritis (OA). OA can affect any joint in the body, but more commonly occurs in the weight-bearing joints of the hips, knees, and spine. OA may also affect the fingers, thumb, neck, toes, and other joints as well. Osteoarthritis pain typically progresses through three stages, although not all people go through each distinct stage.[1] Joint pain is generally referred to as mechanical (Stage 1), meaning it occurs with and is exacerbated by physical exertion, especially weight-bearing activity, and is relieved by rest. As it progresses, pain may become more persistent and begins to manifest itself at rest (Stage 2), usually doing so with an insidious onset. This unremitting pain is often described as deep, aching, and not well localized, and over time, leads to joint stiffness, loss of function, and an inability to perform daily activities (Stage 3). However, people with the same degree of structural damage can experience widely different levels of pain. Prolotherapy injections help strengthen weakened ligaments and eliminate chronic pain, and halt the progression of osteoarthritis.[2]

LIGAMENT LAXITY CAUSES OSTEOARTHRITIS

Osteoarthritis is one of the most common consequences of ligament damage, and subsequent laxity. Traditionally, the pathophysiology of OA was thought to be due to aging and wear and tear on a joint, but more recent studies have shown that ligament injury is one of the initial causes for the development of OA.[3-8] *(See Figure 13-1.)* Joints are composed of two bones covered with articular cartilage, allowing the joint to glide, and ligaments holding the two bones together. Healthy articular cartilage and ligaments enable the two bones to glide evenly over one another when the bones move.

If the ligaments become weak or damaged, the bones will glide over one another in an uneven manner. One area of the bone will bear additional weight on the articular cartilage when the joint is stressed. This uneven distribution of joint

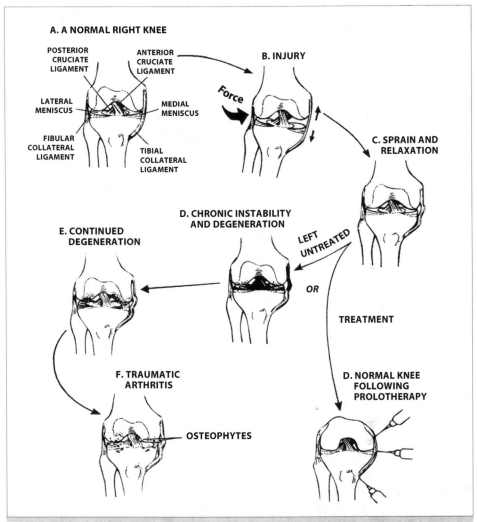

Figure 13-1: How soft tissue injury leads to degenerative arthritis. Following trauma, ligaments become sprained. When healing does not occur, the ligaments become relaxed, resulting in chronic instability and degeneration. When left untreated, post-traumatic "arthritis," or degeneration, follows. This degenerative process can be prevented with appropriate intervention through Prolotherapy.

stress creates an even greater strain on the weakened ligament in order to stabilize this joint. Eventually all of the ligaments of the joint become lax. The more lax the ligaments become, the more unstable the joint. This increases the abnormal weight distribution inside the joint. This continued stress within the joint causes articular cartilage breakdown, which causes the bones to glide roughly over each other producing a crunching noise when the joint is moved. Grinding or crunching is a warning sign that a cortisone shot awaits you at your conventional doctor's office, unless something is done.

At some point in this process, the body realizes the ligaments can no longer stabilize the joint. Muscles and their respective tendons will then tense in an attempt to stabilize the area on the weakened side of the joint, adding to the person's discomfort. As the muscles and their tendons weaken, which will occur over time, they become more painful and unable to stabilize the joint. They will often "knot," producing painful trigger points. When the muscles and ligaments can no longer stabilize the joint, the bony surfaces rub against each other. In a last attempt to stabilize the joint, additional bone begins accumulating where the bones collide. **This bony overgrowth is called osteoarthritis.** Eventually, if the process is not stopped at some point, a stiff joint will form resulting in the eventual development of osteoarthritis.

At any time during this process, the body can quickly stabilize the joint by swelling. Swelling of a joint indicates the presence of some foreign substance inside the joint or that the joint is loose. Microorganisms, such as bacteria, blood, pieces of cartilage, and various bodily breakdown products, can accumulate in the joints and cause swelling. If a tissue is injured inside and around the joint, typically the joint swells as a protective measure so the body can repair the tissue, which may eventually lead to the development of arthritis. *(See Figure 13-2.)*

TREATMENT OF OSTEOARTHRITIS

Acute soft tissue injury, if treated improperly, may begin the cascade resulting in arthritis. As discussed in **Chapter 2**, icing a joint and taking nonsteroidal anti-inflammatory medicines after an acute soft tissue injury, in an attempt to decrease the swelling, inhibits the inflammatory mechanisms that heal the body. Treatments such as Rest, Ice, Compression, and

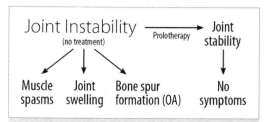

Figure 13-2: Long-term manifestations of joint stability. When left untreated, the body tries to stabilize a joint by causing chronic muscle spasms, joint swelling and eventually bone spur formation and degenerative arthritis. Prolotherapy, by tightening and strengthening the ligaments, causes the joint to stabilize with the resultant resolution of symptoms.

Elevation (RICE) almost guarantee that the joint and the injured tissue will not heal. It is important not to interfere with the body's normal healing mechanism—inflammation—when a soft tissue structure such as a ligament or tendon is injured. Treatment that decreases inflammation after an initial injury will slow and prevent healing, resulting in permanently weak tissue, which may eventually lead to the development of arthritis. Treatments that complement the inflammatory process will enhance the healing process.

A better course of action after a soft tissue injury involving a simple sprain of a ligament or strain of a tendon is Movement, Exercise, Analgesics (painkillers), and Treatment (MEAT). It is preferable to use natural botanicals such as bromelain or cayenne pepper as analgesics. In the case of severe pain, a narcotic, such as codeine, works wonderfully to decrease the pain without decreasing the inflammation necessary to heal the tissue, if used on a short-term basis. When the body experiences pain, it naturally forms its own narcotic, called endorphins. Completely blocking the pain with narcotics is dangerous because the brain does not recognize that a part of the body is injured. For example, dancing the night away on an injured ankle that feels no pain may cause further damage. Natural botanicals, which do not block all of the pain, are preferred.

Treatment, such as ice, that decreases blood flow to the injured area causes a decrease in the flow of immune cells, which hinders the healing process. Treatment that increases blood flow causes an increase in the flow of immune cells to the injured tissue, which triggers the repair process. Movement, exercise, heat, massage, ultrasound, acupuncture, and physical therapy all improve blood flow and have a positive effect on healing.

Attempting to drastically decrease joint swelling after an acute injury is not advisable. The joint swelling is the body saying, "Hey, buddy, I'm hurt. Don't over do it!" Aggressive treatment to decrease the swelling may entice the injured individual to return to action prematurely. The best course of action is to allow the body to heal itself.

To increase the rate of healing and decrease the length of time the joint is swollen, protease enzymes are very helpful. Papain and chymopapain from papaya fruit, bromelain from pineapple, and pancreatin enzyme preparations will encourage the removal of the damaged tissue, thus reducing the swelling.[9]

An injured ligament not allowed to heal will leave the joint unstable and primed for future arthritis. *(See Figure 13-3.)* Prolotherapy blocks the cascade that leads to arthritis by repairing the ligaments that stabilize the joint. The following case study illustrates this scenario.

EXAMPLE OF KNEE OSTEOARTHRITIS

OA of the knee is one of the most common forms of OA. Pain ranges from moderate to "off the charts!" As with any joint, knee OA patients report pain inside, outside, and even behind the knee joint. Pain may worsen with walking up and down stairs and patients may even experience pain at rest. Swelling may or may not be present.

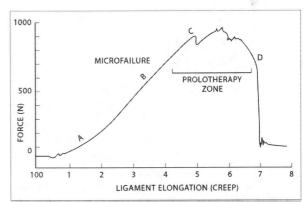

Figure 13-3: Stress-strain curve for ligaments and tendons. Ligaments stretch as force is applied. As additional force is applied to the ligaments, they can return to normal length once the force is removed. If the force is continued past point C, the ligament is permanently elongated unless Prolotherapy is administered to tighten it.

CASE STUDY:
BILATERAL KNEE OA TREATED WITH PROLOTHERAPY

In the February 2009 issue of the *Journal of Prolotherapy*, one of our athlete patients, Alek, shared his story of bilateral knee arthritis treated with Prolotherapy.

Alek has been a bodybuilder since 1962. During the nineties his knee pain became unbearable, for which he took the usual course of anti-inflammatories and had seen his fair share of orthopedists who recommended surgery. After three knee surgeries, his knees were in worse shape than before surgery, and he was suffering from unrelenting pain. Like most people in chronic pain, his sleep was constantly interrupted and depression set in. His personality changed, keeping friends and family at a distance because of his behavior and attitude. He struggled in this

---

MRI OF THE RIGHT KNEE

CLINICAL INDICATION: Knee pain and history of prior right knee surgery.

Multiplanar spin echo images were obtained without contrast material.

There is tricompartmental osteoarthritis with osteophyte formation and Grade IV chondromalacia patella and moderate (Grade II to Grade III) medial chondromalacia.

The cruciate and collateral ligaments are normal and the extensor mechanism is normal.

IMPRESSION:
1. Tricompartmental osteoarthritis with chondromalacia patella and medial chondromalacia.
2. Small joint effusion and popliteal cyst.
3. Deformity of the posterior horn and mid body of the medial meniscus. There is truncation of the posterior horn and I cannot be certain if this represents postoperative changes or in addition a new tear. There is also a displaced meniscal fragment or cartilaginous fragment in the mid knee joint as described above.

MRI OF THE LEFT KNEE

CLINICAL INDICATION: Knee pain.

Multiplanar spin echo images were obtained without contrast material.

There is a small joint effusion. There is Grade IV chondromalacia patella involving the lateral patellar facet. There is moderate medial and lateral chondromalacia. There is an 8 mm osteochondral defect in the posterior medial femoral condyle. There are degenerative changes of the medial knee joint with osteophyte formation.

There is a complex tear of the posterior horn and mid body of the medial meniscus with medial displacement of the meniscus and pseudosubluxation. The lateral meniscus is intact.

The cruciate and collateral ligaments are normal. The extensor mechanism is normal.

IMPRESSION:
1. Tear of the posterior horn of the medial meniscus and mid body of the medial meniscus.
2. Tricompartmental osteoarthritis, most marked medially on the patellofemoral joint.
3. Small joint effusion.

Figure 13-4: Alek's MRI reports.

condition for six years before learning about Prolotherapy while researching an alternative to knee replacement surgery. He was told by a prominent surgeon in Chicago that given his activity level and if he wanted to continue weight lifting, the replacements would last about ten years and that each subsequent replacement would become less successful than the previous. At only 56 years-old, and after already being through three unsuccessful surgeries, Alek was hesitant to jump to knee replacement surgery. But something had to be done. His knees were in constant pain and his MRI backed up the fact that his knees were a mechanical nightmare. *(See Figure 13-4.)* He opted for Prolotherapy.

At the time of his first appointment, he reported being in pain 100% of the time and could only walk one city block. As a bodybuilder, it was unbelievable that his maximum leg extension weight was five pounds. Due to his severe case, we knew he would likely need about a year or two of care. We treated him every four to six weeks for about 7 months and he reported 75% improvement and was able to do 105 pound leg lifts. With every visit, Alek continued to experience more motion, increased strength and less pain. Eight months later he reported minimal pain and maximum function.

His x-rays showed the cartilage improvement as well. So, what did Alek's surgeon think of the results of Prolotherapy? Unfortunately, he was not receptive. The good news is that Alek got his life back![10]

As with Alek's severe knee OA, we have successfully treated many patients not only with knee OA, but also with hip, back, neck, shoulder, wrist, hand, thumb, and toe OA—pretty much any joint in the body!

Let's take a look at the following analogy to help clarify exactly how arthritis develops.

THE HAUSER LOOSE HINGE-JOINT INSTABILITY ANALOGY

The hinge of a door is akin to the peripheral and spinal joints in the body. *(See Figure 13-5.)* The purpose of a hinge

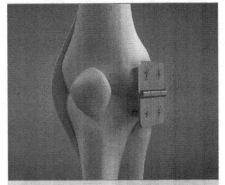

Figure 13-5: The Hinge-Joint analogy. The hinge of a door is akin to the peripheral and spinal joints in the body. A hinge holds the door onto the frame and the screws hold the hinge onto the door. The joint consists of two adjacent bones which are held in place by ligaments.

on a cabinet door is to keep the door in proper alignment as it allows the door to fully open and close. For two adjacent cabinet doors to not touch in the middle, the hinges must be held firmly in place. Assuming that the hinge on a cabinet door has three screws, and one of the screws begins to loosen, what happens to the other screws? There is more pressure transmitted to the other screws, more pressure than they are designed to handle. This eventually leads to the other screws loosening, and the entire hinge becoming loose. As the first hinge becomes loose, what happens to the next hinge? It begins to take on more pressure of the door and its swinging action. However, it was not designed to handle this extra pressure, and thus continues the breakdown of that next hinge as well. At any point in this scenario, the action of the cabinet door will be affected. The door can begin to wobble and hit the adjacent door, beginning the wear and tear process on the cabinet door itself.

To fix the problem of the loose hinge on a cabinet door, what would you attempt first?
• Oil the hinge and hope that stops the wobbling.
• Sand down the door at the point of contact with the other door.
• Replace the door.
• Lower the thermostat to see if a colder room stops the wobbling.
• Stop using the cabinet.
• Hire an architect to come over and assess a redesign of the entire cabinet?
• Ignore it and convince yourself that the door is fine.
• Simply get a Phillips screwdriver and tighten the screws in the hinge.

We bet your first choice would be to use a screwdriver to tighten the screws on the hinge! That would make the most amount of sense. You would probably think all of the other options were a waste of time and money because they are not addressing a simple problem. Perhaps now it makes more sense as to why so many treatments for pain do not correct the problem. Lubricating the joint, seeking out a surgeon to reconstruct or remove tissue from the joint, wrapping the joint, icing the joint, taking NSAIDs to turn off the pain signal, doing nothing... these are all options chosen by people every day that do not deal with the problem of joint instability directly. Our ligaments function similarly to hinges on a cabinet door, creating joint instability when they are loose. **(See Figure 13-6.)** This comparison is apparent in the cases as either a hinge or a joint becomes unstable and begins the degenerative cascade. To fix the hinge, tighten the screws. To fix a joint, tighten the ligaments!

Just like you do not want to deal with a wobbly cabinet door for too long, it is best to heal the ligaments as soon as possible. When the hinge is loose and allowing the door to wobble on a cabinet door, it begins to bang against the other door and eventually the wood of the door will warp and chip off. Similarly, if left unhealed, the lax ligaments become less supportive and allow for abnormal wear and tear on the joint. This causes pressure and destructive changes in the subchondral bone and the cartilage. There is no need to let the deterioration of the joint continue when Prolotherapy is an effective treatment for preventing and eliminating arthritis pain and degeneration in every joint of the body! The more degenerated a joint becomes, the increased need for Stem Cell Prolotherapy, where a person's own cells are placed in the most damaged areas of the joint to induce repair.

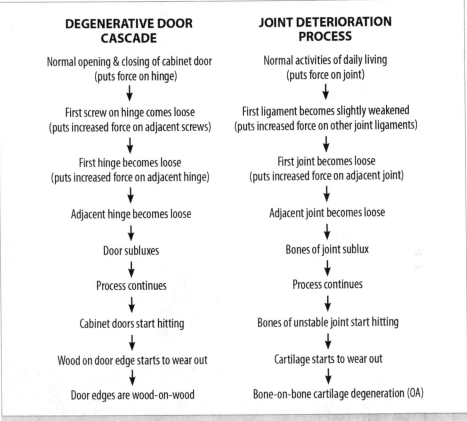

Figure 13-6: Degenerative door cascade compared to the joint deterioration process.

OSTEOARTHRITIS OF THE LUMBAR SPINE

Most people experience some form of back pain by the time they reach middle age. However, athletes who participate in twisting sports such as golf, tennis, and bowling, due to the forces exerted during their sports, are more at risk for developing OA of the spine. Other athletes experience repeated strain on the back due to posture, such as back packing and hiking. We cannot forget, however, the constant poor posture of most Americans as they sit at their desks, slouch on their couches, all the while face down into their computers or mobile devices.

A good portion of the population suffers from daily back pain and ends up choosing back surgery in hopes of alleviating the pain. Unfortunately, many patients are left with even more pain because the surgery that was supposed to strengthen the weak area actually ended up weakening the area to the point that the non–surgerized back was actually stronger. Degeneration occurs in the back due to a weakening of the support structures. Left untreated, this leads to OA with accompanying pain and stiffness.

Aren't degenerated discs the problem? The intervertebral disc is a major component contributing to segmental stability as well as a major load-bearing structure. Disc abnormalities that occur in osteoarthritis, however, are not associated with pain.[11,12] Many patients and athletes are distressed at being told that they are suffering from one or more degenerated discs. Disc degeneration occurs as age advances, but often causes no pain. Thus the other structures in the back are causing the problem.

LIGAMENT LAXITY IN THE LUMBAR SPINE CAUSES INSTABILITY!

Damage to the supporting structures of the spine, namely the ligaments and tendons that hold the spine together, is the cause of lumbar spine OA. The supraspinatus and interspinatus ligaments go from vertebra to vertebra. The iliolumbar ligaments attach along the ilium to sacrum (sacroiliac ligaments). Cumulative injury (without repair) over years of sports or improper movement can result in small tears in these ligaments. Often healing never occurs and people report "chronic nagging back pain." Since the ligaments do not heal, the intervertebral discs do not have the support that they need. This is why there is such a high rate of OA of the spine! Instability and ligament laxity with resultant instability cause chronic low back pain. *(See Figure 13-7.)* Prolotherapy should be administered sooner rather than later to repair the ligament tissues that will then allow the vertebrae to permanently stay in place!

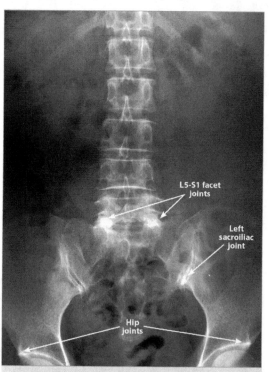

Figure 13-7: AP x-ray of lower back, pelvis, and hips showing areas of sclerosis (arrows). Hardening of the bones or joints (sclerosis) is typically the earliest x-ray sign of joint instability and osteoarthritis. The bone is hardening because of greater pressure on it due to ligament injury causing joint hypermobility or instability. This particular patient was recommended a multi-level fusion, but she chose Prolotherapy instead. She experienced a complete recovery without surgery.

THUMB ARTHRITIS

When you think about osteoarthritis, you may normally think of knee and hip, and maybe even back arthritis. But you cannot discount the growing frequency of osteoarthritis of the thumb, particularly at the base of the thumb. Many people seek relief from a wide array of splints, NSAIDs, hot wax treatments, creams, physical therapy, and the eventual cortisone injection. When none of these treatments cure the problem, patients are left with the option of surgical repair.

The carpometacarpal (CMC) joint is located at the base of the thumb, where the thumb attaches to the hand. Like arthritis anywhere else in the body, the pain comes from joint instability as a result of ligament laxity. Traditional medicine will report that thumb pain is due to cartilage degeneration. But what is the underlying cause of this degeneration? Weakness in the supporting structures leading to joint degeneration (OA). A sea of ligaments in the hand support the thumb! Injury to these ligaments leads to OA of the thumb. Plain and simple. **(See Figure 13-8.)**

Have you ever experienced thumb pain? It can be totally debilitating! We forget how much we use our thumbs just in everyday life! Typing, texting (also likely contributes to the cause of the pain), writing, brushing your hair/teeth, opening a jar, gripping a tool – it's endless.

We see a growing number of thumb arthritis patients at Caring Medical, and we are seeing them at younger and younger ages! Why? Excessive use or trauma that results in an injury that is never healed. Smart phone syndrome is

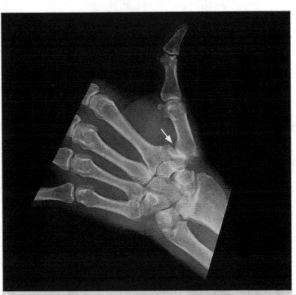

Figure 13-8: Prolotherapy is used to resolve the joint instability that caused the bone-on-bone situation. To rebuild the cartilage, stem (progenitor) cells are injected.

a major contributing factor of overuse, as mentioned in **Chapter 11.** Just like any other joint in the body, thumb OA can be debilitating. Patients develop OA of the thumb as a result of repetitive motion and/or trauma. A fall onto the hand during a sporting event or accident can result in the start of OA of the thumb when left untreated.

The good news is that although traditional literature may not report successful treatment of OA of the thumb, we know that the cause is joint instability as a result of weak supporting structures, namely the ligaments and tendons. Tighten those with Prolotherapy and the patient is well on his/her way to pain-free living. It really isn't that difficult of a concept to grasp when you look at the root cause of the problem!

RESEARCH PROVES EFFECTIVENESS OF PROLOTHERAPY

Prolotherapy research is discussed in much more detail in **Chapter 22**, including some great randomized controlled studies for osteoarthritis by the most well known and respected Prolotherapy researchers today. Many of the patients who participated in our Prolotherapy results studies had chronic pain due to osteoarthritis. In **Chapter 3**, we discussed our published studies using Bone Marrow Prolotherapy for arthritis. At our clinic, we treat osteoarthritis every day, ranging from mild to highly advanced. As the arthritis is advancing and the joint becomes more damaged, we find patients tend to need more aggressive regenerative treatments, which is why Cellular Prolotherapy is often used for these cases.

It is interesting to note that the research and clinical experience shows that Prolotherapy has positive effects on regrowing cartilage.[13-15] This is unheard of in traditional practices because the treatments of NSAIDs and cortisone are degenerative instead of regenerative. It is important to remember that the best patient care is still not based on the results of a scan. A patient with plenty of cartilage can still have pain, and a patient with almost no cartilage can feel pain-free. That said, it is still great to see that Prolotherapy has the power to maintain and regenerate cartilage on x-ray in every joint of the body! *(See Figures 13-9, 13-10, 13-11 & 13-12.)*

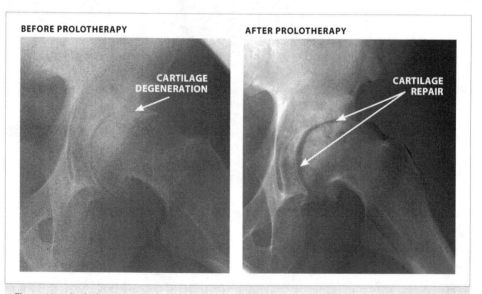

Figure 13-9: Prolotherapy regeneration of hip cartilage. Prolotherapy can bring a significant amount of pain relief and healing in severely degenerated joints. Note the increase in joint space after Prolotherapy.

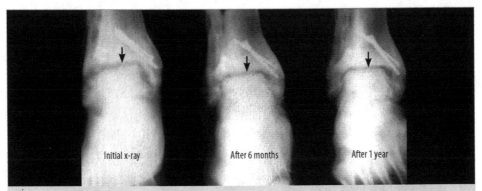

Figure 13-10: Improvement of ankle x-rays with Stem Cell Prolotherapy. This patient received several Lipoaspirate Prolotherapy treatments between x-ray studies. These studies showed a gradual improvement in the ankle joint articular cartilage (arrows), which correlated to reduced pain and range of motion improvement.

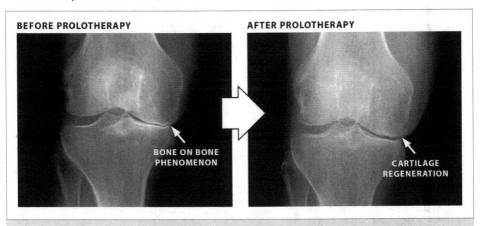

Figure 13-11: Standard weight-bearing knee x-rays before and after Prolotherapy. The widening of the medial joint space width indicates that cartilage regeneration has taken place.

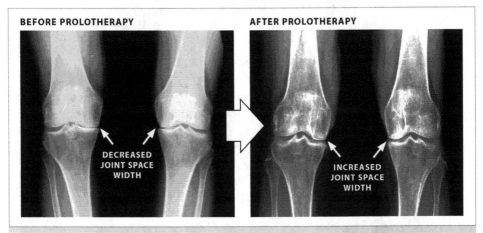

Figure 13-12: Standard weight-bearing bilateral knee x-rays before and after Prolotherapy. The widening of the medial joint space in both knees indicates that cartilage regeneration has taken place.

RHEUMATOID AND INFLAMMATORY ARTHRITIS

Inflammatory arthritis, or rheumatoid arthritis (RA), is a totally different kind of arthritis and generally occurs when the body attacks itself by making antibodies against itself. Antibodies are proteins, made by the immune system, that fight microorganisms such as bacteria that invade the body. In these instances, this inflammation is counterproductive because the body is reacting against its own immune system.

Autoimmune disorders are not a prednisone or NSAID deficiency. Correcting the underlying cause of why the body is attacking itself is key to reversing these conditions. This can include investigating the possibility of leaky gut syndrome, poor diet, food sensitivities, heavy metals, fatty acid or other nutrient deficiency, underlying infection such as Lyme disease or mycoplasma, and unresolved trauma. Treatment may involve a comprehensive approach to diet and supplements, hormones, IV nutrients, oxygen therapies, mind-body therapies, and more. It is for this reason that people suffering from these painful chronic conditions should seek the care of a Natural Medicine physician so the cause of the condition can be treated.

Although inflammatory arthritis pain is not an appropriate application for Prolotherapy, people who have this systemic condition can suffer an injury that would be appropriate for Prolotherapy. For instance, in a patient with very well-controlled rheumatoid arthritis who sustains a shoulder injury while playing tennis, Prolotherapy is the ideal treatment.

BONE DESTRUCTION

It is unfortunate that some people do not hear about Prolotherapy until their bones are actually destroyed and they are faced with joint replacement surgery.

We occasionally see patients where the bone has deformed due to unresolved joint instability with continued joint usage. In a ball and socket joint, such as the hip, the head of the femur bone should be round. But as the ligament damage allows for more joint instability the bone continues to take the brunt of each step, flattening and producing bony overgrowths. This is why we wish people who suffer a sports injury or trauma, and want to stay active, would seek a Prolotherapy consultation sooner rather than later. Prolotherapy has the potential to save your joint from being destroyed. However, if the injury is not repaired and degenerative arthritis sets in, Prolotherapy cannot make a flattened bone round again. These cases end up requiring joint replacement surgery because they waited too long to do something about the problem. *(See Figure 13-13.)*

THE CHOICE IS YOURS: OSTEOARTHRITIS OR PROLOTHERAPY?

Osteoarthritis is not the result of aging. *See Figure 13-14*, which dispels the myths about arthritis and aging. Why, however, do people develop arthritis in many body parts as they age? Part of the reason for this is decreased levels of chondroitin and glucosamine sulfate levels with OA, which is the basis for their supplementation for this condition.

Otherwise, the answer is simple: Arthritis is the result of an injury to a joint that was never allowed to heal. Trauma is the number one cause of ligament, tendon, and labrum injuries, resulting in non-repair and joint degeneration with resultant OA. Many mechanisms exist to explain this, but we believe that joint instability is the primary cause which leads to increased pressure on the articular cartilage and sheer

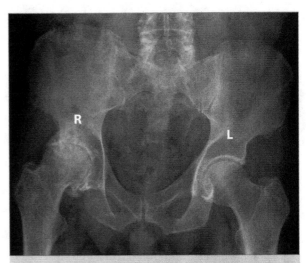

Figure 13-13: Hip x-ray showing advanced osteoarthritis with spur development. While the left hip has good joint space and cartilage in most of the joint, the right hip has severely advanced osteoarthritis with minimal joint space and multiple bone spurs lining both acetabulum and femoral head. The patient was referred to orthopedic surgery for total hip replacement or resurfacing. Do not wait until it is too late!

forces, both of which have been shown to cause chondrocyte cell death (apoptosis) and dysfunction (altered metabolism).[16-20] Consider the pharmacological (drugs) approach to this as the old view and stimulating repair of the ligaments and structures that stabilize the joint with Prolotherapy as the new view. *(See Figure 13-15.)*

The best way to prevent formation of arthritis in ANY joint in the body— if you participate even in the most brutal of sports, such as boxing, martial arts fighting, rugby, or football— is to make sure that your injuries heal. Heal the injury and the likelihood of having a long and prosperous pain-free life is excellent. This means doing the MEAT treatment after the injury. MEAT includes movement, exercise, analgesics, and specific treatments such as heat, ultrasound, massage,

Comparison of changes in articular cartilage in aging vs osteoarthritis		
Criterion	**Aging**	**Osteoarthritis**
Water content	Decreased	Increased
Glycosaminoglycans and chondroitin sulfate	Normal or slightly less	Decreased
Glucosamine	Increased	Decreased
Keratan sulfate	Increased	Decreased
Hyaluronate	Increased	Decreased
Proteoglycans aggregation	Normal	Diminished
Link protein	Fragmented	Normal
Proteases	Normal	Increased

Figure 13-14: The joint composition in aging and osteoarthritis are opposites. Chondroitin and glucosamine content are lower in osteoarthritis. Thus, these patients often require supplementation.

Adapted from The Biology of Osteoarthritis. Herman, D. *The New England Journal of Medicine.* 1989, Vol. 20, pp. 1322-1329, Table 2.

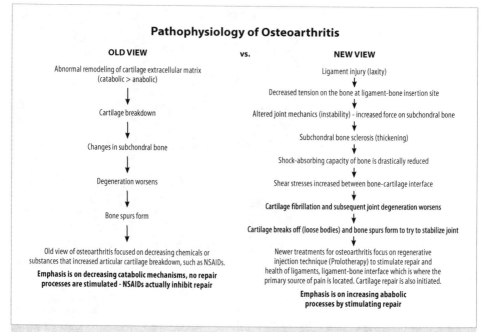

Figure 13-15: The old vs. new view on formation of osteoarthritis. NSAIDs and other drugs focus on decreasing cartilage breakdown, while newer more effective treatments, such as Prolotherapy stimulate repair.

and Prolotherapy. Do not allow your injuries to be treated with RICE, anti-inflammatories, cortisone shots, and arthroscopy. It is our hope that traditional pain management will continue to come around in its understanding of the pathophysiology of osteoarthritis. If this happens, more people will never have to know the chronic pain and disability of osteoarthritis because regenerative techniques, like Prolotherapy, would be part of the first-line treatments, halting the progression of osteoarthritis altogether.

SUMMARY

Ligament laxity is normally the cause of degenerative arthritis, also known as osteoarthritis. The weak ligaments, if not repaired by Prolotherapy, will eventually lead to loose joints. The muscles and tendons tighten in an attempt to stabilize the joints and stop the progression. When this fails, the articular cartilage deteriorates on one side of the joint. The bones begin rubbing on that side of the joint. This causes an overgrowth of bone, called osteoarthritis. Prolotherapy injections to strengthen the joint stop this arthritis cascade. If osteoarthritis has already formed, Prolotherapy will relieve the pain but cannot reverse the bony overgrowth that has already occurred. ∎

CHAPTER

14

PROLO YOUR SPORTS INJURIES AWAY!

One of the most common reasons patients seek our clinics is Prolotherapy for sports injuries. This is an excellent treatment option for getting an athlete back to sports quickly and safely. We covered most conditions in the previous chapters, organized by body area. In this chapter, we will put to rest some of the popular sports myths that keep injured people sidelined or on the fast-track to surgery, and kissing their favorite sports good-bye. For any athlete, coach, or trainer who is interested in exploring this in greater detail, we authored a 900 page book devoted to sports: *Prolo Your Sports Injuries Away!*

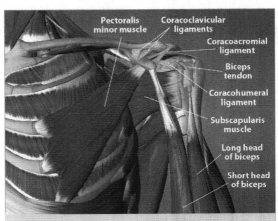

Figure 14-1: Anterior view of the shoulder joint. A vast majority of athletic injuries involve the muscles, ligaments, and tendons.

MYTH NUMBER 1: REST IS GOOD

Yes, rest is necessary between workouts for recovery. Rest from athletics is even suggested after Prolotherapy for a few days. What we are talking about here is resting injured joints over long periods of time without any other regenerative treatment being done. How many times do we hear people with a simple sprain say "I was told to rest it for a few weeks." What?! And lose all that time you could be healing and getting back to activities? *(See Figure 14-1.)* Resting injured areas just encourages stagnation of blood and damaged tissue, resulting in increased swelling and scar tissue formation. The longer an athlete restricts movement after an injury, the longer it will take to heal. For each day of non-movement, two days are added to the length of rehabilitation. Walk around and move the injured limb.

MYTH NUMBER 2: IMMOBILIZE THE INJURED AREA

Immobilization can be detrimental to ligament healing and should not be done casually, though it is sometimes necessary under medical supervision. In our office, it may be used early in the treatment course for more severe cases of instability. Immobilization is generally discouraged for most cases because it can cause the following changes:

- proliferation of fatty connective tissue within the joint
- cartilage damage and necrosis
- scar tissue formation and articular cartilage tears
- increased randomness of the collagen fibers within the ligaments and connective tissues
- ligament weakening with a decreased resistance to stretch.[1-3]

A study performed on animals revealed that after several weeks of immobilization, the strength of the ligament tissue was reduced to about one-third of normal.[2-5] Immobilization also significantly decreases the strength of the fibro-osseous junction, the bone-ligament interface.[2] Eight weeks of immobilization produced a 39% decrease in the strength of the fibro-osseous junction of the anterior cruciate ligament of the knee.[6,7] Other researchers have shown that even partial immobilization (restricted activity) has similar deleterious effects on ligament insertion sites.[1]

Immobility causes decreased water content, decreased proteoglycans, increased collagen turnover, and a dramatic alteration in the type of collagen cross-linking of the ligaments, producing a weak ligament.[2,8] Immobility is one of the primary reasons ligaments heal inadequately after an injury.

MYTH NUMBER 3: ICE IS NICE

Ice is nice if you are having a cool lemonade on a hot day, but it has no place around most sports injuries. Ice decreases circulation to the area of injury, thereby allowing fewer immune cells to clean up the injured site and lay down new collagen tissue needed to repair ligaments, tendons, and muscles.[9-12]

Immobilization (rest), ice, compression, and elevation, decreases blood flow, resulting in reduced immune cell production

HEAT vs. ICE in Healing Sports Injuries

Effects	Heat	Ice
Arterioles	Dilate	Vasoconstrict
Blood supply to connective issues	Increased	Decreased
Metabolic rate	Increased	Decreased
Number of immune cells to the injured area	Increased	Decreased
Joint collagen effects	Relaxation	Stiffness
Net effect	Anabolic	Catabolic

Figure 14-2: HEAT vs. ICE in healing sports injuries. HEAT promotes connective tissue growth and has a net anabolic effect. ICE is catabolic, inhibiting connective tissue growth and repair.

necessary to remove the debris from the injury site. This produces formation of weak ligament and tendon tissue. *(See Figure 14-2.)* Swelling is the physical manifestation of inflammation, and is evidence that the body is working to heal itself. It has been shown that as little as five minutes of icing a knee can decrease both blood flow to the soft tissues and skeletal metabolism.[13] Icing an area for 25 minutes decreases blood flow and skeletal metabolism another 400%. Healing is hindered by a decrease in blood flow and metabolism to the area. Regular use of ice increases the chance of incomplete healing by decreasing blood flow to the injured ligaments and tendons.

MYTH NUMBER 4: ANTI-INFLAMMATORY MEDICATION IS GOOD

After an athlete rests an injured limb, he/she will likely wrap it with ice, and then start popping ibuprofen to decrease the swelling. This technique masks the pain, only to decrease the athlete's chance of complete healing after the injury. Why is the foot swollen? The body is trying to heal the area. When animals are injured do they run to the drug store? No, they start limping. *(See Figure 14-3.)*

Sometimes animals are smarter than people! By retarding the healing process, anti-inflammatory medications make re-injury much more likely in the future. Anti-inflammatory medications mask the pain and do nothing to help the injured tissue repair itself. Athletes have a choice: anti-inflame the pain to stay or Prolo the pain away!

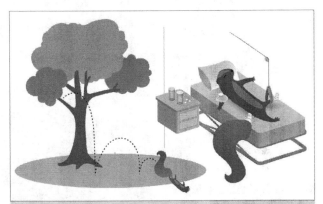

Figure 14-3: Nature does not use R.I.C.E. When a squirrel falls from a tree it doesn't start putting ice on its injury, elevating its leg, or popping anti-inflammatory pills right?

MYTH NUMBER 5: CORTISONE SHOTS HELP

Corticosteroids, such as cortisone and prednisone, have an adverse effect on bone and soft tissue healing. Corticosteroids inactivate vitamin D, limiting calcium absorption by the gastrointestinal tract and increasing urinary excretion of calcium. Bone also shows a decrease in calcium uptake, ultimately leading to weakness at the fibro-osseous junction. Corticosteroids also inhibit the release of Growth Hormone which further decreases soft tissue and bone repair. Ultimately, corticosteroids lead to a decrease in bone, ligament, and tendon strength.[14-19]

Corticosteroids inhibit the synthesis of proteins, collagen, and proteoglycans in articular cartilage by inhibiting chondrocyte production—the cells that comprise the articular cartilage. The net catabolic effect (weakening) of corticosteroids is inhibition of fibroblast production of collagen, ground substance, and angiogenesis (new blood vessel formation).

Cortisone, even one shot, may cause irreversible damage to the joint and cartilage. Imagine what two, three, or 10 shots will do.

A patient who came to our Florida office was a former basketball player who had been drafted to an international team. He had received dozens of cortisone injections for his chronic shoulder pain. By the time he was in his late 20s, the pain was so bad that he was referred for surgery. When the surgeon looked at the joint, he noted that the patient's shoulder resembled that of someone twice his age. Had the patient originally received medical care from a Prolotherapist who prioritized the long-term strength of the joint, he could have avoided surgery and saved his career. Instead, so many players are subjected to treatments that help them play the game today, but leave them with irreparable damage that can prematurely end their careers.

As discussed in greater detail in **Chapter 2**, cortisone permanently weakens tissue, including cartilage. Prolotherapy strengthens it. The choice is yours. Mask your pain with cortisone or cure it with Prolotherapy. *(See Figure 14-4.)*

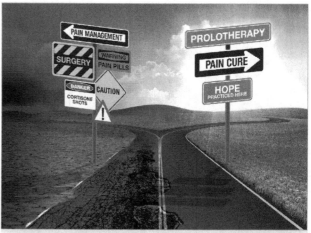

Figure 14-4: Many roads lead to pain management, but only one road leads to pain cure...Prolotherapy.

MYTH NUMBER 6: "SURGERY WILL FIX THE PROBLEM"

Surgery, except for a complete tear of a ligament or tendon, does not fix problems, it creates them. Taking a scalpel and slicing open muscles and fascia, and removing disc, cartilage, and ligament tissue weakens the injured joints. The knife treatment should always be the last resort for an athlete. How many big-time athletes do you see come back and compete at the same level after the surgeon has touched them? Any athlete who consents to exploratory surgery without receiving an evaluation for Prolotherapy is playing Russian roulette with his/her career. Arthroscopy, and the cutting, burning, or shaving that goes with it, leaves the athlete in a weakened state. Very few come back. Prolotherapy, if fully utilized, would stop about 80% of the orthopedic surgeries in this country for chronic pain. Prolotherapy gets at the root cause of athletic injuries: joint instability. By strengthening the tendons, ligaments, and other supporting structures of the joints, Prolotherapy strengthens the injured areas. Is this not what the athlete desires?

MYTH NUMBER 7: "AFTER A LITTLE BIT OF REHAB, YOU'LL BE BACK TO PLAYING"

Every athlete should read this book and other books on the predicted rehabilitation course after surgery. Very rarely is an athlete back to playing shortly after surgery. An ACL repair or elbow tendon transfer generally requires about one year of rehabilitation for an athlete to achieve full function, if this ever does occur. After an athlete experiences a torn ACL, one week after surgery the athlete is usually given a brace to wear and is confined to no activity. A tennis player would be lucky to be hitting tennis balls again by five months after the ACL repair. Compare this to the athlete who received Prolotherapy to the knee. Within a few days, most are hitting tennis balls and playing at full speed in a week or two, not months.

MYTH NUMBER 8: "IF I WEAR MY KNEE BRACE, I WILL BE FINE"

It is amazing how many athletes are wearing knee braces, taped elbows, and the infamous ankle wraps. There are some times when sports tape may be helpful between treatments, or if a person is doing a more extreme event than normal that may require assistance. But for a person to need a brace to perform a moderate workout means the joint is not strong enough. The joint structures, namely the ligaments, need to be strengthened. We prefer the long-term strengthening of a joint to the long-term use of a brace. In more extreme cases of joint instability or in those where tissue like the meniscus was fully removed via surgery, the person may need to brace occasionally for more demanding sports. Our goal for most athletes is to get them back to the point of not needing a brace, though it may be necessary while the tissue is repairing during the Prolotherapy treatment series.

MYTH NUMBER 9: "THE TEAM EMPLOYEES HAVE MY BEST INTEREST AT HEART"

This is the mistake that most of the big professional athletes make. What most of them do not realize is that everyone has an ego. Say you are an athletic trainer, chiropractor, physical therapist, acupuncturist, or another specialist, and Michael Jordan walks into your office to become a patient. How likely would you be to refer him to someone else, even if your treatments were not working? The likelihood is not too great! The reason is you can now say that you are the athletic trainer to Michael Jordan. This is what happens. The more famous the athlete, the less likely he/she is going to be referred for the most appropriate treatments. Do not put all the blame on the athletic trainers. If they have an athlete where the usual and customary treatments are not working, guess what they have to do? Send the athlete to the team physician. Unfortunately, most teams do not have a team physician; they have a team surgeon. It is imperative for the athlete to research what treatment is best for him/her. Relying solely on your athletic trainer, chiropractor, orthopedist, or physical therapist could be dangerous to your career.

Telling stories always helps better illustrate the point. As a youngster, Dr. Hauser wanted to grow up to be like Jack Nicklaus. He played golf and dreamed about becoming a pro golfer. He followed Jack's career closely. When he became a doctor, he followed Jack's injuries closely. When Jack turned 50 years-old, Dr. Hauser knew Jack had the ability to have a great career on the senior tour. He won 70 tournaments and 21 majors, including two U.S. amateurs, while on the regular PGA tour. One of his elders, Lee Trevino, for example, won 27 tournaments on the regular PGA tour, but has won 28 tournaments on the senior tour. Well, Jack just did not win very much on the senior tour because of back and hip trouble. Being the faithful fan that he is, Dr. Hauser sent him information on Prolotherapy in 1993. **(See Figure 14-5.)** He graciously replied with a personally signed note. Unfortunately, we will never know if Prolotherapy would have helped him because in early 1999 he ended up having a total hip replacement for his degenerative arthritis in his left hip. He, like a lot of people with chronic pain and sports injuries, had tried a lot of different treatments, just not Prolotherapy.

Athletes: when are you going to realize that the team, the coaches, and their helpers are paid employees? They do what is best for the owner of the team. Please, do what is best for you.

If the athlete exhausts all the conservative treatments (including Prolotherapy) and still has pain, then and only then would a referral be made to an orthopedist. Surgery should always be a last resort. Why teams have surgeons as the first resort we will never know.

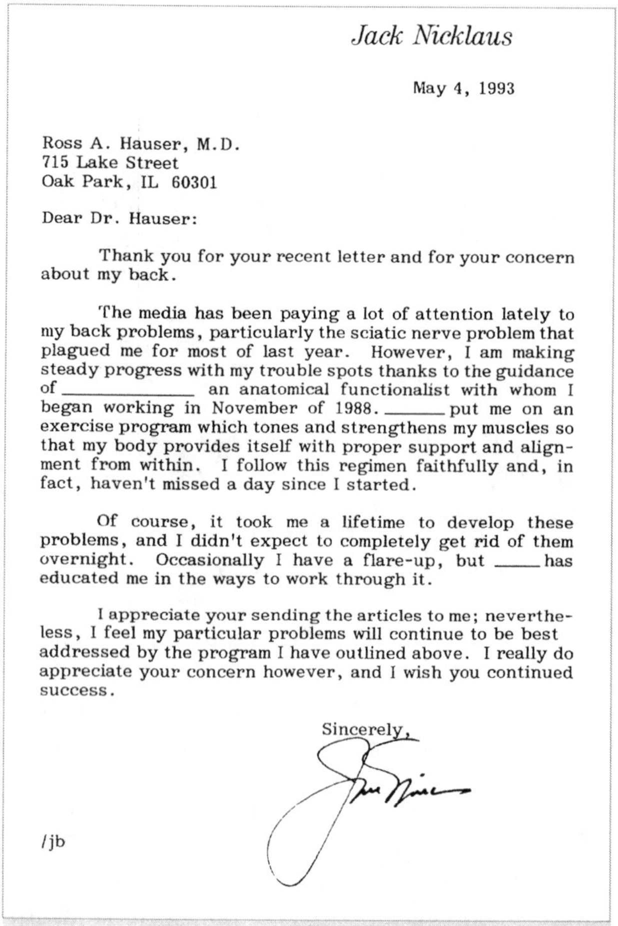

Jack Nicklaus

May 4, 1993

Ross A. Hauser, M.D.
715 Lake Street
Oak Park, IL 60301

Dear Dr. Hauser:

Thank you for your recent letter and for your concern about my back.

The media has been paying a lot of attention lately to my back problems, particularly the sciatic nerve problem that plagued me for most of last year. However, I am making steady progress with my trouble spots thanks to the guidance of _____ an anatomical functionalist with whom I began working in November of 1988. _____ put me on an exercise program which tones and strengthens my muscles so that my body provides itself with proper support and alignment from within. I follow this regimen faithfully and, in fact, haven't missed a day since I started.

Of course, it took me a lifetime to develop these problems, and I didn't expect to completely get rid of them overnight. Occasionally I have a flare-up, but ____ has educated me in the ways to work through it.

I appreciate your sending the articles to me; nevertheless, I feel my particular problems will continue to be best addressed by the program I have outlined above. I really do appreciate your concern however, and I wish you continued success.

Sincerely,

/jb

Figure 14-5: Letter to Dr. Hauser from Jack Nicklaus.
Unfortunately, Jack did not choose Prolotherapy.

MYTH NUMBER 10: "ATHLETICS, ESPECIALLY RUNNING, WILL GIVE YOU ARTHRITIS"

Properly performed, athletics does nothing but help a person become physically, emotionally, and mentally stronger and happier. As long as crunching in the joints and pain do not occur, athletes can keep going. If an athlete begins to hear a new crunching sound in a joint, or has bouts of pain during the sport, it is time to see the Prolotherapist. Athletics, including long distance running, does not cause cartilage injury or arthritis. Only injury to joints, ligaments, and tendons cause cartilage injury or arthritis. Ligaments provide stability to the joints. Once these are injured, pain occurs. The healing process begins when the person receives Prolotherapy. If the route of anti-inflammation is chosen, such as a prescription for NSAIDs (non-steroidal anti-inflammatory medications), then further ligament injury occurs with resultant joint laxity (weakness). Joint laxity or weakness manifests itself by clicking in the joint. To stabilize the loose joint, the body overgrows bone. This overgrowth of bone is called arthritis. **(See Figure 14-6.)** Joint, ligament, or tendon weakness causes arthritis, not running, jumping, or throwing a javelin. By treating the cause of arthritis, Prolotherapy can stop the downhill process.

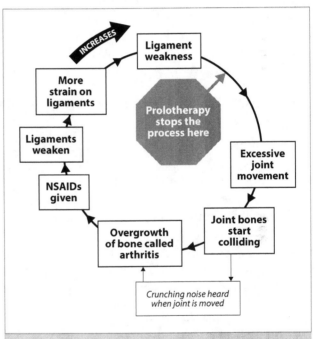

Figure 14-6: How weakened ligaments lead to arthritis. Prolotherapy stops arthritis from forming by healing the ligament weakness that started and perpetuates the cascade.

MYTH NUMBER 11: "JUST QUIT, YOU ARE NOT GOING TO GET BETTER"

This is the myth that prompted the writing of the sports injuries book. A Big Ten basketball player came to our office. "I was told that I can no longer play," he said dejectedly. "What position do you play?" Dr. Hauser asked. "Power forward." "Do want to play pro?" "Yes, sir." He further explained that he was diagnosed with degenerative disc disease in his lower spine and had to sit out the season because of the pain. We discussed the high success rate of Prolotherapy in treating this condition in our office. Not only could his pain be relieved, but he had an excellent chance of playing as much basketball as he desired. Needless to say, he jumped on the table.

He was seen for a total of four visits at four-week intervals. After the second visit, he was feeling much better. At this point, Dr. Hauser advised him to start playing. At his fourth appointment, he was doing great, but still experienced slight discomfort. He again received Prolotherapy to his back and was cleared to play full time. We did not hear from him again, but did get a jingle from the "team physician," Dr. Orthopedist from the university. The physician said that this player was back to playing, but he needed a letter written to the NCAA for the player to obtain a sixth year of eligibility. We were sure he was playing, and probably playing very well.

Other patients from his hometown were in our office a few months later. Somewhere along the way we started talking about sports. They were all excited that the star player from their alma mater was back to playing basketball. Of course, they were discussing the patient who had been seen in our office. To the athletes out there: do not give up your dreams.

MYTH NUMBER 12: YOUR FOOTWEAR IS THE PROBLEM

Many people spend hundreds or thousands of dollars on the best shoes and orthotics to try and fix their pain. We like to try new running shoes just like any other athlete, but it's not all about the shoes or orthotics, especially when it comes to injuries. Shin splints are a common reason why people go through shoe after shoe, trying to find relief. Shin splints, also known as medial tibial stress syndrome, is the catch-all term for lower leg pain that occurs below the knee either on the front outside part of the leg (anterior shin splints) or the inside of the leg (medial shin splints). They are the bane of many athletes, runners, tennis players and even dancers. The condition typically involves only one leg, and almost always the athlete's dominant one. If the athlete is right-handed, he or she is usually right-footed as well. Thus, the right leg of this individual would be more susceptible to shin splints. Physical examination of the patient with shin splints reveals a diffuse area of tenderness over the posterior medial edge of the tibia. The pain is occasionally aggravated by contractions of the soleus, posterior tibialis, or flexor digitorum longus muscles. We find the most reliable sign, though, is to poke on the area with the thumb to reproduce the athlete's exact pain.

There are several causes and theories for why shin splints occur. Tightness in the posterior muscles that propel the body forward places additional strain on the muscles in the front part of the lower leg, which works to lift the foot upward and also prepares the foot to strike the running surface. Hard surface running as well as worn or improper shoes increase the stress on the anterior leg muscles. The lower leg muscles suffer a tremendous amount of stress when a runner lands only on the balls of the feet (toe running), without normal heel contact. The muscles of the foot and leg overwork in an attempt to stabilize the pronated (rotated in and down) foot, and the repeated stress can cause the muscles to tear where they attach to the tibia. Another possible cause is ligament damage. Both the "spring," or plantar calcaneonavicular ligament, and the posterior talofibular ligament may be weakened or injured during running, again leading to painful shin splints. *(See Figure 14-7.)*

Shin splints often plague beginning runners who do not build their mileage gradually enough, as well as seasoned runners who abruptly change their workout regimen by suddenly adding too much mileage or switching from running on flat surfaces to hills, to cite just two examples.

Since shin splints are felt as intense pain in the leg, traditional treatment usually involves rest. This is after other measures, such as taping the arches, using heal cups in the athletic shoes and applying muscle pain-relieving topical gels and creams. The problem with this approach is that extended resting of the muscles and the periosteum, or the bone covering, will further weaken the already weak structures. It does not repair the weakened "spring," or

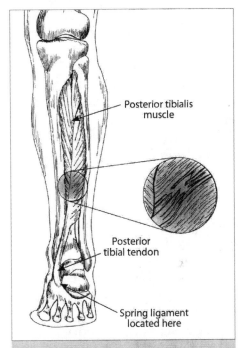

Figure 14-7: Shin splints. Periostitis of the bony attachment of the posterior tibialis muscle can occur because of tension caused not at the shin, but at the medial arch. Spring ligament laxity necessitates the posterior tibialis tendon to provide more arch support which increases tension on the posterior tibialis muscle origin. Prolotherapy to the spring ligament, along the posterior tibialis muscle origin and tendon is one of the treatments for arch pain and shin splints. This is a better approach for a runner than cutting back training!

plantar calcaneonavicular ligament, or the posterior talofibular ligament, both of which take a considerable beating during running, the activity that is the most common cause of shin splints. Additionally, most athletes wish to get back to running as soon as possible. We have found that shin splints respond very well to Prolotherapy. As the ligament and tendon attachments strengthen, the athlete can continue to get back to working out without dreaded shin splints.

REASONS FOR SPORTS INJURIES

Most sports injuries are soft tissue injuries involving ligaments, tendons, and muscles.[20] Sports injuries occur when the repetitive strain of the athletic event is too much for a particular ligament, tendon, or muscle to withstand, resulting in a strain—an injured weakened tendon—or a sprain—an injured weakened ligament.

The customary treatment for such injuries, as discussed in *Chapter 2*, is RICE which refers to treating soft tissue injury with Rest, Ice, Compression, and Elevation. This treatment regimen decreases inflammation when the injured area needs it most, resulting, unfortunately for the athlete, in decreased healing of the injury.[14-18] Consequently, many sports injuries do not heal completely and are easily re-injured.

A better approach is the treatment known as MEAT—Movement,

	RICE	MEAT
Immune system response	Decreased	Increased
Blood flow to injured area	Decreased	Increased
Collagen formation	Hindered	Encouraged
Speed of recovery	Delayed (lengthened)	Hastened (shortened)
Range of motion of joint	Decreased	Increased
Complete healing	Decreased	Increased

Figure 14-8: RICE vs. MEAT. The RICE protocol hampers soft tissue healing whereas MEAT encourages healing.

Exercise, Analgesics, and specific Treatments. Specific treatments that aid in the healing process include ultrasound, heat, and massage, because they increase blood flow. If an injury has not healed after six weeks, more aggressive treatments, including Prolotherapy, should be considered. Prolotherapy can be done immediately after an injury because it has been found to speed recovery. *(See Figure 14-8.)*

Stretching, body balancing or body work, chiropractic or osteopathic manipulation, and other physical modalities do help correct problems with posture, tight muscles, and other factors that contribute to sports injuries. Sometimes the patient's technique needs to be improved with coaching or lessons. *(See Figure 14-9.)*

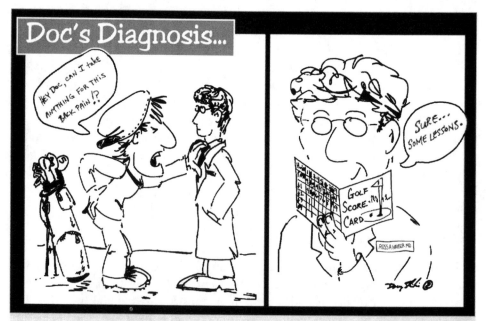

Figure 14-9: The golfer with back pain. Some sports injuries need more help than Prolotherapy can provide...

The fact remains that sports injuries occur when an area of the body is weak. Sports injuries, whether an ankle sprain or rotator cuff tendonitis, occur because a muscle, ligament, or tendon is not strong enough to perform the task the athlete requires of it. For this reason, the best curative treatment for a sports injury is to strengthen the weakened tissue.

Many sports injuries are muscle strains. Such injuries cause muscle pain when the injured muscle is contracted. Muscles enjoy a constant blood supply, which brings them necessary healing ingredients. As a result, muscles are usually quick to heal—regardless of the treatment.

We know that ligaments and tendons have poor blood supply and are thus more prone to incomplete healing after an injury. The goal in sports injury therapy should not be pain relief but restoring normal tissue strength, in other words, complete healing of the injured body part.

INJECTIONS NOW OR LATER: EVERY INJURED PERSON WILL NEED INJECTIONS

The skeletal muscles are the largest organ system of the human body and account for nearly 50% of the body weight.[21] Not counting heads, bellies, and other divisions of muscles, the *Nomina Anatomica* reported by the International Anatomical Nomenclature Committee, under the Berne Convention, lists 200 paired muscles, or a total of 400 muscles in the human skeletal system.[22] *(See Figure 14-10.)* The majority of these have tendons that allow the muscles to move the joints. All of the joints that are moved contain articular cartilage, so the joint surfaces glide easily over each other. The joints stay in place by the stabilizing effects of the joint capsule and

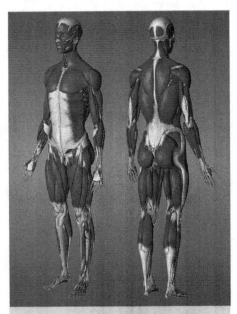

Figure 14-10: Muscles of the body. There are 400 muscles in the body. Each can have trigger points that cause pain.

ligaments. For instance, even for the modern 21st century athlete who desires to excel, over 50% of the body weight consists of soft tissue and, most assuredly, will be injured at some time.

Potential injuries await many people, especially athletes. It is not a matter of "Will the athlete be injured?" but "When will the athlete be injured?" *Figure 14-11* lists 62 of the more common injection sites for sports injuries that are lurking every day for athletes and others.

Possible Injection Sites Grouped by Body Part

Elbow
Annular ligament
Collateral ligaments
Cubital tunnel
Intra-articular joint
Lateral epicondyle
Medial epicondyle
Olecranon bursa

Foot
Interdigital nerve
Metatarsophalangeal joint
Plantar fascia
Sinus tarsi
Spring ligament
Tarsal tunnel

Hand
Collateral ligaments
Flexor tendon cyst
Flexor tendon sheath
Metacarpal joints

Hip
Greater trochanteric bursa
Intra-articular joint
Lateral femoral cutaneous nerve
Piriformis tendon

Knee
Bakers' cyst
Biceps femoris tendon
Collateral ligaments
Cruciate ligaments
Intra-articular cartilage
Patellar tendon
Pes anserine bursa
Pre-patellar bursa

Leg and Ankle
Achilles tendon
Anterior tibialis
Medial tibial tendo-osseous junction
Pre/post Achilles bursae
Posterior tibialis
Talofibular ligament
Tibiotalar joint

Lumbosacral
Erector spinae
Lumbar and spinous process
Lumbar facet joints
Quadratus lumborum
Sacroiliac joint

Neck
Annular ligament
Cervical facets
Cervical transverse process
Cervicothoracic muscles
Collateral ligament
Costovertebral junctions

Pelvis
Adductor tendon
Hamstring tendon
Ischial bursa
Pubic symphysis

Shoulder
Acromioclavicular joint
Glenohumeral ligament
Longhead biceps sheath
Rotator cuff tendon
Subacromial bursa

Wrist
Carpal tunnel
Carpometacarpal joint
De Quervain sheath
Ganglion cyst
Radiocarpal joint
Ulno-carpal joint

Figure 14-11: Possible injection sites grouped by body part. In the case of athletes, it's not a matter of if, but when they are going to get injected. A more important question is: Injected with what? We recommend Prolotherapy. Adapted from: *Injury Clinic: Injection Techniques and Use in the Treatment of Sports Injuries*, Warren A. Scott © 1996.

TREATMENT FOR SPORTS INJURIES

Prolotherapy is the best treatment to help cause permanently strong tissue to form where a weakened sports injury exists. Prolotherapy stimulates the healing process and, therefore, decreases the length of time it takes for soft tissue sports injuries to heal. Prolotherapy, because it triggers the growth of normal collagen tissue, causes stronger ligaments and tendons to form. Consequently, the athlete returns to his or her game stronger. After Prolotherapy treatments, not only is the athlete able to return to the sport, but often the particular area that was injured will be stronger than before the injury and performance will be enhanced.

FREQUENCY OF PROLOTHERAPY FOR SPORTS INJURIES

Because injured athletes often desire to return to their game as soon as possible, Prolotherapy injections may be given once every one to two weeks instead of every four to six weeks. This is because athletes do not have the time to wait to grow tissue. They desire tissue growth and they want it now! Sometimes stronger solutions are used to help increase the speed of the healing process. This is not the ideal situation, however. A preferred treatment regimen is for athletes to receive Prolotherapy treatments during their off-season so that by the start of the season the injury is healed.

PERSONAL EXPERIENCE WITH PROLOTHERAPY

Dr. Hauser has personally experienced the success of Prolotherapy for a number of sports injuries he has sustained over the years. Dr. Hauser has completed five Ironman triathlons. An Ironman race is a marathon in three sports – 2.4 mile swim, 112 mile bike, and a 26.2 mile marathon run all in the same day. The training for this is rigorous to say the least.

Dr. Hauser threw out his back just weeks before his second Ironman race due to an improper bike fitting. He could not even sit or stand upright. He had been training for this race for nearly a year, so you can imagine the disappointment he felt. He received Prolotherapy to his back and sacroiliac joints twice before the race. Fortunately Prolotherapy saved him and he was able to complete the race, improving his time one hour compared to his previous race!

Marion has experienced her share of Prolotherapy treatments as well for a wide array of sports injuries, including shin splints, meniscal tears, and IT band injuries. We are personally familiar with the healing power of Prolotherapy for sports injuries. Many professional, as well as amateur athletes have come through our office doors, most importantly, leaving with the ability to return to playing their sports. It saddens us when we read in emails or in the news about athletes who undergo surgery for a sports injury without trying Prolotherapy. Surgery often ends or severely limits an athletic career!

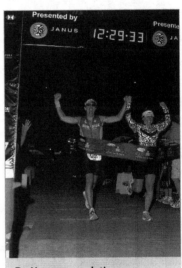

Dr. Hauser completing an Ironman with Marion running alongside him for the final push.

SUMMARY

In summary, sports injuries are caused because muscle, tendon, or ligament tissue is too weak to perform a particular task. Treatment regimens for soft tissue injury, such as taking ibuprofen and applying ice to the area to reduce inflammation, or undergoing surgery to remove tissue, often provide pain relief but cause incomplete healing, making the athlete prone to re-injury.

A better approach to treatment of sports injuries, more than just pain control, is complete healing of the injured tissue. Prolotherapy, because it stimulates the growth of ligament and tendon tissue, helps sports injuries heal faster. While surgery causes tissue to become weaker, Prolotherapy helps form stronger tissue.

Because athletes want to continue playing their sports without a reduction in ability or fear of reinjury, many are choosing to Prolo their sports injuries away! ■

CHAPTER

15

PROLO YOUR KID'S INJURIES AWAY!

PROLOTHERAPY FOR INJURIES IN YOUNG ATHLETES

There is nothing that makes a Prolotherapist happier than seeing a teenager or a young person come in for Prolotherapy. Children, adolescents, and young adults are growing collagen so rapidly that they usually require just one or two Prolotherapy treatments to heal their injuries. This is why we felt it was necessary to include a chapter on young people's pain. When we're talking about young athletes who are at risk of missing a whole season, forgoing athletic scholarships, or not being able to compete, these missed opportunities can alter one's life path forever. At Caring Medical, we have had the honor to see joy return to the faces of many young athletes and their parents after Prolotherapy has helped get their athletics back on track. Whether it is a soccer injury resulting in an ACL tear, pain from osteochondritis dissecans in pitchers, Osgood-Schlatter disease, or a host of other injuries, Prolotherapy should be considered a first-line treatment.

GROWING PAINS: THEY ARE FOR REAL

Younger athletes suffer many of the same injuries as their adult counterparts. However, there are also some significant differences in the type of injuries sustained by adolescents because of the differences in the structure of growing bone compared with adult bone. The other significant fact is that bone growth occurs at a different rate than ligament, tendon, and muscle growth; which in a young person, can produce its own set of problems. *(See Figure 15-1.)*

The differences between adult bone and growing bone include the following:

1. The articular cartilage of growing bone is of greater depth than that of adult bone and is able to undergo remodeling at a faster rate.

2. The junction between the epiphyseal plate and metaphysis is vulnerable to disruption, especially from shearing forces.

3. Tendon and ligament attachment sites, the apophyses, are cartilaginous plates that provide a relatively weak cartilaginuous attachment, predisposing the young athlete to the development of avulsion injuries.

SITE	MECHANISM	INJURY IN ADULT	INJURY IN CHILD
Thumb	Valgus force as in "skier's thumb"	Sprain of ulnar collateral ligament	Fracture of proximal phalangeal physis
Distal interphalangeal joint of finger	Hyperflexion injury	Mallet finger	Fracture of distal phalangeal epiphysis
Hand	Punching injury as in boxing	Fracture of metacarpal head	Fracture of distal epiphysis
Shoulder	Fall on point of shoulder	AC joint sprain	Fracture of distal clavicle epiphysis
Shoulder	Abduction and external rotation force	Dislocated shoulder rotator cuff tear	Fracture of proximal humeral epiphysis
Thigh/Hip	Acute flexor muscle strain or extensor strain	Quadriceps strain or hamstring strain	Apophyseal avulsion of anterior inferior iliac spine
Knee	Overuse injury	Patellar tendonitis	Osgood-Schlatter disease
Knee	Acute trauma (e.g., skiing injury)	Meniscal or ligament injury	Fractured distal femoral epiphysis
Heel	Overuse	Achilles tendonitis	Sever's apophysitis

Figure 15-1: Comparison of injuries that occur with similar mechanisms in adults and children.

4. The metaphysis of long bones in children is more resilient and elastic, withstanding greater deflection without fracture, compared to adults. Thus, children tend to suffer incomplete fractures of the greenstick type, which do not occur in adults.

5. During rapid growth phases, bone lengthens before muscles, tendons, and ligaments are able to stretch correspondingly and before the musculotendinous complex develops the necessary strength and coordination to control the newly lengthened bone. This may lead to muscle, tendon, and ligament injuries, or to a reduction in coordination.

6. In adults, the weakest link of the ligament-bone junction is the ligament, whereas in younger athletes, the ligament attachment to bone is relatively strong compared to the apophysis. Thus, the younger athlete is more likely to injure cartilage and bone or completely avulse an apophysis than to have a significant ligament sprain.[1]

Of special note is the area of the young, growing bone called the epiphysis. Growth areas called epiphyses occur at both ends of long bones in children and adolescents. *(See Figure 15-2.)* Bone grows from this area to make the child's bones longer. This is what allows the child's arms and legs to grow to the appropriate normal length. These epiphyses areas "close" at an average age of 14.5 years for girls, and 16.5 years for boys. These are the ages when most people just about reach their adult height. An important fact to note is that these areas are the weakest

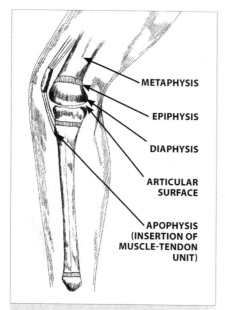

Figure 15-2: Different parts of the growing bone. The metaphysis, the epiphysis, the diaphysis and the articular cartilage are common sites of sports injury in the young athlete.

Labels in figure:
- METAPHYSIS
- EPIPHYSIS
- DIAPHYSIS
- ARTICULAR SURFACE
- APOPHYSIS (INSERTION OF MUSCLE-TENDON UNIT)

parts of the bone. The ligaments are 300% stronger than the epiphyseal area in a Tanner Stage 3 child (period of maximum growth). It is this weak area that is prone to injury in active children and adolescents.[2]

CLASSIFICATION OF GROWTH PLATE INJURIES

The Salter and Harris classification of growth plate injuries is commonly used to describe injuries to the growth plate. The Salter 1 injury is a nondisplaced fracture. The x-ray is often normal and according to traditional orthopedic teaching, this can cause the examining practitioner to miss the diagnosis. The diagnosis should be based on clinical findings of point tenderness over the epiphyseal area.[3] Types 1 and 2 have excellent prognoses for prompt healing and no residual problems or growth disturbance. Types 3 and 4 require open reduction and internal fixation (surgery) and have a more guarded prognosis. Lastly, Type 5 can go unrecognized and has the potential to lead to major growth disturbances. *(See Figure 15-3.)*

The traditional orthopedic surgeon's recommendation for a young athlete with a normal x-ray and palpatory tenderness is rest. However, the RICE treatment (Rest, Ice, Compression, Elevation) is detrimental not only to the ligaments and tendons, but also to articular cartilage. Diminished weight-bearing has been shown to lead to degeneration of the articular cartilage.[4] Activity and weight-bearing are necessary to maintain the biochemical and structural integrity of ligaments and tendons, as well as cartilage growth.[5,6] We feel that a much better approach for the young athlete is MEAT (Movement, Exercise, Analgesics, and specific Treatments, such as Prolotherapy). There are many situations where this choice can mean the difference between a life in sports or a life in pain.

OSTEOCHONDRITIS DISSECANS

Osteochondritis dissecans (OD) is a localized injury or condition affecting an articular surface of a joint, that involves separation of a segment of cartilage and subchondral bone. It is found most commonly in the knee although other joints can be affected, notably the elbow, ankle and hip. OD affects two distinct populations of patients as differentiated by the status of the physes (growth plates). Children and adolescents between the ages of five and approximately 16 years-old,

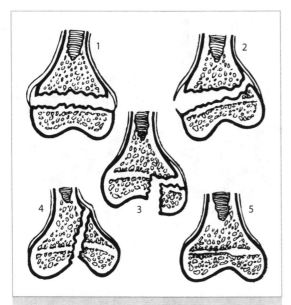

Figure 15-3: Salter-Harris classification of growth plate injuries. Used with permission: Peter Brukner. *Clinical Sports Medicine.* McGraw-Hill, New York City, NY, 1995, p.524.

who have open physes, are classified as having the juvenile form of the disease. Older adolescents, who have closed physes, and adults are classified as having the adult form.[7] Repetitive microtrauma is thought to be the primary mechanism responsible for the development of OD, however, other causes including acute trauma, ischemia, ossification abnormalities and genetic factors have also been proposed.[8,9]

In the February 2011 issue of the *Journal of Prolotherapy (JOP)*, we reported two studies of osteochondritis dissecans in young baseball players.[10] The first case was a 13 year-old pitcher with osteochondritis dissecans of the knee. He had been following the usual rest and ice recommendations from his other doctor, and was unable to return to sports for months. After only two Prolotherapy treatments, J.C. reported a 75% improvement, and was back to running and jumping. In total, he needed four treatments to get back to sports 100%. He continued to be very active in sports through his college years. We shudder to think that J.C. might have had to give up all athletics through high school, college, and beyond had it not been for Prolotherapy.

The second case published in *JOP* was that of another 13 year-old pitcher, L.M. His MRI revealed osteochondritis dissecans of the capitellum. **(See Figure 15-4.)** He had not been able to pitch for six months by the time he came to Caring Medical, after having an orthopedist tell him that he will never pitch again. Lucky for L.M. his family continued to

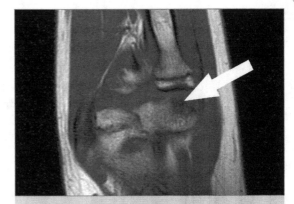

Figure 15-4: MRI right elbow without contrast, prior to Prolotherapy. The arrow points to the evolving osteochondral defect involving the capitellum typical of osteochondritis dissecans. The defect is stable without evidence of in situ loose body.

search for better options. We worked with L.M. over the course of three Prolotherapy treatments, in which he was able to increase his time spent pitching, in addition to weight lifting, swimming, and running. On repeat MRI, resolution of the osteochondritis dissecans was revealed. *(See Figure 15-5.)* More importantly, L.M. has been able to pitch and participate in sports without restriction after Prolotherapy. Isn't that fantastic? We think so too!

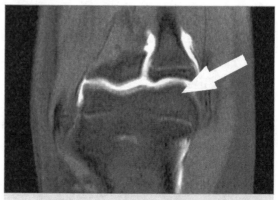

Figure 15-5: MRI right elbow with intra-articular contrast, after Prolotherapy. Arrows show resolution of the articular cartilage fraying, as well as the subchondral cystic changes. Improvement of the subchondral edema with almost complete resolution of the osteochondral lesion.

OSGOOD-SCHLATTER DISEASE: APOPHYSITIS OF THE KNEE

Chronic knee pain may develop in young people, especially teenage boys, and is often due to Osgood-Schlatter disease, a condition whereby the tibial tubercle becomes painful where the patellar tendon attaches to the tibia. *(See Figure 15-6.)* Pain occurs because the tendon attaches to the same area of the tibia that is growing. The pain is exacerbated by physical activity, especially running and jumping, and often limits participation in sports, resulting in the young athlete's physician recommending cessation of playing sports. Needless to say, this advice is not popular. A better treatment is to strengthen the fibro–osseous junction of the patellar tendon onto the tibial tubercle, eliminating the problem.

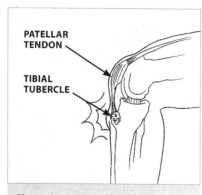

Figure 15-6: Osgood-Schlatter disease. Patellar tendon weakness leads to tibial tubercle swelling that is characteristic of Osgood-Schlatter disease.

PATELLAR TENDON

TIBIAL TUBERCLE

In a small study published in 1993, Prolotherapy was 83% effective in eliminating the pain of Osgood-Schlatter disease.[11] In this study only one to two treatments were needed to resolve the problem.

Topal et al. conducted a double-blind randomized, placebo-controlled study of 54 subjects with Osgood-Schlatter disease.[12] The participants were randomized into injections of either dextrose with lidocaine (38), lidocaine (13), or usual care, i.e., supervised exercise (14). Injections were given at zero, one, and two months. At one year from the start of the study, the group with the best scores (0 on the Nirschl Pain Phase

Scale, NPPS) for asymptomatic sport were the dextrose-treated knees (32 of 38), compared with only lidocaine (6 of 13) or usual care (2 of 14).

LIGAMENT LAXITY: A FORGOTTEN ENTITY IN CHILDREN

Joint laxity, or the looseness of a joint, can create a fine balance between an athlete's ability to excel in sport and the likelihood of injury. A good example of this is gymnastics. The greater the joint laxity in the child, the more likely that child will be able to do all of the required contortion movements in gymnastics. Hypermobile joints are exhibited by being able to do things such as bending the elbow or knee past the point of neutral, doing the splits, touching the floor with the palm while bending forward at the waist, or touching the thumb to the forearm. While these antics are often used for entertainment by flexible children, repetition can lead to sustained laxity and injury down the line. *(See Figure 15-7.)*

As we have been noting throughout the book, ligament laxity creates joint instability, which leads to osteoarthritis, chronic pain, bone spurs, etc... Applying this knowledge to young people can help save them a lifetime of those events. Excessive joint laxity is the main risk factor for recurrent ligamentous injury.[13] Pathologic joint laxity, especially about the knee and shoulder, are the main risk

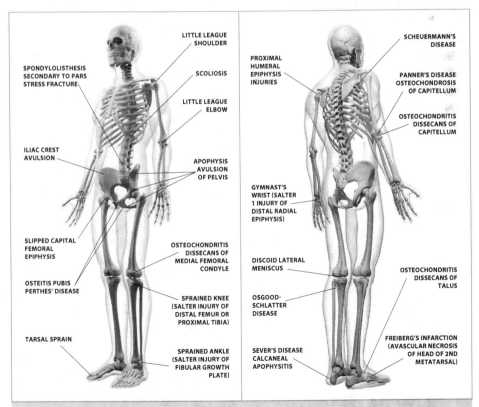

Figure 15-7: Common sites of musculoskeletal injuries in adolescent athletes.
Prolotherapy can help all of these injuries heal quickly!

factors for young athletes for recurrent problems in these areas.[14-16] If the joint laxity is not addressed, joint dislocations occur with the end result being osteoarthritis.[17,18] As a young person continues to dislocate, their chance of developing osteoarthritis as an adult increases.

CHOOSING REGENERATIVE MEDICINE AT A YOUNGER AGE

We have seen patients in their 20s who have already been recommended for a joint replacement. The reason for such dramatic recommendations is due to the effect of cortisone injections, RICE, pain prescriptions, and other traditional treatments done at a young age. Parents and young patients need to understand that the traditional methods are not always the best idea in the long-term. As we've discussed, RICE and NSAIDs are detrimental to a child's long-term musculoskeletal health. If those methods fail and then orthopedic surgery is done with poor results, you cannot undo that surgery. It can begin a string of additional surgeries trying to chase the pain. On the other hand, seeking a practitioner who understands joint laxity and restoration, along with sports mechanics, can take the young athlete down a more curative path. *(See Figure 15-8.)* Most physicians do not know how to adequately examine a patient for joint mobility and ligament laxity. Therefore, consulting a Prolotherapy practitioner is a wise idea, and is especially important when a young person has chronic dislocations. Prolotherapy is a win-win for athletes, because they are able to continue exercising longer and harder as the body continues to heal over time. What's more is children typically need fewer treatments than adults with similar injuries.

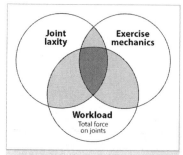

Figure 15-8: Risk factors for developing musculoskeletal injuries in adolescent athletes. Traditional sports medicine tries to modify workload (rest) and throwing mechanics in little league elbow for instance, but it does nothing to address the elbow joint laxity. Prolotherapy is successful at curing this and other growth plate and musculoskeletal injuries in young athletes because it strengthens the injured structures, specifically the ligaments which stabilize the lax joints.

SUMMARY

Children and teens respond extremely well to regenerative medicine treatments because they are in the growth phase of life: hormone levels, growth factors, and healing nutrient levels are very high. Kids often require only one treatment to achieve complete healing. Prolotherapy is a must for those kids involved in high level athletics who sustain sports injuries. It provides a fantastic method for young athletes to continue in their sports without a black mark on their sports resumes. For kids with congenital loose ligament issues, Prolotherapy helps them lead a normal life. They no longer need to stay home because they are in too much pain to be out with their friends. Do not underestimate the power of Prolotherapy for the young patient with an injury or painful condition! ■

CHAPTER

PROLO YOUR NERVE PAIN AWAY!

Joint instability and ligament injury are almost always the missing diagnoses, even in patients with nerve pain from such conditions as neuritis, neuroma, nerve entrapments, neuralgia, and unusual nerve syndromes. Nerves alert the brain of the presence of an injury or problem because they themselves are either being inflamed or undergoing neurogenic inflammation; entrapped or experiencing compression by nearby bone or myofascial tissue; or encountering excessive stretch.

As in other chronic painful conditions, patients seek all sorts of suppressive, ablative or surgical therapies for relief of nerve irritations not realizing that these treatments are actually causing more harm than good. **It is often not understood that ALL pain has a nerve component.** As in other sensations, pain is carried by nerves to the central nervous system ultimately to be interpreted and experienced by the brain. To understand how Prolotherapy and other natural injection therapies such as Lyftogt Perineural Injection Therapy™ and Nerve Release Injection Therapy (NRIT), can resolve, correct, decompress, and cure, the various nerve pain disorders, it is necessary to provide an overview understanding that pain comes from four different sources. Once you understand this key concept, it is very simple to understand why the curative treatment of nerve pain must be in the realm of natural regenerative injection therapies because only these treatments can truly resolve neurogenic inflammation, nerve entrapment, and the excessive stretching of nerves by tightening ligaments and restoring joint stability, whether directly or indirectly!

The four primary causes of almost all painful conditions are excessive stretch of a primary ligament, the many harmful effects of joint instability, neurogenic inflammation, and nerve entrapment. *(See Figure 16-1.)*

Four Causes of Almost All Chronic Pain

1. Ligament laxity
2. Manifestations of joint instability
3. Neurogenic inflammation
4. Nerve entrapment

Figure 16-1: Four primary causes of almost all painful conditions.

LIGAMENTS ARE WHY WE HAVE PAIN

While ligaments are predominantly known as the stabilizing agents of the joints, they have an equally important role as a sensory organ for the joint. They contain many nerve endings (called Ruffini, Pacician and Golgi free-nerve endings) that are very sensitive to stretch. The brain is notified if they (or the joint) are under too much tension. If the tension is too great, then they stimulate muscle contraction via the ligamento-muscular reflex. *(See Figure 16-2.)* The muscles contract to preserve joint stability. The sharp pain experienced during activity or trauma is from the ligament being stretched too much, but the low level long-term pain is from the chronic muscle spasms.

THE MANY PAINFUL EFFECTS OF JOINT INSTABILITY

A myriad of consequences from joint instability unfold once a ligament becomes injured besides just the nerve endings within the ligament firing to produce pain. Once a joint begins excessively moving, the body will compensate in almost all of the structures involved in that particular joint, including the other

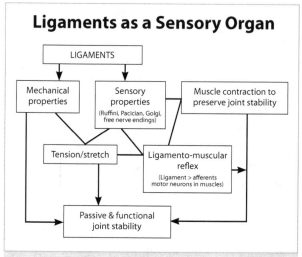

Figure 16-2: Ligaments as a sensory organ.
Basic organizational plan adapted from Johansson H, Sojka P. A Sensory Role for the Cruciate Ligaments. *Clinical Orthopaedics and Related Research.* 1991; (268): 161-178.

ligaments, tendons, muscles, and other stabilizing structures such as menisci, discs, labrum, as well as the nerves that supply the joints. These compensatory changes initially produce beneficial effects to temporarily stabilize the joint and disperse the forces more evenly across the joint by tightening various muscles and swelling the joint. This process works fine for a few days, a week, possibly a few weeks, but it was never meant to be the long-term solution. If you think about it, at this point, the injured patient has three sources of pain: the original ligament injury, the muscle spasms, and the joint swelling.

At this point, patients are at a crossroad and need to decide on one of two paths: the path of healing or the path of destruction. *(See Figure 16-3.)* The correct path, the one that ends with a healthy, stable joint, involves undergoing Prolotherapy by an experienced comprehensive Prolotherapist. Think of that person as a joint mechanic! Mechanics fix things. By obtaining Prolotherapy at this early stage, complete healing is most likely only going to require one or two visits! Unfortunately, some injured patients go to practitioners who suppress the many manifestations of the joint instability, such as muscle spasm and joint swelling. Once these treatments are received, such as anti-inflammatory medications, corticosteroid injections, and muscle relaxants, the joint is put in an unprotected, unstable state making it very vulnerable to worsening and further injury. This then leads down the path of joint destruction and often leads to various potentially harmful surgeries.

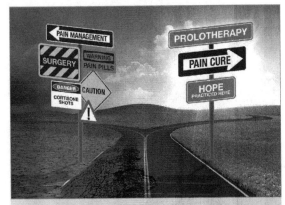

Figure 16-3. The crossroads of pain therapy. Every person has a choice to go down either road. One ends in joint replacement. The other leads to enjoying your favorite activities pain-free.

COVERING UP PAIN IS NEVER GOOD

Think about it, if your house was on fire and the smoke detectors were sounding, would it be in your best interest to remove the batteries in the smoke detectors so the alarms stopped blaring or should you actually put out the fire or call the fire department? When patients receive pain suppressing therapies, such as corticosteroid shots, anti-inflammatory, narcotic or muscle relaxation medications or receive radiofrequency ablation or neurectomy and other pain sensation removing therapies, they are, in essence, not allowing the body to "sound the pain alarms."

For a family to go about their normal business during a fire, just because the alarm is not sounding would be absolutely deadly! The same is true when an athlete suppresses the pain of an injury. Playing tennis or performing other exercises or activities while pain is blocked could, in essence, be doing the same thing to the injured area as the fire did to the house!

Pain protects the body from further harming itself. Anyone who receives pain suppression therapies runs the risk of increasing the joint damage to such a point that even Prolotherapy will not be able to work! We recommend not removing the batteries when the alarm is going off and running, not walking, to the nearest experienced Comprehensive Prolotherapist!

JOINT INSTABILITY IS ALWAYS A PROGRESSIVE DISORDER!

The long term manifestations of joint instability include the following: autonomic nervous system dysfunction, radiculopathies, tendinopathies, recurrent joint swelling, chronic muscle spasms, accelerated joint degeneration, myofascial restrictions, nerve entrapments, and neurogenic inflammation. As the scenario is likely to be repeated in the next adjacent joints, it is really easy to understand that unresolved joint instability can progress very quickly to severe chronic disabling

pain and joint degeneration.
(See Figure 16-4.)

When thinking about all
of the various pain treatments
utilized, including botulism
injections, medications or
supplements, radiofrequency
ablation, electrothermal
coagulation, massage
therapy, electrical stimulation
treatments, exercise, and
epidural injections, it makes
sense that these have little hope
of *curing* pain, on account that
they treat the manifestations,
not *the cause* of the pain, which is joint instability.

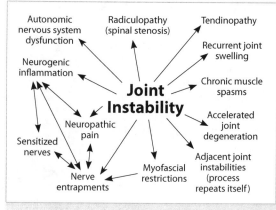

Figure 16-4. The many painful long-term manifestations of joint instability.

Unresolved long-term joint instability causes forces to be concentrated on the same side of the primary injury, accelerating articular cartilage, tendon, meniscus, labrum, or disc injury on that particular side of the joint. **(See Figure 16-5.)** As the unresolved process lingers, muscles and tendons fatigue, no longer able to limit joint motion. A subtle change in bony anatomical alignment results, on the order of 1-2 mm. This small change causes microinstability of the joint which leads to myofascial restrictions, as well as irritation to the local milieu of nerves. This subtle microinstabilty can directly and/or indirectly cause inflammation, entrapment, and excessive stretching of the nerves. These nerves become hyperirritable,
swollen, and inflamed, causing the
symptoms of allodynia and hyperalgesia
which are characteristic of neuropathic
pain. Allodynia occurs when a non-
painful stimulus, like a very gentle
touch or stretch, is extremely painful.
Hyperalgesia involves an exaggerated
pain response to something that is
minimally painful.

This stretchability of the nervous
system has normal and abnormal
limits. Under normal conditions, nerve
fibers are able to comply with low
to moderate strain or compression
associated with physiological (normal)
joint movements. When nerves are
healthy no pain signals are produced
with normal motions or stretch.

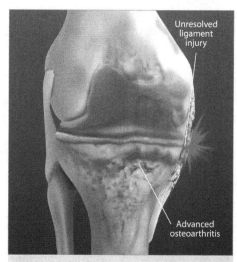

Figure 16-5. Accelerated articular cartilage degeneration from unresolved joint instability. Joint deterioration is typically worse on the side of the primary ligament injury.

A normal nerve can stretch approximately 6% without any damage or resultant symptoms. Mechanotransduction is the process whereby the nerves tell the body what is going on with regard to a force. A normal pressure or motion is not painful; however when local inflammation occurs in a nerve, then normal physiological pressures and motions can cause significant pain. This is called pressure mechanosensitivity and can be documented by local tenderness over the nerve with palpation or various movements. *(See Figure 16-6.)* This occurs due to neurogenic inflammation. Once these small nerves are inflamed, they can produce a pain signal with as little as only 3% stretch, which occurs with just normal motions.[1]

When normal motions and pressures produce significant symptoms, the diagnosis is neuropathic pain. This can accompany ligament injury and joint instability or be present by itself. This sounds bad, doesn't it? However! There is hope! We have a solution! The small nerve inflammation can be easily turned off by injecting 5% dextrose around the nerve, a process called Lyftogt Perineural Injection Therapy (LPIT)!

Perhaps the most underappreciated but most profound long-term manifestations of joint instability are nerve entrapments, radiculopathy (spinal stenosis), and autonomic nervous system dysfunction. The body will do whatever it takes to protect the spinal cord, spinal nerves, and peripheral nerves, even

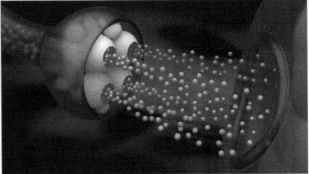

Figure 16-6. Sensitized inflamed small nerve. An inflamed nerve releases substances that not only cause pain at rest, but also allodynia, the hallmark of neuropathic pain. Allodynia is a type of pressure mechanosensitivity where a very soft pressure on the skin, where the nerve is located, causes excruciating pain.

encasing them in bone (spinal vertebrae), or having them run close to bone or in bony tunnels. The course through which all nerves run to get to their final destination contains only 1-2 mm of extra space.

Another way to look at this: at some point a nerve is within 1-2 mm of a bone or bony prominence as it zig zags from its origin through the myofascial plane between muscles, through bony tunnels to its end point. *(See Figure 16-7.)* As a person with stable joints goes about their daily activities, including exercise and sports, adjacent bones normally move about 1-2 mm. This extremely small space is what prevents the bone from hitting the nerve. When the joint is unstable, however, the bones that make up the joint move excessively resulting in the nerve being hit or compressed producing zinging pain and/or numbness. *(See Figure 16-8.)* The compression (inflammation) of the nerve can also be documented with ultrasound. *(See Figure 16-9.)* The key characteristic finding to determine that the nerve irritation is coming from joint instability is that the main

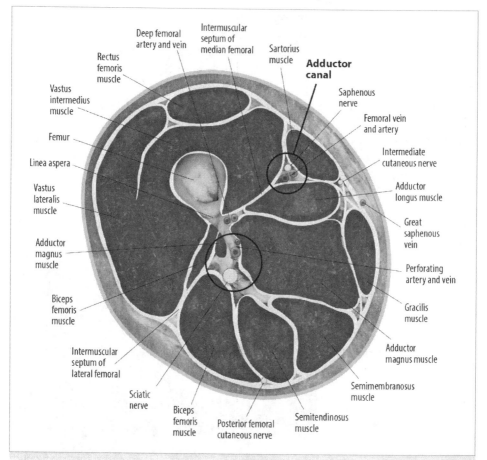

Figure 16-7. The nerve highway. As can be seen by this cross-section of the thigh, the nerves, arteries, and veins often run together between the muscles in what is called the myofascial planes.

symptom is *positional*. This can be any kind of symptom, including numbness, or even more unusual or bizarre symptoms such as tremors, dystonia, temperature changes in your limbs, torticollis, vertigo, dizziness, ringing in the ears, numb tongue, swallowing difficulties, burning mouth, unexplained muscle spasms, or unexplained stiffness in the body. When symptoms can be decreased or increased significantly by a certain movement or position, then joint instability is most likely an instigating cause of the condition and will need to be treated for long-term resolution.

When a nerve is compressed but the body wants it to stretch because the rest of the body is moving, the nerve will release a painful nerve impulse and if the compression goes on for too long, the tissues the nerve supplies can actually start to die and muscle atrophy and loss of sensation can result. So when a large nerve is compressed, such as a nerve root or the sciatic nerve, the condition needs to be taken very seriously as *irreversible* nerve damage may occur. Any type of nerve irritation should be addressed sooner rather than later. Determining which nerve compressions or entrapments require a Prolotherapist for treatment and which need a surgeon is extremely important!

When a patient can eliminate or significantly reduce a symptom by placing himself in a particular position, such as lying down, or placing his arm or leg in a certain position, then almost assuredly the underlying cause of that symptom is joint instability. Even a patient who has been diagnosed with a pinched nerve in the neck or low back will normally report the ability to get into a comfortable position when lying down, where the arm or leg pain is significantly reduced. Generally, pinched nerves in the neck feel better when looking down (versus looking up at the sky); whereas pinched nerves in the lower back feel better when the patient sits down vs standing or walking. This improvement of neck pain and arm pain with the head facing down and the improvement of low back pain and leg pain vanishing when sitting down are clues that the symptoms are positional and should respond to Prolotherapy!

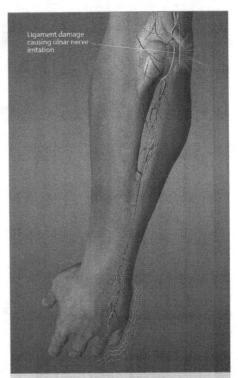

Figure 16-8. Ulnar collateral ligament (UCL) injury causing ulnar neuritis. UCL injury causes valgus instability of the elbow which can cause the humerus and/or ulna bones to touch and irritate the ulnar nerve. Prolotherapy, by correcting the elbow instability, resolves this cause of ulnar neuritis.

If we could view the nerve when the patient is in the **asymptomatic** position, we would see that the nerve is not being compressed or touched by any bone in

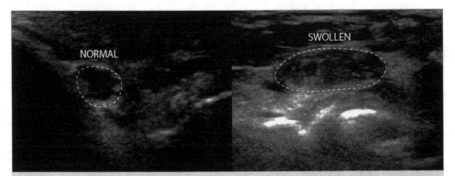

Figure 16-9. Normal and swollen ulnar nerve at elbow. Ultrasound can show nerve entrapments, such as this one in a patient with ulnar nerve entrapment of the elbow, or cubital tunnel syndrome.

Modified from: Soo-Jung Choi, et al. Ultrasonography for nerve compression syndromes of the upper extremity. Ultrasonography. 2015;34(4):275-291. Figures 8 & 9.

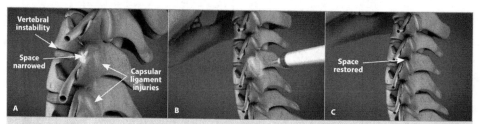

Figure 16-10. Resolution of nerve space in intervertebral foramen. Prolotherapy resolves pinched nerves by stabilizing joint movement as ligaments tighten. **A.** Capsular ligament injury. **B.** Prolotherapy to the cervical facet joints. **C.** Restoration of nerve space in intervertebral foramen.

that position! Likewise the nerve space narrows when microinstabilty is present, while taking on other positions or movements which produce symptoms. We call this process dynamic (with movement) nerve compression. The treatment of choice for this latter condition is Comprehensive Prolotherapy to resolve the joint instability and keep the space for the nerve open. *(See Figure 16-10.)*

We must point out that dynamic nerve compression even applies when the patient has been given diagnoses of degenerative arthritis, osteophytes, or spinal stenosis. If symptoms are aggravated by a certain position or movement, then they have a dynamic quality, and are thus most likely going to be successfully treated with Prolotherapy. If the symptom(s) is constant, which is called static compression, signifying symptoms 24/7 and in all positions and activities, then most likely joint instability is **not** the cause and a decompression surgery may be necessary.

NERVE SYNDROMES

The nerve entrapment and unusual pain syndromes (and its various names) are classified according to the anatomical part affected as facial, trigeminal, occipital, intercostal and according to the cause as in diabetes. *(See Figure 16-11.)* Thus, a nerve pain in the location of the trigeminal

Nerve	Place	Condition
Abdominal cutaneous nerve	Abdominal wall	Abdominal cutaneous nerve entrapment syndrome
Common peroneal	Fibular neck	Peroneal nerve compression
Digital	Metatarsal head	Morton's neuroma
Femoral	Inguinal canal	Femoral nerve entrapment syndrome
Iliohypogastric	Lower abdomen	Iliohypogastric nerve entrapment
Lateral femoral cutaneous nerve	Inguinal ligament	Meralgia paresthetic
Medial plantar	Navicular bone	Jogger's foot
Obturator	Obturator canal	Obturator nerve entrapment
Pudendal	Pelvis	Pudendal nerve entrapment
Saphenous nerve	Adductor canal	Saphenous nerve entrapment
Sciatic	Piriformis	Deep gluteal syndrome (piriformis syndrome)
Super gluteal	Piriformis	Superior gluteal nerve entrapment syndrome
Tibial	Tarsal tunnel	Tarsal tunnel syndrome

Figure 16-11. Common lower limb, abdomen and pelvis nerve entrapments.

nerve would be called trigeminal neuralgia. All trigeminal neuralgia means is nerve pain in the nerve distribution of the trigeminal nerve. It actually does not tell a person anything about what is causing the condition. When a physician and a patient believe that a nerve is getting compressed it is easy to see why a surgery would be recommended. Unfortunately, when joint instability is the cause of the neuralgia, the surgery does not help relieve the pain. When a person has peripheral neuropathy from diabetes it is called diabetic neuropathy. Even diabetic peripheral neuropathy is helped when the compressed nerves are released.[2]

Many nerve syndromes have joint instability (and thus ligament injury) as their underlying etiology. *(See Figure 16-12.)* The easiest of these to understand is when a nerve is entrapped in a tunnel such as the median nerve in the carpal tunnel. These bony tunnels are designed to protect key structures such as arteries and nerves, but again the space is pretty crowded. Nerves often traverse through tunnels or narrow bony canals. At their limiting (smallest) height, depth or width the most common nerve tunnels including the cubital, carpal, and tarsal tunnels are less than 10mm.[3-5] This amount of space is decreased by certain positions and movements.[6-8] When the space in the tunnel becomes reduced, the nerve is compressed, the pressure inside the nerve rises which compromises its microvascular blood supply and leads to focal ischemia of the nerve. This in turns leads to demyelination (disruption of outer coating of the nerve), which disrupts nerve signal transmission; prolonged compression can lead to more permanent damage to the neurons themselves, including degeneration distal to the point of compression. The neurogenic inflammation and ischemia also leads to fibrosis (scarring), which can further tether the nerve and lead to more traction (stretch) injury during motion.

Nerve Syndromes and Associated Joint Instabilities

Medical condition	Nerve	Joint instability	Ligaments involved
Carpal tunnel syndrome	Median	Wrist and/or elbow	Dorsal wrist (radial collateral) & lateral elbow (annular)
Cervical radiculopathy	Cervical nerve root	Cervical facet joint	Capsular
Cubital tunnel syndrome	Ulnar	Elbow	Ulnar collateral
Intercostal neuralgia	Intercostal	Thoracic spine	Costotransverse, capsular
Lumbar radiculopathy	Lumbar nerve root	Lumbar facet joint	Capsular
Occipital neuralgia	Upper cervical	Cervical facet	Capsular
Peroneal neuralgia	Peroneal	Knee	Lateral, collateral, arcuate
Piriformis syndrome	Sciatic	Sacroiliac	Sacroiliac
Pudendal neuralgia	Pudendal	Pelvis	Sacrotuberous, pubis, sacroiliac
Tarsal tunnel syndrome	Tibial	Ankle	Deltoid
Trigeminal neuralgia	Upper cervical	Cervical facet	Capsular

Figure 16-12: Nerve irritation and entrapment syndromes and their associated joint instabilities. These painful conditions respond well to Prolotherapy when the underlying cause is joint instability.

The ability of peripheral nerves (and also ligaments) to stretch and slide is of paramount importance to maintain ideal neural function. Like ligaments, nerves can stretch to a certain degree. **When a nerve becomes sensitized, meaning injured and neurogenic inflammation sets in, the nerve is no longer stretchable and will produce severe stinging pain when stretched even a little.** In the office, when a patient asks on the first visit, "Please don't move my leg, or touch these specific spots because they are so sensitive," we know that a neurogenic inflammation in some of the nerves is present. Healthy nerves do not elicit pain with normal movement. When a nerve is irritated with normal movements or pressure, you know that the nerve is experiencing neurogenic inflammation.

Pain from a sensitized nerve may be treated with four different types of regenerative injections: Cellular Prolotherapy, Hackett-Hemwall Prolotherapy, Lyftogt Perineural Injection Therapy (LPIT), and Nerve Release Injection Therapy (NRIT). *(See Figure 16-13.)* When joint instability is the primary etiology of the neuropathic pain (nerve being sensitized) then either Cellular or Hackett-Hemwall Prolotherapy is given. When the nerve is located superficially or is larger and easy to identify then LPIT is given. When the nerve involved is deep and/or entrapped, then an ultrasound-guided nerve release injection technique (NRIT) is used.

To better understand why certain natural nerve injection techniques are used it is important to understand how a nerve travels from the lower back to the tips of the toes, or the neck to the tips of the fingers without normally becoming compressed. As nerves traverse from deep within the body to their final destinations, they travel between the muscles in fascial tissues along with the arteries and veins. This is how a person can lift heavy weights and contract muscles and not compress the nerves. Nerves, however, can get compressed in

Natural Injection Therapies and Proposed Mechanism of Action	
Type of Injection Therapy	**Mechanism of Action**
Cellular Prolotherapy	Injection of biologics (cells) to stimulate repair in cellular deficient tissue
Hackett-Hemwall Prolotherapy	Injection of nonbiologics (dextrose) to enhance soft tissue repair to resolve joint instability
Lyftogt Perineural Injection	Restore normal function of sensitized peptidergic nerves
Nerve Release Injection Therapy	Release entrapped nerves from underlying tissue

Figure 16-13: Natural injection therapies and proposed mechanism of action.

the fascial layers by various constrictions in the fascia, especially where bony prominences or places where the nerve has to change direction. These places are said to cause a chronic constriction injury to the nerves causing them to swell and become painful. These sensory (peptidergic) nerves pierce the fascia to get to the subcutaneous tissues including the ligaments, tendons, and skin. Once the pressure in the nerve rises about 30mmHG, axonal flow within the nerve can stop. Since these nerves are involved in the health maintenance and renewal of the tissues they innervate, including ligaments, it is best for everyone that they remain healthy!

We often treat nerves along with the ligaments when a person has joint instability, with the hopes of speeding healing! Often repetitive motions or repetitive strains pinch the peptidergic nerves as they exit the fascia. LPIT is done at the sites of nerve restriction and inflammation, relieving the constriction and restoring homeostasis to the nerve. **(See Figure 16-14.)** LPIT was discovered by a family physician from New Zealand, John Lyftogt, MD, who published several papers on it, demonstrating its efficacy.[9-11] One interesting fact is the term inflammation neuritis was used in several papers by Dr. George Hackett, the inventor of Prolotherapy. He felt that neurogenic inflammation also could lead to a myriad of medical conditions including ligament weakness and bone decalcification.[12-16] As it turns out, he was right!

NERVE ENTRAPMENT

There are many nerve syndromes, such as carpal tunnel syndrome, that clearly involve entrapment of a certain nerve. The median nerve which supplies many of the muscles and sensations in the hand resides in the carpal tunnel of the wrist. The carpal tunnel walls are lined by bone on the sides and bottom and a tough fibrous tissue on the top called the transverse carpal ligament. The bones that comprise the walls of the carpal tunnel (as in

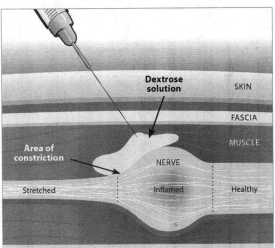

Figure 16-14: Chronic constriction injury of a nerve. The dextrose solution used during Prolotherapy draws excessive fluid out of the inflamed nerve, via osmosis, to resolve the constriction.

other bony tunnels) are connected to other bones which make up the wrist. When a person sustains a wrist ligament injury, the adjacent bones can move too much, thus narrowing the carpal tunnel. In this instance, Prolotherapy would decompress the nerve and open up the space by limiting the wrist bone movement through joint stabilization. **(See Figure 16-15.)**

A key clue that a nerve entrapment syndrome such as carpal tunnel syndrome stems from joint instability is associated cracking, popping, or clicking in the joints near the bony tunnel. On physical examination, other clues include excessive motion or soft joint end feel compared to the non–symptomatic side, as well as tenderness when the ligaments of the nearest joint are palpated and stressed. When these signs or symptoms are not present, the cause of the nerve entrapment is most likely not joint instability, thus a different type of natural injection therapy should be utilized: Nerve Release Injection Therapy (NRIT).

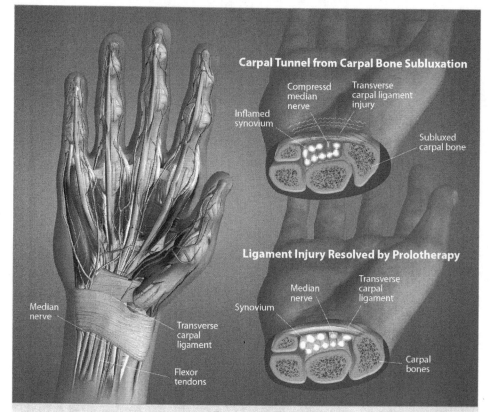

Figure 16-15. Carpal tunnel syndrome. One cause of median nerve compression is subluxation of the carpal bones from ligament injury. Prolotherapy decompresses the nerve by improving wrist joint stability and bony alignments.

NERVE RELEASE INJECTION THERAPY (NRIT)

NRIT involves the injection of natural substances to mechanically release the nerve (also called hydrodissection) but also to nourish and restore homeostasis. NRIT is done under ultrasound guidance to direct the solutions to the exact nerve entrapment location. **(See Figure 16-16.)** Because the nerve entrapment is resolved and the health of the nerve is immediately restored, the symptom–relieving effects are often felt instantly, right there in the office.

How many treatments of LPIT or NRIT are required? Sometimes just one, but often, approximately three to six visits are needed for permanent resolution of the nerve irritation and entrapment. Thus it is best to get in to see a Comprehensive Prolotherapist as soon as symptoms begin. People with long–term nerve entrapment may not fully recover. Do not delay!

Dr. Hauser's experience is a good example of this exact situation. One weekend he planted two trees in the back yard, which necessitated digging large holes with a shovel. As the clay ground in the back yard was not easily broken, he had to exert tremendous force with his foot onto the shovel in order to dig the holes. He developed an incredibly painful small spot on the medial side of his heel making

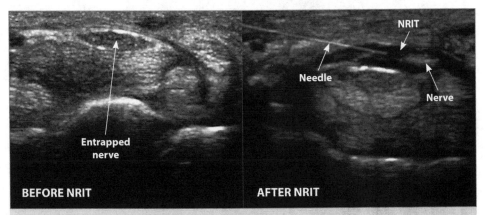

Figure 16-16. Ultrasound showing Nerve Release Injection Therapy (NRIT). You can clearly see the entrapped nerve in the before image. The median nerve is released in the after image.

walking very painful. The pain was in a very specific area on the medial side of his heal and increased in intensity over the day and became exquisitely point tender! Two days later, one of the Prolotherapists at the clinic, diagnosed him with inferior calcaneal neuralgia and treated him with NRIT. Four days later he was running hill repeats at almost 100% effort without pain! When nerve entrapment occurs without joint instability, it can be quickly relieved and treated just with NRIT!

CAUSES OF NERVE COMPRESSION/ENTRAPMENT

Any nerve in the body can become entrapped or compressed. The three main causes, from most to least prevalent, are joint instability, direct trauma, and degenerative arthritis. Far and away, the most common reason for nerve entrapment in the spine, whether the neck or the back, affecting the spinal nerve roots or autonomic nervous system is joint instability. It is common when patients come to our office to already have seen 5 or more doctors and been given diagnoses such as spinal stenosis, cervical radiculopathy, lumbar degenerative disc disease, and been told that they need various surgeries such as decompressive laminectomy with or without spinal fusion to decompress the compressed nerve and/or spinal cord. Again we cannot emphasize this enough, if the symptom is not present in a significant manner 24/7 and specific activities reduce the symptoms such as sitting or lying down, then dynamic joint instability is the correct diagnosis and Prolotherapy is the correct treatment. If the degenerative process is well-advanced, and it is causing a significant narrowing of the nerve canal and it is strangling the nerve 24/7, then clearly no motion or position will relieve symptoms. This type of static compression does affect nerve transmission and significant symptoms are normally present. If the nerve transmission is not going to your skin, you get a true numbness, and the same goes for muscles, as weakness and atrophy are seen. When these are present, and an MRI shows narrowing of the appropriate spinal nerve root from excessive bone spurring and arthritis, then surgical consultation is what is needed.

When given a diagnosis of any of the nerve pain conditions which commonly end with the words neuritis, neuralgia, neuroma, or syndrome, a person should **run**, not walk, to the nearest Prolotherapist and run, not walk, **away** from any neurologist or orthopedic surgeon! Most of these conditions are easily treated with one of the four natural injection therapy techniques described in this chapter. Yes, that means common conditions such as intercostal neuritis, occipital neuralgia, Morton's neuroma, as well as thoracic outlet or piriformis syndrome. If the syndrome involves an irritated, compressed, or sensitive (to stretch or touch) nerve, most likely a simple in-office natural injection technique is needed to restore the nerve to health along with all of the tissues it innervates!

THE CENTRAL NERVOUS SYSTEM

The nervous system of the body is akin to an electrical grid. At any point in the grid a blockage or short can occur. Everything we do, including our very thoughts, is related to the nervous system. Nerves connect your brain and spinal cord to everything in the body, including muscles, ligaments, skin, and organs, providing movement and feeling. Nerves are primarily responsible for the transmission of communication between cells and even between organs or joints and the brain. The function of the nerve is to deliver a message from one cell to another cell. In that sense, cells can function independently, as well as cooperatively. Rest assured, however, the local environment of the cell takes a priority compared to the organism as a whole. What does that mean? Let's take knee joint instability as an example. The nerves in and around the knee will be sensitized to this instability. They know something is wrong locally and will notify the brain by sending out pain signals. These sensitized nerves in the area of an injury, including joint instability, are said to have neurogenic inflammation, whereby the compressed nerves themselves release inflammatory substances such as substance P, histamine, interleukins, and cytokines that can cause significant local pain. Nerve homeostasis fortunately can be restored with natural injection therapy such as Lyftogt Perineural Injection Therapy. *(See Figure 16-17.)* If the injury is due to nerve compression, an interruption in the transformation of information occurs to the soft tissue end organs such as local muscles, ligaments, and skin. This can produce far-reaching effects to organs and even physiological changes in the central nervous system (brain and spinal cord) including the autonomic nervous system, which controls everything that happens in the body automatically such as breathing, heart rate, and blood flow. As you can see, these types of injuries need to be taken very seriously and treated as soon as possible.

The cervical spine can be thought of as the main passage way through which the central nervous system connects to the peripheral nervous system. Cervical instability may affect both the peripheral and central nervous systems, resulting in many unusual and often bizarre symptoms and syndromes. Caring Medical Regenerative Medicine Clinics has seen the following syndromes and symptoms

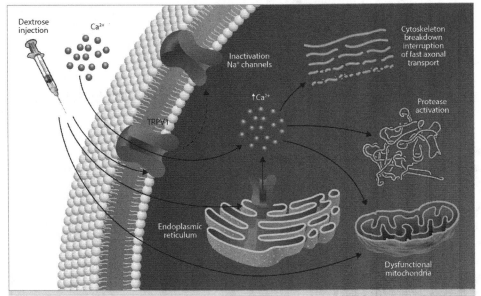

Figure 16-17. Lyftogt perineural injection into sensitized peptidergic nerve. The injections are felt to restore the normal function of the TRPV1 receptor on sensory neurons of the pain pathway. These nerves then help restore the tissues they innervate back to health.

from cervical instability: burning mouth syndrome, myoclonic storms, swallowing difficulty, small fiber neuropathy, fibromyalgia, hand tremor, cervical dystonia, torticollis, migraine headache, occipital neuralgia, adrenal fatigue, severe nausea, continuous belching, chronic sinusitis, and many others. Unfortunately, many of these patients have spent a lot of money to see a myriad of practitioners with little to no resolution of the problem. Not until the underlying cause of the problem is addressed can patients with these symptoms find complete healing. We have been blessed to help many people find hope again and go on to live normal lives.

THE AUTONOMIC NERVOUS SYSTEM

The body's homeostatic mechanisms are primarily run by the autonomic nerve system (ANS) which is divided into two parts: sympathetic nervous system (SNS) and parasympathetic nervous system (PNS). *(See Figure 16-18.)* They run everything in the body that happens automatically and are absolutely involved with every injury to the body. The sympathetic nervous system revs up the body to handle stress and the parasympathetic repairs the damage from the stress, producing relaxation of the body.

The main nerve cell centers for both the SNS and PNS reside in the neck. The three cervical sympathetic ganglions are just anterior to the vertebral bodies and the main PNS nerve, the vagus nerve, is anterior to the upper cervical vertebrae. Anyone with any types of symptoms from ANS involvement should consider the possibility of a structural cervical cause of their instability. *(See Figure 16-19.)* This argument is made stronger when headaches and/or neck pain are present, along

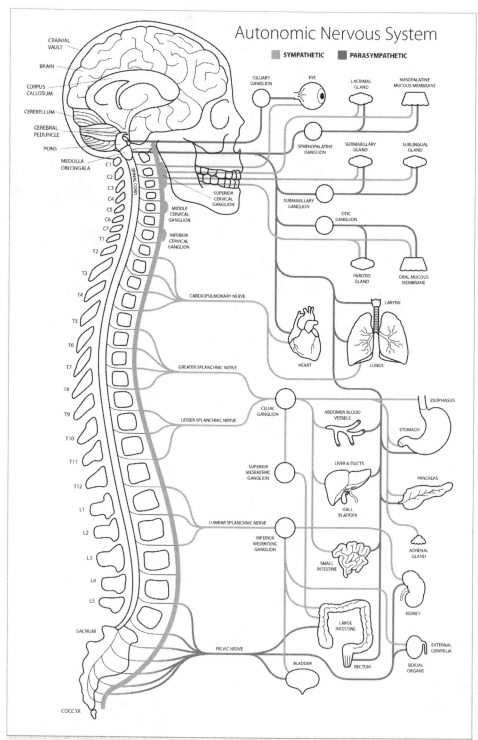

Figure 16-18. Autonomic nervous system.

with a history of neck popping, cracking, or grinding with or without a lot of chiropractic or self-manipulation. If cervical instability is the cause of the ANS symptoms then Prolotherapy is the cure. *(See Figure 16-20.)*

Since all nerves from the whole body (electrical grid) must pass through the neck, many different mechanisms by which cervical instability produces symptoms may occur. These include referral pain patterns, subluxations affecting muscles and nerves, disruption of the autonomic and peripheral nerve conduction, convergence of nerves in the trigeminocervical nucleus, vagus nerve compression, blockage of cerebrospinal fluid

Symptoms from Autonomic Nervous System Involvement

- Aches and pains
- Anxiety
- Blurred vision
- Changed appetite
- Chronic fatigue
- Cognitive impairment
- Difficulty concentrating
- Difficulty sleeping
- Dizziness
- Ear pain
- Eyeball pain
- Flushing (vasodilatation)
- Generalized loss of muscle strength
- Headaches
- Increase in heart rate
- Irritability and impatience
- Lacrimation (tearing)
- Lightheadedness
- Loss of interest and enjoyment in life
- Memory problems
- Muscle tension
- Neck pain/stiffness
- Paresthesia (face)
- Photophobia (sensitivity to light)
- Rhinorrhea (runny nose)
- Ringing in the ears
- Sinus congestion
- Suboccipital headache
- Sweating
- Sweaty hands
- Tinnitus
- Trembling
- Vertigo
- Visual disturbances
- Withdrawal

Figure 16-19: Symptoms from autonomic nervous system involvement.
Adapted from: Magee D. *Orthopedic Physical Assessment.* 6th Edition. St. Louis, MO: Saunders; 2014.

flow, interference of blood flow through the vertebral arteries, dural tension, and biomechanical alterations of the temporomandibular joint. *(See Figure 16-21.)* Cervical instability affects the functioning of not only the cervical nerves that innervate the muscles and skin of the arms and hands, but also the autonomic nerves that control blood pressure, heart rate, digestion, immune system function,

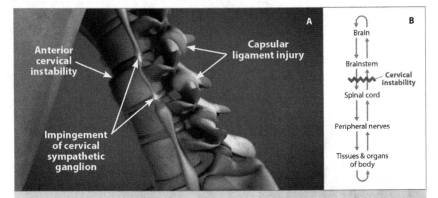

Figure 16-20. Cervical instability etiology of whole body systems. The body's electrical grid travels through the neck to reach the main electrical transmission center, the brain. **A.** Capsular ligament laxity (weakness) causes anterior cervical instability with neck flexion, producing impingement of the cervical sympathetic ganglion. Cervicocranial syndrome accounts for many of the seemingly odd array of symptoms post neck trauma. **B.** Disruption of nerve input and output is caused by cervical instability.

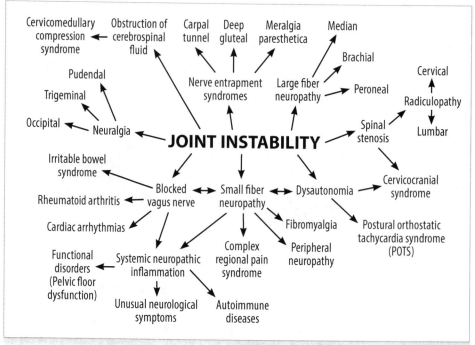

Figure 16-21. Joint instability etiology of various nerve entrapments and unusual pain syndromes.

breathing, and energy levels, as well as neurons involved in the central relay systems in the brain that are involved with vision, proprioception (balance and 3-D perception), hormone levels, and even concentration, memory, emotions, and happiness. A stable cervical spine plays a vital role in allowing us to live vibrant productive lives! Fortunately when the cervical spine and surrounding nerves are injured, Prolotherapy, sometimes in combination with LPIT and NRIT, restores stability, relieves pain, and gives many grateful patients back their normal lives!

SUMMARY

All pain has a nerve component. Nerves alert the brain to the presence of an injury or problem because the nerves are inflamed, entrapped, or encountering excessive stretch. The hallmark sign of nerve irritation is neurogenic pain which produces significant symptoms including sharp pains when an extremity is moved or touched in a normal non-painful way. This symptom is called allodynia.

The most common cause of all nerve pains is ligament injury leading to joint instability. Ligaments are the sensory organs of the joints. When a ligament is injured, the nerves within it experience excessive stretch and start firing. If the ligament injury is not addressed with Prolotherapy, joint instability develops which results in the development of many long term manifestations including tendinopathies, recurrent joint swelling, chronic muscle spasms, accelerated joint degeneration, myofascial restrictions, nerve entrapments, neurogenic inflammation, autonomic nervous system dysfunction, radiculopathy, and spinal stenosis, which may lead to the same processes occurring in adjacent joints as well!

When a symptom is improved or worsened by motion or activity, the symptom is said to be dynamic. Dynamic symptoms arise from joint instability. Many nerve entrapment conditions and syndromes including carpal tunnel syndrome, occipital neuralgia, thoracic outlet syndrome, piriformis syndrome, cervical and lumbar radiculopathy, and even spinal stenosis occur as a result of joint instabilities. Because the extra space for nerves, including vertebral foramina or tunnels, is only 1 to 2 mm, microinstability of joints, can cause bones to move enough to compress nerves. When this happens, positions or movements where the tunnel or foramina is open may occur, thus temporarily eliminating the nerve compression, so symptoms abate. Other positions or movements may cause the nerve space to narrow and symptoms increase. This dynamic (changing) component of the symptomatology is a sign that joint instability is the cause and Prolotherapy is the cure.

Neuropathic pain from neurogenic inflammation caused by nerve entrapment or excessive nerve stretch occurs because of joint instability and requires Prolotherapy to resolve the symptoms long-term. One of the common causes of neurogenic inflammation is chronic constriction injury in the fascia where nerves become entrapped. When joint instability is not present, other natural injection therapies may be provided directly to the nerve: Lyftogt Perineural Injection Therapy (LPIT) and Nerve Release Injection Therapy (NRIT). Both of these treatments involve the injection of natural solutions, including 5% dextrose, to release nerve entrapments and restore health and homeostasis to the inflamed nerves. These small peptidergic nerves are involved in the health maintenance and renewal of tissues such as ligaments, thus LPIT and NRIT are often given in conjunction with Prolotherapy. NRIT requires ultrasound guidance to direct the injection of fluid to release (hydrodissect) the nerve from entrapment, which often occurs in the nerve highways, which are the myofascial layers between muscles. It also occurs in various tunnels, like the carpal tunnel. As the entrapped nerve is released immediately, symptoms may often improve or resolve instantaneously. Sometimes several sessions may be required to produce long-lasting resolution of the nerve pain and symptoms.

Perhaps the least appreciated nerve irritation is that which involves the autonomic nervous system (ANS). Because both the sympathetic and parasympathetic components of the ANS reside just anterior to the cervical spine, cervical instability may produce a wide array of symptoms including blurred vision, tinnitus, dizziness, swallowing difficulties, ear and eyeball pain, tachycardia (fast heart rate), lacrimation (tearing), memory loss, paresthesia, suboccipital headache, sweating, trembling, migraines, and neck pain. When these symptoms are associated with neck popping, cracking, or grinding with or without a history of chiropractic or self-manipulation, cervical instability can be assumed and the best treatment is Prolotherapy. ∎

CHAPTER

17

CONNECTIVE TISSUE DEFICIENCY CONDITIONS

Connective tissues comprise 50% of the body weight, muscles being 40% and the rest coming from ligaments, tendons and fascia. Each day connective tissue itself, along with the cells that make it, need to be replenished. When catabolic (breakdown) processes exceed anabolic (build-up) ones, a connective tissue deficiency or weakness occurs. Diagnoses such as fibromyalgia syndrome, myofascial pain syndrome and symptoms such as whole body pain or achiness and plain-ol' just feeling awful occur. When the connective tissue weakness is genetic, similar symptoms can arise but these are well established disorders including joint hypermobility syndrome (JHS) and Ehlers-Danlos syndrome (EDS). While symptoms can range from mild in those who are sedentary to moderate for more active individuals, symptoms are generally severe after strenuous activity. As in all conditions, the goal is to get at the root cause of the problem and then resolve it! Prolotherapy is an excellent option to strengthen the weakened ligaments in the spine and other painful joints that are causing pain throughout the body! It provides hope and pain relief in some of the most painful, and often hopeless, conditions. The body has tremendous regenerative capabilities, but one must never forget the fact that many different factors affect connective tissue healing. *(See Figure 17-1.)*

JOINT HYPERMOBILITY SYNDROME (JHS)

Joint hypermobility syndrome (JHS) is a largely under-recognized, hereditary connective tissue disorder which manifests in a variety of different clinical presentations. JHS, also called benign congenital hypermobility (a milder variation of EDS, occurs with prevailing gross joint laxity throughout the body.

While hypermobility is a feature common to them all, they are all believed to be caused by a defect in collagen, the essential connective tissue protein responsible for tensility and integrity of skin and joints tissues.[1,2] When a defect such as the one found in EDS is present, collagen fibers become weakened, allowing tissues to become more elastic. In the case of JHS and hypermobility type EDS, the weakened collagen fibers affect the integrity of ligaments in the joints. The weakness of these

FACTORS AFFECTING HEALING OF CONNECTIVE TISSUES

- Age
- Blood supply
- Degree of hypoxia (systemic and local)
- Dietary intake
- Electrical fields
- Gender
- Growth factors, cytokines, eicosanoids
- Hormonal influences
- Mechanical-load forces
- Metabolic and cell turnover rates of connective tissues
- Mobility (local and whole-body)
- Muscular strength and forces
- Nutritional status
- Overall health status
- pH and lactate concentration
- Pharmacological agents (drugs)
- Psychological influences (placebo effects and psychoneuroimmunological links)
- Severity of injury
- Structural (physical) deformities
- Temperature
- Timing and return to physical activity
- Type of injury
- Type of onset (acute or chronic)
- Type of tissue(s) affected
- Underlying disease processes

Figure 17-1: Factors affecting the healing of connective tissues. Reversing connective tissue deficiency syndrome involves many different factors including diet, medications, and other metabolic factors. It is not just a simple fix. Adapted from *Nutrition Applied to Injury Rehabilitation and Sports Medicine* by L. Bucci, CRC Press, Boca Raton, FL © 1995

ligaments is what allows joints to hyperextend beyond the normal physiological limits.

Hypermobile joints are exhibited by bending the elbow or knee past the neutral position, touching the floor with the palm while bending at the waist, and touching the thumb to the forearm. In subtler cases, this condition can only be determined by a physical examination—one of the reasons it is not diagnosed by most physicians, since they are not trained to adequately examine for joint mobility and ligament laxity. As we have been discussing, when ligaments are weak, joints become loose and unstable. Affected individuals over 40 years of age typically have recurrent joint problems and almost universally suffer from chronic pain. The end result of this condition is often diffuse osteoarthritis.[3]

While hypermobility may be generalized or extreme in a small number of joints, it is important for pain physicians to recognize when it is present. Comparing a patient's joint range of motion with normal ranges for age and sex can point the clinician toward the presence of joint hypermobility signs and symptoms. Other common clues in children, adolescents, and adults that suggest joint hypermobility is present includes recurrent joint dislocations, frequent ankle sprains, child with poor ball catching and handwriting skills, premature osteoarthritis, as well as laxity in other supporting tissues and structures. *(See Figure 17-2.)*

It is not uncommon for patients with JHS to go 10 years or more before receiving an appropriate diagnosis.[4] One reason for this is doctors and other health care providers are trained to examine for *reduction* of joint mobility rather than for an *increased* range, so that hypermobility is commonly missed. When hypermobility *is sought* it is the most common finding among patients presenting to a rheumatologist, but more often than not, is overlooked.[5] Nearly one-half of rheumatologists are skeptical about the significant impact that JHS has on people's lives, and about three-quarters are skeptical about a significant contribution to the overall burden of rheumatic diseases.[6] That is unfortunate for this resilient and brave patient population who trudge on, despite disabling pain, to try and lead normal lives. The tremendous mental and physical effort needed to perform everyday functions, such as walking, cooking, or bending down to pick something up, without hurting or dislocating joints can be mind-boggling to anyone who does not suffer from JHS-related conditions. Besides arthralgias, generalized

In children and adolescents[*]
- Coincidental congenital dislocation of the hip
- Joint dislocations
- Late walking with bottom shuffling instead of crawling
- Poor ball catching and handwriting skills
- Recurrent ankle sprains
- So called growing pains or chronic widespread pain
- Tiring easily compared with peers

In adults
- Autonomic dysfunction, such as orthostatic intolerance (dizziness or faintness) or postural tachycardia syndrome (in this form of dysautonomia, in 60° upright tilt the blood pressure remains constant while the pulse rate rises by a minimum of 30 beats/min)
- Functional gastrointestinal disorders (sluggish bowel, bloating, rectal evacuatory dysfunction)
- Increase in pain or progressive intensification of pain that is largely unresponsive to analgesics
- Joint dislocations
- Laxity in other supporting tissues – for example, hernias, varicose veins, or uterine or rectal prolapsed
- Multiple soft tissue (including sporting) injuries
- Non-inflammatory joint or spinal pain
- Premature osteoarthritis
- Progressive loss of mobility owing to pain or kinesiophobia (pain avoidance through movement avoidance)

Figure 17-2: Common clues suggesting joint hypermobility syndrome (based on observations, expert opinion, and case series). *Ross J, et al. Joint hypermobility syndrome. BMJ. 2011;342:c7167.*

joint laxity, the hallmark of the heritable disorders of connective tissue (HDCT), including JHS, is a significant risk factor for conditions such as joint dislocations, temporomandibular disorders, pathologic disc degeneration, diffuse idiopathic skeletal hyperostosis, osteoarthritis, as well as joint injury during sports.[7-11] This is often the point when these patients learn about our clinic and how Prolotherapy can help by strengthening the ligaments, thereby improving joint stability.

While hypermobility with arthralgias (joint pain), may sound rather benign, JHS is typically a multi-system disease that can be quite disabling. In one study out of the University of Manchester involving 125 children with JHS, 74% presented with arthralgia, 13% speech difficulties, 14% learning difficulties, 12% urinary tract infections, 10% subluxation/dislocations of joints, while 48% experienced limitations of school-based physical education activities, and 67% difficulties in other physical activities.[12] Because of deconditioning, children with JHS have been found to have a significantly decreased maximal exercise capacity compared with age and gender-matched control subjects.[13] Another study linked an increased prevalence of migraine headaches with JHS.[14]

DIAGNOSING VARIOUS DEGREES OF JOINT HYPERMOBILITY SYNDROME

People who are hypermobile without symptoms are merely people with hypermobility. Those with symptoms attributable to their hypermobility may have JHS if they conform to the Brighton criteria. Joint hypermobility is diagnostically evaluated according to the Brighton criteria, which utilizes the Beighton score. The names sound similar but serve different purposes for a clinician. Determining the Beighton score is essential for making the diagnosis of JHS because it measures generalized joint laxity. The Beighton score measures the ability to perform certain hyperextensive functions, including significant flexion of the thumb and fifth finger, hyperextension of both knees and elbows greater than 10 degrees, and the ability to place the palms on the floor with the knees fully extended, by assigning a point to each of these functions. *(See Figure 17-3.)* The Brighton criteria were developed to establish diagnostic criteria for JHS. Using these criteria helps physicians to distinguish JHS from other connective tissue disorders.[15] According to the Brighton criteria, a Beighton score of four or higher indicates generalized joint laxity and this along with athralgia in four or more joints for longer than three months signifies joint hypermobility syndrome.[16,17] *(See Figure 17-4.)* Typically a Beighton score of five or higher is used as the cut-off for Ehlers-Danlos syndrome.

While there is still some debate on the necessary criteria for making the diagnosis of Ehlers-Danlos syndrome (EDS), a Beighton score of 5 is indicative of EDS, a score of 4 does not preclude the diagnosis. Generally the diagnosis is made by a family history of the condition and the clinical evaluation. Genetic testing and muscle and skin biopsies confirm the connective tissue (collagen) disorder. Other diagnostic testing such as an echocardiogram, MRI and/or CT scan can be used to confirm blood vessel, valvular, organ, and connective tissue problems seen in the various types of EDS.

Beighton 9-Point Scoring System for Joint Hypermobility

Dorsiflex the 5th metacarpophalangeal joint (pinky finger) to the ≥ 90° (1 point for each side, left and right)

Score: _____

Oppose the thumb to the volar aspect of the ipsilateral forearm (1 point for each side, left and right)

Score: _____

Hyperextend the elbows to ≥ 10° (1 point for each side, left and right)

Score: _____

Hyperextend the knees to ≥ 10° (1 point for each side, left and right)

Score: _____

Place the hands flat on the floor with knees fully extended (1 point)

Score: _____

Total Score: _____

A score of ≥ 4/9 is usually indicative of generalized hypermobility

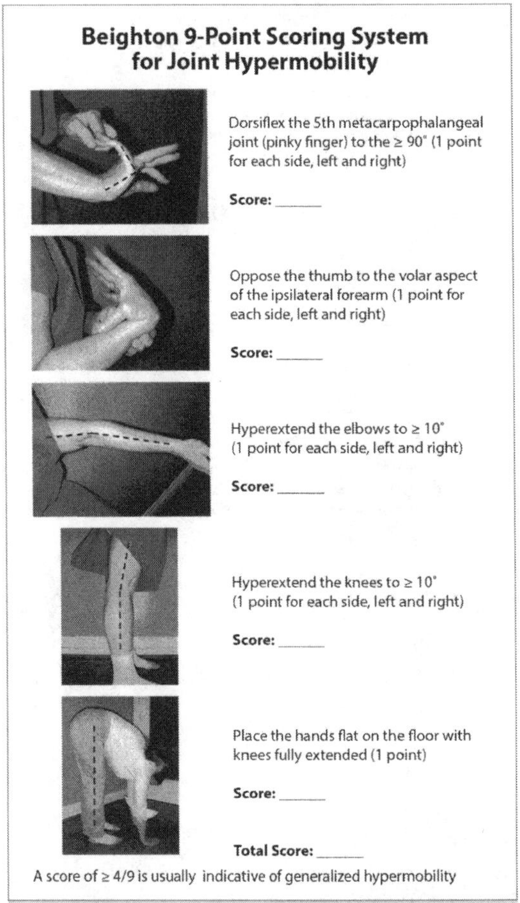

Figure 17-3: Beighton 9-point scoring system for joint hypermobility. A score of 4 or greater is indicative of generalized joint hypermobility.

A small proportion of patients with generalized joint hypermobility will have one of the more serious conditions such as Ehlers-Danlos syndrome, Marfan syndrome or Osteogenesis Imperfecta. When these more serious conditions are considered, a referral is made to a geneticist or other clinician for genetic testing, skin biopsy or diagnostic tests, such as an echocardiogram to look for valvular defects, or diagnostic tests on other organs to search for signs of a multisystem connective tissue disorder. It is important to differentiate JHS from the vascular Ehlers–Danlos syndrome, for instance, to prevent life threatening vascular hemorrhages from arterial ruptures in the latter condition.

EHLERS-DANLOS SYNDROME

Ehlers-Danlos syndrome is caused by defects in the biogenesis of collagen, the major structural protein of the body. The condition can be either inherited from a parent with the defect or caused by a genetic mutation. EDS is generally inherited in an autosomal dominant pattern, though an autosomal recessive type exists. EDS is collectively believed to affect one in every 5,000 children at time of birth, although this

Brighton Criteria

Major Criteria
- Arthralgia for longer than 3 months in 4 or more joints
- Beighton score of > 4

Minor Criteria
- Arthralgia (> 3 month duration) in one to three joints or back pain (> 3 month duration) or spondylosis, spondylolysis/spondylolisthesis
- Beighton score of I, II, or III
- Dislocation or subluxation in more than one joint, or in one joint on more than one occasion
- Marfanoid habitus (tall, slim, span greater than height (> 1.03 ratio), upper segment less than lower segment (< 0.89 ratio), arachnodactyly)
- Mitral valve prolapse
- Ocular signs: drooping eyelids, myopia, antimongoloid slant
- Skin striae, hyperextensibility, thin skin, or abnormal scarring
- Three or more soft tissue lesions (eg, epicondylitis, tenosynovitis, bursitis)
- Varicose veins, hernia, or uterine or rectal prolapse

Requirements for Diagnosis
Any one of the following:
- Four minor criteria
- One major plus two minor criteria
- Two major criteria
- Two minor criteria and unequivocally affected first-degree relative in family history

Figure 17-4: Brighton criteria for joint hypermobility syndrome. Keer R and Grahame R. *Hypermobility syndrome: recognition and management for physiotherapists.* London: Butterworth Heinemann; 2003.

number is a rough estimate due to the fact that EDS is widely underdiagnosed in the general population.[18,19] At present, there are six primary known classifications of EDS: Classic, Hypermobility, Vascular, Kyphoscoliosis, Arthrochalasia, and Dermatosparaxis. (See Figure 17-5.) The hypermobility type, which is found to be the most common, is estimated to affect one in every 10,000 to 15,000 individuals.[20]

DIFFERENTIATING EHLERS-DANLOS SYNDROME FROM JOINT HYPERMOBILITY SYNDROME

Ehlers-Danlos syndrome should be considered in the evaluation of every hypermobile patient who has a pain complaint. A key characteristic for diagnosis and differentiation of EDS from JHS is the addition of skin findings.[21]

Classic	Hypermobility	Vascular
• Extensive atrophic scarring • Extensive bruising • Joint hypermobility • Skin hyperelasticity • Smooth/velvety skin	• Chronic joint pain • Recurrent joint dislocation • Vertebral subluxations	• Arterial fragility • Extensive bruising • Intestinal fragility • Tendon/muscle rupture • Uterine fragility
Kyphoscoliosis	**Arthrochalasia**	**Dermatosparaxis**
• Arterial rupture • Atrophic scars • Excessive bruising • Kyphoscoliosis • Osteopenia	• Congenital hip dislocation • Joint hypermobility • Kyphoscoliosis • Recurrent joint dislocation • Tissue fragility	• Extensive bruising • Hernias • Premature rupture of membranes • Severe skin fragility

Figure 17-5. The six primary known classifications of Ehlers-Danlos syndrome (EDS).

EDS type 1 and type 2, previously known as EDS classic type, has skin that extends easily and snaps back after release. *(See Figure 17-6.)* The skin is fragile, as manifested by splitting of the dermis following relatively minor trauma, especially over pressure points (knees, elbows) and areas prone to trauma (shins, forehead, chin). Wound healing is delayed, and the stretching of scars after apparently successful primary wound healing is characteristic. While EDS type 4, vascular type, can have all of the above, besides easy bruising and hematoma formation in areas of trauma, the skin is translucent (visible veins on the chest).[22] These skin findings are in contrast to EDS type 3, hypermobility type, which has soft skin with normal or only slightly increased extensibility.[19] All forms of EDS, like JHS, affect the joints, causing hypermobility, and as a result, individuals are more susceptible to dislocations, subluxations, sprains, strains, and sometimes fractures. While there is no distinguishing feature of the joint and neuromuscular symptoms of EDS versus JHS, EDS is often more disabling.[23,24]

The results of one study showed that 1) chronic pain in EDS is highly prevalent and associated with regular use of analgesics; 2) pain is more prevalent and more severe in the hypermobility type; 3) pain severity is correlated with hypermobility, dislocations, and previous surgery; 4) pain is correlated with low nocturnal sleep quality; and 5) pain contributes to functional impairment in daily life, independent of the level of fatigue. The authors concluded, "Therefore, treatment of pain should be a prominent aspect of symptomatic management of EDS."[25] In our opinion, the best treatment for pain caused by EDS hypermobility is Prolotherapy!

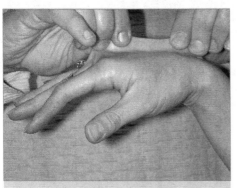

Figure 17-6: Patients with EDS type 1 and type 2 demonstrate skin that extends easily and snaps back after release.

CASE STUDY: 21 YEAR-OLD FEMALE WITH EHLERS-DANLOS SYNDROME, HYPERMOBILITY TYPE

Ellie first began experiencing the symptoms of Ehlers-Danlos syndrome, Hypermobility type in the fifth grade, when one of her knees subluxed. Over the next 12 years, the pain and joint subluxations spread to other joints including the other knee, elbows, shoulders, and spine. Ellie tried many different forms of therapy including physical therapy, massage, ultrasound, taping, and compression braces which managed her pain well enough to perform daily activities as well as gymnastics, track, and cross country. At the age of 19, she tore the meniscus in her right knee and underwent surgical meniscus repair.

Following the operation, she experienced intense pain, and subsequently underwent a second operation. While the symptoms in her knee appeared to be resolved, pain in her other joints persisted. During this time, Ellie also began experiencing other health issues including hypothyroidism, eczema, chest pains, food allergies, irregular menstrual periods, and degenerative disc pain in her neck and back.

In the search for a treatment for her joint pain, Ellie found Prolotherapy, which she felt was needed for the pain in her neck, thoracic, low back, knees, and shoulders. During this time, she continued physical therapy, and managed her pain with multiple medications. After a year and a half of minimal improvement, her pain doctor referred her to Caring Medical for Prolotherapy. As a 21 year-old college student, Ellie was living with constant joint pain, which disturbed her ability to exercise, study, and sleep. She contemplated dropping out of school. By this time, she also suffered from joint dislocations in her shoulders and elbows causing its own amount of excessive pain and stiffness. Her spine, including the neck, thoracic, and lumbar regions, would also "freeze," sending shooting pain up and down her back.

Ellie's first Prolotherapy treatment included injections to her neck, spine, both scapulas, low back, and knee. Within a week of her first visit, Ellie reported a decrease in her thoracic and scapular pain and improved physical stamina and energy. A month later, she began running again and no longer required treatment to her knee. By her second visit, Ellie had discontinued all use of pain patches, and only required occasional Tylenol for pain and muscle relaxers to help her sleep.

For the next six months, Ellie continued to receive monthly treatments to her neck, thoracic, and shoulders, showing gradual improvement of pain and well-being. After eight months of treatments, Ellie no longer required any pain medications, was no longer experiencing any joint dislocations, and was back to running and gymnastics. She was seen an average of once per year throughout her college and Masters program. After that, she went on to receive a PhD in her chosen profession. It is now many years after her Prolotherapy treatment series. Ellie continues to lead a full life, without daily pain or disability. She has no limitations while exercising most days. Prolotherapy has the power to drastically improve the lives of EDS patients!

WHEN BEING "DOUBLE JOINTED" HURTS

Patients with JHS often say that they are "double jointed" or that they can contort their bodies into strange shapes (i.e. voluntary subluxations) or do the splits. Many JHS patients have signs and symptoms suggestive of fibromyalgia and are usually misdiagnosed.[26] These patients present with a wide variety of readily identifiable traumatic and overuse lesions, such as traction injuries at tendon or ligament insertions, chondromalacia patella, rotator cuff lesions, or back pain due to soft tissue injury or disc herniation. Others suffer the effects of joint instability, such as flat feet, recurrent dislocation or subluxation–notably of the shoulder, patella, metacarpophalangeal joints, or temporomandibular joints. Others still, develop a chronic degenerative arthritis that may be a direct complication of JHS **(See Figure 17-7.)**

For those who suffer from dislocation of joints, the pain can be immense, and sometimes is the first indication a patient has hypermobile joints. Many hypermobile patients also experience myofascial pain, which may be explained by the extra stress placed on muscles to compensate for lax joints as the muscles attempt to stabilize the joints. One of the more serious long-lasting affects of joint laxity is chronic joint degeneration. The increased mechanical stress caused by ligament laxity leads to chronic joint instability, making them more susceptible to soft tissue injuries. Continual instability and injury leads to an earlier onset of degenerative joint disease in hypermobile and other patients with ligament injuries than in the normal population.[20,26-28]

Types of Hypermobility

Example:	**Example:**	**Example:**
A shoulder, knee, or elbow is lax or prone to dislocation.	Joint hypermobility syndrome	Ehlers-Danlos syndrome, Hypermobility Type Marfan syndrome Osteogenesis Imperfecta
Ligament laxity occurs in a single joint or multiple joints independent of each other. Only symptoms are hyperextension and arthralgia.	Hypermobility of four or more joints occurs in the absence of any rheumatologic disease, characterized by joint hyperextension, arthralgia, and joint dislocation or vertebral subluxation.	Hypermobility is congenital and caused by an inheritable defect. Effects are multisystemic and can include cardiac, optical, uterine, gastrointestinal, respiratory, spinal, integumentary, and joint abnormalities.
Beighton score: 1-3	**Beighton score: > 4**	**Beighton score: > 5**
	Brighton criteria: 2 major criteria or 1 major and 2 minor criteria, or 4 minor criteria	**Brighton criteria:** 2 major criteria, 1 major and 2 minor criteria, or 4 minor criteria

Figure 17-7: Types of hypermobility, by severity, using the Beighton score.

OVER-MANIPULATION SYNDROME

You may not have heard of over-manipulation syndrome, but it is one of the most common conditions we help every day with Prolotherapy in our clinics. Over-manipulation syndrome (OMS) is defined as a musculoskeletal condition characterized by a constellation of symptoms ranging from chronic pain to muscle spasms due to ligament laxity and joint instability, induced by musculoskeletal manipulation performed by practitioner, and/or self-manipulation. *(See Figure 17-8.)*

Excessive manipulation causes the cervical and spinal supportive ligaments to become stretched as the manipulation continues, leading to more and more joint instability.[29] This has become an epidemic in the offices of any practitioner treating chronic pain patients, but often goes unidentified.

• Anxiety	• Memory problems
• Blurred vision	• Nausea
• Cognitive impairment	• Neck pain/stiffness
• Dizziness	• Numbness in face and tongue
• Ear pain	• Pain radiating down arms
• Facial pain	• Paresthesia in upper extremities
• Headaches/migraines	• Tinnitus
• Insomnia	• TMJ pain
• Light sensitivity	• Vertigo
• Lightheadedness	

Figure 17-8: Over-manipulation syndrome symptoms.

The neck and back are most commonly affected by over-manipulation syndrome. These are frequent target areas for high velocity manipulations. A high velocity manipulation consists of a violent thrust and contortion of the spine to achieve the audible popping sounds or cracking of the cervical, lumbar, or even thoracic spine in an attempt to realign or adjust the spine. *(See Figure 17-9.)* The resultant spinal instability responds great to Comprehensive Prolotherapy.

UPPER CERVICAL INSTABILITY FROM OMS

George came in just like most folks. "Doc, my neck pain and stiffness is terrible. It is just getting worse and worse. It now involves my whole spine." He had tried physiotherapy, various injection therapies, and chiropractic care, but no surgeries. His MRIs showed bulges and mild degeneration here and there, but nothing that would account for such terrible spinal pain. When asked, "Do you self-manipulate?" he immediately said, "Yes, all the time!" After several Prolotherapy sessions and the admonition to stop self-manipulating his neck and spine, he calculated approximately how many times he had self-manipulated his spine in his life time. He came up with 677,000 times! That is the record at Caring

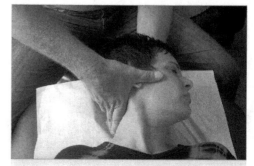

Figure 17-9: High velocity manipulation.

Medical. Do you think someone who has sustained 677,000 high velocity spinal "cracks" might experience ligament laxity and joint instability? You have by now learned the answer is an emphatic "yes!"

We see a large number of hypermobility cases where the patients present with a history of excessive chiropractic manipulations. Don't get us wrong. We like chiropractors. And in many instances chiropractic is very helpful. A short course of manipulation to relieve pain or tension is understandable. However, patients who sign up for long-term chiropractic packages that include thrusting manipulations often find themselves even more unstable after the treatment course. Good chiropractors treat each patient individually and conservatively.

High velocity thrusts can hurt someone, especially if the muscles are in spasm. The greater the muscle spasm present, the more force that has to occur to "crack" your neck. Ligaments in the neck, for instance, can be injured by as little as 10 newtons of force and high velocity thrusting can cause forces greater than 1000 newtons.[30-35] The chiropractors we go to make sure that the muscles are relaxed before any manipulation (if needed) is done. The force required to move a subluxed vertebrae or bone into place, should be minimal. Muscle spasms are often a complaint of people who suffer from loose joints, and those who have been diagnosed with over-manipulation syndrome.

The capsular ligaments, which hold the cervical, thoracic and lumbar vertebrae in place are typically injured with a rotational force. When a person self-manipulates or receives a high velocity thrust by a health care practitioner before the muscle stiffness or spasm has been addressed a supraphysiological rotation force is applied. This is the exact mechanism by which capsular ligaments are injured.[36-40] Then the muscles have to overcompensate in order to stabilize the joint, leading to tight muscles and muscle spasms. So it is easy to see how this can become a vicious cycle of pain, ligament laxity, muscle spasms, more pain, etc...

We estimate that approximately 7% of new patients that come and see us at Caring Medical have OMS. It has been evident for many years that patients who continue to self-manipulate or receive high velocity manipulations either need many more sessions than other people receiving Prolotherapy for the same condition that did not manipulate, or they simply do not get better. When receiving Prolotherapy, you should not manipulate the body part receiving Prolotherapy or have anyone else do it either!

Some of our neck patients claim to have never had neck issues until after seeing a chiropractor for an unrelated condition. The chiropractor insisted upon giving them high velocity neck manipulation. This then began a pattern of receiving continued adjustments for chronically subluxing and suffering for years until they found out about Prolotherapy. By the time they reach our office, they had all the same symptoms as whiplash-associated disorder (from cervical instability): neck pain, stiffness, vertigo, dizziness, ringing in the ears, swallowing difficulty, stress, anxiety, racing heart, severe fatigue and memory issues. This is a serious problem in our experience. There is no reason to be receiving 100-200 high velocity manipulations in your neck. Great chiropractors can generally get people significantly better in five visits. For those getting 20+ adjustments, our experience has been that at least one of those will be too forceful or aggravate cervical instability.

WHAT'S SO BAD ABOUT CRACKING YOUR SPINE AND OTHER JOINTS?

The anatomical dangers can clearly be understood if we consider the movement of a joint. Our muscles move a joint from neutral to a certain point, which is called active movement. This is the movement that we can make using just our own muscle strength. Passive movement includes the same range of motion as active movement plus a little more. Think of this as turning your head to the right, but then taking your hand to push your head a little further to look over your right shoulder. Beyond active movement and passive movement is the anatomical limit, which is where the joint should stop due to the ligament becoming taught. It's your body's way of saying "This is as far as we go. End of the line." But high velocity adjustments continually pushing to or past those anatomical limits begin

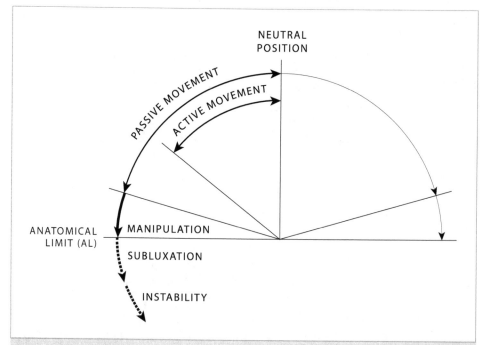

Figure 17-10: What is too much movement? Neutral position occurs when a person lays down with hands at the sides. Active movements are those movements performed using muscular power, such as turning the head. Passive movement occurs when someone else gently pushes the head further to one direction. When a supraphysiological force (force greater than a passive movement) is applied, additional motion can occur, as in a high velocity thrust. If this force is too great and goes beyond the anatomical limit (AL) subluxation and/or instability may result, due to the ligamentous structures becoming too lax or loose. Prolotherapy may be required to repair the damage.

Adapted from Figure 22.3 in Maigne R. *Diagnosis and Treatment of Pain of Vertebral Origin*, 2nd Edition. 2006 Taylor & Francis Group, LLC. Boca Raton, FL.

to allow overstretching of the ligaments, and thus, joint instability. **(See Figure 17-10.)** Attempting realignment with manipulations that will not hold, only further stretches the ligaments, even more extensively potentiating the symptoms of over-manipulation syndrome.

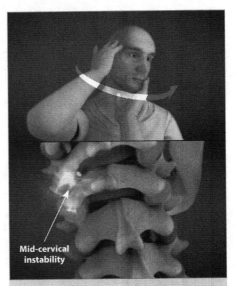

Mid-cervical instability

Figure 17-11: Self-manipulation causing mid-cervical instability. To allow the ligaments the opportunity to repair, self-manipulation of joints must stop.

Repeated adjustments for a hypermobile patient is not helpful because it will worsen the hypermobility and instability. If after numerous adjustments, the joint is still not staying in place after manipulation, then there is an obvious ligament injury. Manipulation should stop at this point. Treatment to stabilize the vertebrae by strengthening the ligaments is necessary. Prolotherapy is the treatment of choice that strengthens and repairs injured ligaments.

Self-manipulation of the spine refers to high velocity manipulation achieved by contorting and thrusting one's own spine to achieve the cracking and supposed adjustment of the spine. **(See Figure 17-11.)** In our office we see patients who are frequently cracking their ankles, wrists, fingers, or any other joint routinely. It is not uncommon for patients to tell us they routinely pop their joints back in place 10 or more times per day. Generally, this cracking is not a one-time event. Self-manipulation often becomes excessive and habit-forming and may lead to the development of over-manipulation syndrome.

A high velocity thrust to the C1, C2 area can cause this joint to become unstable. The thrust injures the cervical ligaments that stabilize these cervical vertebrae. There are no discs between the head and C1, or between C1 and C2, and thus the vertebrae are suspended by ligaments alone. The force of a high velocity thrust in this area puts a lot of stress on these ligaments, causing the ligaments to become stretched.

The ligaments in the spine called the capsular ligaments hold the joints of the spine or facet joints in place. Capsular ligaments are very small, therefore they are easily torn if stretched more than a centimeter. As you can see, it does not take much of a stretch for these ligaments to weaken or become lax. This is why we recommend exercising caution when receiving chiropractic manipulations. Not all chiropractors are created equal.

Continuous stretching and torquing to ligaments, such as from excessive high velocity manipulations, will cause them to elongate and deform. The stretched out cervical and capsular ligaments of the spine will cause instability. Joint instability is actually a contraindication to receiving manipulation. **(See Figure 17-12.)** However, this does not translate to what our experience has been with patients coming in with obvious over-manipulation syndrome. Realize that when this manipulation/subluxation cycle goes on for too long, the ligaments stretch to the point of no return, and are unable to hold the vertebrae in place. The vertebrae shift and start to cause pain and other symptoms of joint instability. Prolotherapy is the only treatment that can break this cycle and stabilize the vertebrae or other joints permanently, thereby eliminating the pain and symptoms related to joint instability, as well as the need for additional manipulations.

Cautions against manipulation	Contraindications to manipulation
• Acute inflammation	• Active collagen disease
• Atypical patterns of restriction	• Active rheumatic disease
• Bone disease	• Ankylosed joint
• Coagulation problems	• Hyperacute pain
• Congenital anomalies	• **Joint instability**
• Dizziness/vertigo	• Multiple nerve root involvement
• History of cancer in the area	• Spinal cord lesions
• History of poor response to manual techniques	• Vertebral artery symptoms
• Neurotic patient	
• Non-mechanical reason for hypomobility	
• Osteoporosis	
• Pending litigation	

Figure 17-12: Cautions and contraindications to joint mobilization (and/or high velocity manipulation) of the cervical spine.
Adapted from: Maigne R. *Diagnosis and Treatment of Pain of Vertebral Origin*, 2nd Edition. CRC Press. 2005.

DIAGNOSIS OF FIBROMYALGIA

When a fibromyalgia patient first seeks help for pain, a diagnosis such as tendinitis is generally given. When the pain continues, an MRI scan or some such study will be ordered. The diagnosis then changes to a "disc problem." After more unsuccessful treatments, the pain sufferer will be sent to a pain center where the diagnosis of depression will be made. After several thousands of dollars of treatment, diagnostic tests, and a lot of frustration and misery, the person will be given that all-inclusive, "so everyone will know I'm not crazy" diagnosis: fibromyalgia. Nearly anyone who has had pain long enough and seeks enough medical opinions will eventually be labeled with this diagnosis.

It is important to remember that nothing of the etiology is revealed when a physician gives a patient a "diagnosis" with the word "syndrome" on the end of it. A "syndrome" is what physicians call a constellation of symptoms for which the actual cause is unknown. A good example of this is what we call the "couch potato syndrome." This syndrome typically describes a balding, middle-aged man with a "basketball-belly," who enjoys watching, talking, and reading about sports, but couldn't walk around the block without getting chest pain. People with this syndrome typically reside in a lounge chair that envelopes the body upon contact and a remote is a must. You see, the physician "diagnosed" "couch potato syndrome," but this says nothing about the etiology of the condition. It is much more important to know the cause of pain than to have a label placed on it. The diagnosis of fibromyalgia, chronic pain syndrome, or myofascial pain syndrome does not determine the etiology and, thus, the cure for the condition.

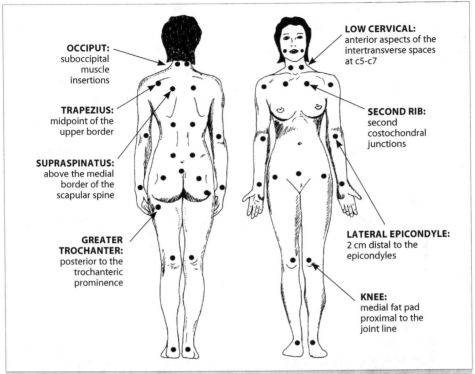

OCCIPUT: suboccipital muscle insertions

TRAPEZIUS: midpoint of the upper border

SUPRASPINATUS: above the medial border of the scapular spine

GREATER TROCHANTER: posterior to the trochanteric prominence

LOW CERVICAL: anterior aspects of the intertransverse spaces at c5-c7

SECOND RIB: second costochondral junctions

LATERAL EPICONDYLE: 2 cm distal to the epicondyles

KNEE: medial fat pad proximal to the joint line

Figure 17-13: Fibromyalgia tender points. General locations of the 18 tender points that make up the criteria for identifying fibromyalgia. Adapted from: *Primer on the Rheumatic Diseases*, Tenth Edition, © 1993, the Arthritis Foundation.

Traditional medicine will label someone with fibromyalgia if certain diagnostic criteria are met.[41] Unfortunately, the criteria are somewhat vague. The main criterion is the presence of aches or pains at more than four sites, for more than three months, with no underlying condition causing the pain. This is why we believe this "diagnosis" is erroneous because a cause for chronic pain can **almost always** be found. Other symptoms revealed by a patient's medical history that lead to a fibromyalgia diagnosis may include pain in at least 11 of 18 specific tender points, a "hurt all over" feeling, anxiety or tension, poor sleep, general fatigue, and/or irritable bowel syndrome.[42] *(See Figure 17-13.)*

THE IMPORTANCE OF SLEEP

Upon falling asleep, a person enters stage I and stage II sleep, which is a very light sleep. After approximately 90 minutes, the person will enter stages III and IV, or deep sleep. It is during deep sleep that hormones, like Growth Hormone, are secreted. *(See Figure 17-14.)* Growth Hormone is one of the anabolic hormones that the body needs to repair itself. If a person does not enter the deep stages of sleep, the ability to repair injured tissue is hampered. More than 50% of body weight is muscle tissue. It is imperative that the body is able to repair this muscle tissue from

its daily use. The body does
its repair during the deep
stages of sleep. If this is not
accomplished, the end result
is muscle aching. Do you
see the cycle? A person has a
localized pain, such as neck
pain, that does not resolve.
Eventually, the chronic pain
causes chronic insomnia. The
chronic insomnia causes a
decrease in the body's ability
to repair itself. This causes
pain to move to other parts
of the body, causing more
insomnia. A vicious cycle continues.

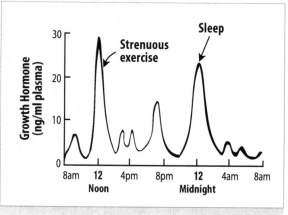

Figure 17-14: Growth hormone secreted during sleep.
Adapted from: *Textbook of Medical Physiology*, by A. Guyton and J. Hall, © 1996, W.B. Saunders Co., Philadelphia.

In a 1976 study, Harvey Moldofsky, MD, solicited healthy volunteers and allowed them to sleep only in stages I and II. Dr. Moldofsky put electrodes on their heads and gave them a little zap, not enough to wake them but enough to keep them from achieving stage III or IV sleep, the deep stages of sleep.[43] Guess how long it took before the previously healthy volunteers had diffuse body aches, tender points, and symptomatology exactly mimicking fibromyalgia? **Seven days!** In other words, after seven days of non-restful sleep, these previously healthy people met all the criteria for fibromyalgia, except for the chronicity of the problem.

We all know what this is like. For two days your throat feels scratchy, but you tell yourself, "Nah, I'm not sick." You work another 12-hour day. You mow the lawn, clean out the garage, and do the grocery shopping. The next day you say, "Yeah, I'm sick," as you lay in bed looking for sympathy. After a few days of laying in bed fighting a fever and runny nose, your entire body hurts. It's stiff, sore, and you are exhausted. Do you have fibromyalgia after this? Of course not; you have a cold. Chronic insomnia is the number one reason people have diffuse body aching. To cure diffuse body aching, the cause of the chronic insomnia must be found.

FIBROMYALGIA HAS A CAUSE

The most common reason for chronic pain is joint instability caused by chronic ligament laxity. The second most common reason is chronic insomnia. Other causes of diffuse chronic body pain are multiple chemical sensitivities, hypoglycemia, hypothyroidism, hypoadrenocortisolism, viral infection, yeast infection, increased gut permeability, nutrient deficiency, and poor tissue oxygenation. To cure fibromyalgic-type complaints, these conditions must be evaluated and treated. For this reason, it is recommended that the person suffering from diffuse body pain see a Natural Medicine physician. Prolotherapy is an effective treatment for people suffering from diffuse body pain when tenderness is elicited over muscle, ligament, and tendon attachments to the bone.

Prolotherapy is not an isolated treatment. The physician must investigate all possible factors which may be involved with a person experiencing diffuse body pain.

To make the diagnosis of fibromyalgia, one of the cardinal features is tenderness over specific points on the body. The diagnosis is made when at least 11 of the 18 points are tender. The unilateral sites are the occiput (insertion of the suboccipital muscles), inter-transverse ligaments C5 through C7, trapezius muscle, origin of the supraspinatous muscle, second costochondral junction (ligament), lateral epicondyle (wrist extensor muscle insertions), gluteal area (gluteus maximus muscle), greater trochanter (gluteus medius muscle insertion), and the medial fat pad of the knee (medial collateral ligament). In essence, 14 of the 18 points are located where either a ligament, tendon, or muscle inserts and the remaining four are in the middle of a particular muscle. **(Refer to Figure 17-13.)** Prolotherapy grows ligament, tendon, and muscle tissue where they attach to the bone, thus eliminating trigger points and the pain of fibromyalgia.

Whether a patient has been given the label of fibromyalgia, myofascial pain syndrome, or post-surgical pain syndrome, the hallmark feature typically is very sensitive trigger point areas. The person often feels a knot in the muscle in that area. These areas are called "trigger points" because they trigger a person's pain if compressed and palpated and cause the positive "jump sign." Trigger points also refer pain to a distal site that becomes painful. In a study published in 1994, K. Dean Reeves, MD, showed that even in people with severe fibromyalgia, Prolotherapy caused a reduction in pain levels and increased functional abilities in more than 75% of patients. In 38% of the patients, Prolotherapy was the only effective treatment they ever received. An additional 25% said that Prolotherapy was much more effective than any previous treatment. The study showed that overall, 90% of the severe fibromyalgia patients benefited from the Prolotherapy injections.[44] Prolotherapy is a powerful treatment for alleviating fibromyalgia pain!

MYOFASCIAL PAIN SYNDROME

Fibromyalgia and myofascial pain syndrome are often diagnosed in the same patient. Myofascial pain syndrome (MPS) is a common painful muscle disorder caused by taut bands or trigger points in the muscles.[45] Myofascial trigger points are tender areas in muscles causing local and referred muscle pain. Trigger points may cause the tight muscles and tight muscles may cause trigger points.

Between 85-93% of musculoskeletal pain sufferers exhibit trigger points.[46,47] Interestingly enough, about 50% of us have latent trigger points just waiting to be activated! That is right! When studies are done on asymptomatic people, about 50% of them have these trigger points that refer pain when palpated and are just primed to start causing pain![48-50] This high percentage of latent trigger points in asymptomatic people explains why some people who sustain small "fender-bender" collisions end up with severe, significant, non-healing pain. This also explains why small "fender-bender" type accidents can lead to unrelenting pain syndromes.

Trigger points cause pain that is often poorly localized and of aching quality. The pain is often referred to a distant site, along with numbness or paresthesias (prickly feelings). When the trigger point is palpated, the pain may sharpen and the referral pain pattern becomes more distinct.

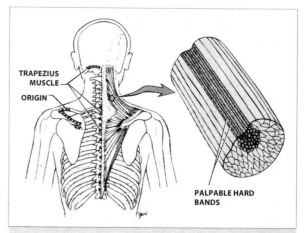

Figure 17-15: Trapezius muscle trigger point. Palpation on the trigger point is not only tender but can refer pain to distant sites. In this case, the trigger point is causing headaches.

(See Figure 17-15.) Autonomic problems can also arise from trigger points because of dysfunction of the autonomic nervous system. This is the part of the nervous system that functions automatically, controlling functions such as breathing, balance, circulation, and blood flow. Symptoms of autonomic dysfunction that can occur because of trigger points include abnormal sweating, persistent lacrimation (tearing), persistent coryza (allergic runny nose), excessive salivation, imbalance, dizziness, tinnitus (ringing in the ears), and cold hands and/or feet.[48]

THE MYOFASCIAL PAIN THEORY

Janet Travell, MD, championed the now traditionally accepted Myofascial Pain Theory, describing the pain experienced in the fascia (tissue) surrounding the muscles. Janet Travell published some 40 papers on trigger points between 1942 and 1990 and coined the term myofascial pain syndrome.[51, 52] She published the first volume of *The Trigger Point Manual* in 1983 and the second in 1992.[48] The main tenets for her theory on the muscular origin of pain are from a 1952 report by her and J. Rinzler, in which the pain patterns of trigger points in 32 skeletal muscles were depicted in the medical journal *Postgraduate Medicine*, entitled in one article, "The Myofascial Genesis of Pain."[53]

Janet Travell, MD, and her proteges believe that the main sources of chronic pain are the trigger points, and that the primary pathology causing the trigger points is in the muscle itself or in the small nerves to the muscles. The evidence for this was derived from scientific information where some abnormalities in the excitability of the endplates (nerves) to the trigger points were found, and some biopsy specimens showed evidence of muscle fiber degeneration. The problem with this is that even the text, entitled *Travell & Simons' Myofascial Pain and Dysfunction, The Trigger Point*

Manual, published in 1999, states, "In muscles accessible to palpation, a myofascial trigger point is consistently found within a palpable taut band. Theoretically and clinically, the taut band is a basic criterion of a trigger point. However, by itself it is an ambiguous finding. Taut bands are found in asymptomatic subjects with no evidence of tender nodules or trigger points." In regard to taut bands...It is difficult to measure with accuracy, specificity, and reliability. Studies indicate that palpable taut bands can be present in normal muscles without any other indication of abnormality such as tenderness or pain."[50]

The Myofascial Pain Theory is based on the premise that the basic underlying problem is in the muscle or within the electrical activity of the muscle itself. This so-called abnormality causes a taut band in some muscle fibers, which is felt as a taut band or nodule and, thus, a trigger point develops. Treatment is, therefore, directed at correcting this taut nodule through specific treatments to cause trigger point release. The main treatments used are spray and stretch, myofascial release massage, osteopathic techniques such as strain-counterstrain, skin rolling, biofeedback, heat and ice, ultrasound, iontophoresis, electrical stimulation, posture work, and our favorite—injections.

TREATING TRIGGER POINTS

Since the condition is caused by a supposed muscle problem, and the trigger points typically involve taut bands or nodules, then it would make sense to stretch those nodules to get them to relax. Those who espouse the myofascial pain syndrome theory point out, "The key to treating trigger points is to lengthen the muscle fibers that are shortened by the trigger point mechanisms."[54] The main way that myofascial therapists do this is by a spray-and-stretch technique. Vapocoolant sprays are dispensed in a fine stream onto the skin, and then the muscle is slowly stretched. This technique is generally done by physical therapists. Each muscle is stretched in a particular manner.[48,54] Other techniques are also utilized to try and stretch the muscle to get rid of the trigger points. This is usually the goal of each session of physiotherapy.

While the contributions made by Janet Travell, MD, and her associates have been monumental, unfortunately, traditional physical therapy and myofascial therapy often do not resolve the problem. Most people with trigger points obtain pain relief with traditional physical therapy modalities such as massage, ultrasound, and stretching; however, the results diminish on their way home from the therapist's office. Traditional medical doctors who treat people with trigger points will give various kinds of injections into these areas.[55] If, after months of therapy and muscle trigger point injections, the pain has not subsided, most likely the etiological source of the trigger point has not been addressed. The true etiology of the problem is in the ligament, not the muscle. When there is joint instability, the body will do one of three things: swell the joint, overgrow bone, or overuse the muscles to keep the joint stabilized. This is why some people have chronic trigger points and are labeled with myofascial pain syndrome. A better diagnosis would be chronic ligament laxity, and the better treatment is Prolotherapy. As the ligaments repair and the joints stabilize, the muscles no longer continuously work to stabilize the joint and can relax.

POSTURAL ORTHOSTATIC TACHYCARDIA SYNDROME (POTS)

One of the main functions of the autonomic nervous system is the control of heart rate and blood pressure. **POTS is what occurs when the system goes awry!** The defining symptom of POTS is an excessive heart rate, characterized by a marked rise of 30 beats per minute or greater within 10 minutes of standing from supine, or greater than 120 bpm while upright. This is often accompanied by a mild decrease in blood pressure. POTS symptoms manifest due to the body's inability to make the necessary adjustments to counteract gravity when standing up. Symptoms range from mild to a severely incapacitating disease. POTS sufferers often present with numerous musculoskeletal conditions, as POTS is frequently associated with hypermobile conditions such as EDS.[56] Joint instability causes overactivity of the sympathetic nervous system that has systemic ramifications. The more energy wasted on autonomic fluctuations during the day, along with increasingly disrupted sleep, the more exhausted a patient becomes—a vicious cycle.

SMALL FIBER NEUROPATHY

Some patients with connective tissue pain disorders, including fibromyalgia and EDS, have small fiber neuropathy that can be documented through small skin punch biopsy.[57,58] Studies have shown that about 50% of patients diagnosed with fibromyalgia have small fiber neuropathy.[59,60,61] It is believed that small fiber neuropathy is likely to contribute to some of the pain symptoms of fibromyalgia.[62] Classic symptoms of small fiber neuropathy are burning, stabbing, and tingling, in contrast to the typical deep muscular and aching pain seen in fibromyalgia.[63] Other symptoms of small fiber neuropathy include vague disturbances of sensation in the feet though some can have full-blown numbness. Though it does not explain all the symptoms of fibromyalgia it may help explain the hyperalgesis, allodynia and autonomic dysfunction seen in some patients.[64] What is not as appreciated is the concept of small fiber neuropathy potentially being caused by ligament laxity. As discussed in the previous chapter, the autonomic nervous systems function in health and disease cannot be overemphasized. The autonomic symptom improvement with Prolotherapy is generally very good in these patient populations and should be included as part of a comprehensive approach to treating connective tissue disorders.

SUMMARY

For patients suffering from full body pain, loose joints, and chronic subluxations, Prolotherapy is the ideal treatment to help strengthen the ligament junctions. Ligaments are made up of a very high amount of collagen. When these collagen cells mature, the ligaments get thicker and stronger. Strong ligaments allow the joints to properly glide through their normal range of motion without constantly subluxing and causing body pain and triggering autonomic nervous system symptoms.

Over-manipulation syndrome can begin after high velocity adjustments from a chiropractor or through self-manipulation. While chiropractors provide wonderful care in many cases, there is a risk of damaging the ligament structures and causing joint instability with continued high-velocity adjustments. If these manipulations are done over and over to the point where the area is continuously subluxing, it proves that the ligaments are overstretched and must be addressed. Prolotherapy should be sought to repair the ligaments and stabilize the joints. Additionally, it is important for the patient to stop receiving and performing manipulation of the joint, especially while receiving Prolotherapy.

There are varying degrees of congenital joint hypermobility that can be diagnosed according to the Beighton score and the Brighton criteria, in addition to other diagnostic tests as necessary for more severe cases. For all degrees of joint hypermobility syndrome, including the hypermobility type of Ehlers-Danlos syndrome, Prolotherapy provides an excellent treatment to strengthen ligaments, which can lessen or eliminate painful subluxations and chronic pain. This allows patients suffering from these debilitating conditions an improved chance at living an active lifestyle.

Fibromyalgia and myofascial pain syndrome may be diagnosed in the same patient due to their overlapping and vague descriptions, both involving pain throughout specific tender areas or trigger points that cause both local and referred pain. Digging a little deeper into a patient's health can help the clinician and the patient understand if the pain is due to issues that can be helped with Natural Medicine, such as food sensitivities, low hormones, poor sleep, and/or infections, among others. On the other hand, the physical exam may demonstrate undiagnosed joint instability in the areas exhibiting tender muscles and trigger points. The latter cases have remarkable success with Prolotherapy as a standalone treatment. Oftentimes, a combined approach is necessary to help the patient fully recover. As the joints repair, the muscles can relax and the pain is alleviated. With the pain-relief, sleep is improved and the vicious cycle is stopped! ■

CHAPTER

18

WHY YOU DON'T HEAL

In order for the body to optimally heal, people need to change. The health care providers need to change their thinking from providing "band-aid" approaches that actually worsen the degenerative process; and patients need to change their thinking to focus on what the body needs to heal itself. We summarize this point in what we call the Hauser Corollary: "If nothing changes, nothing changes." If patients with injuries continue through the traditional cascade of treatments starting with RICE, then NSAIDs, graduating to steroid shots, and finally getting promoted to arthroscopies and ending up with knee, hip, or other joint replacements, then, yes, nothing will change!

We encourage you to take health matters into your own hands. Make decisions based on what is best for your body. If a treatment prescription does not make sense to you or does not seem to focus on healing, we encourage you to ask more questions. Do not receive treatments based solely on what your insurance company will cover or what the so-called "expert" health care provider tells you. Realize that there are other options available. You do not have to accept "surgery is your only option" or "you need a cortisone shot" or "take these anti-inflammatory medications, you'll feel much better."

The other part of the Hauser Corollary that is vitally important to optimal health and healing from injuries is related to the part that you play in taking responsibility for your own health, particularly as it relates to avoiding things in your life that could be hurting the healing process.

THE HAUSER COROLLARY

Jenny is a good example to illustrate this point. Jenny was an avid athlete, playing several sports. She had all the answers before she came in to see us for ankle pain. After evaluating her, it was determined that she was suffering from significant ligament laxity in her ankles, which was the cause of her pain. Perhaps even more important was the fact that she had no specific incident where she could remember injuring her ankles. Jenny also exhibited tenderness on various parts of her body in addition to her ankles. This appeared to be related to nutritional factors. When delving into her history, we discovered that her ankle pain started a couple of years prior to her visit in our office, just after she had started taking the birth control pill because of painful, irregular menstruation. The medication she was taking contained an analogue of estradiol. Her diet consisted of nearly 100% carbohydrates, very small amounts of protein, and she was averse to taking vitamins. Yes, she was a good candidate for The Hauser Corollary.

Jenny was, however, open to receiving Prolotherapy on her ankles, but not to correcting the multiple factors that were related to her systemic connective tissue deficiency problem. She had multiple signs and symptoms that confirmed this diagnosis, such as non-healing sports injury with no overt trauma causing the original pain; multiple tender points in other parts of her body, especially about the knees and hips; dry skin; brittle nails and hair; menstrual problems; improper diet for her metabolism; and finally, taking synthetic estradiol. In order for the Prolotherapy to be maximally effective, we needed to address Jenny's inability to heal and convince her that she needed to do something about this in order to make the Prolotherapy worth enduring the shots! Reasoning alone would be insufficient. A visual graphic of The Hauser Corollary would help Jenny understand.

THE HAUSER COROLLARY: A GRAPHIC REPRESENTATION

Prolotherapy is a treatment that stimulates the body to repair painful areas. To put it another way, it is a treatment that causes the body to grow strong connective tissue. This connective tissue is primarily collagen, which makes up ligaments and tendons. Thus, Prolotherapy causes the growth and strengthening of ligaments and tendons. When a person's injury lingers beyond the usual healing time, it typically involves the ligaments and tendons. A weakening of the connective tissue graphically represents this. Prolotherapy injections reverse this by stimulating the connective tissues to heal. As the connective tissue grows and strengthens after Prolotherapy, the person reaches the eventual point where the pain has ceased. For the patient with a strong immune system, no more treatment or additional medical care is needed. Prolotherapy was indeed a cure for this individual. *(See Figure 18-1.)*

The person with systemic connective tissue deficiency, on the other hand, experiences no specific traumatic event to start the pain because the condition itself is weakening the connective tissues. In such an instance, all (or a majority) of the body's connective tissues are weakening. This process occurs normally with age, but with a systemic connective tissue deficiency (perhaps more appropriately called The Hauser syndrome) a person experiences an accelerated decline in connective tissue strength. This may result in sagging of the skin, thinning of the hair, and a myriad of other symptoms, the most prominent of which is pain. The first area to become painful will typically be the one used the most. For the pitcher it will be the shoulder, for the runner the knee, for the golfer the back, and so on. Just because a golfer gets back pain does not mean that golf is causing the injury. It could be primarily a systemic connective tissue deficiency problem. If the golfer, in

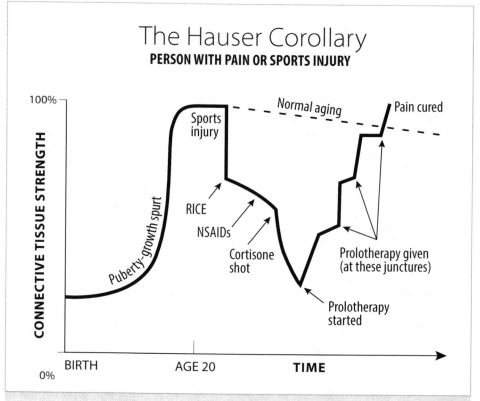

Figure 18-1: Graph of progress of a sports injury cured with Prolotherapy. The typical healthy Prolotherapy patient achieves a curative result after approximately 4 visits.

such an instance, just receives Prolotherapy, the pain relief from Prolotherapy will only last a certain amount of time. Once the connective tissue strength decreases below the pain-threshold point, the pain will recur. A cure will only be obtained when the person receives Prolotherapy **along with** additional treatments to correct the connective tissue deficiency problem. *(See Figure 18-2.)*

THERE ARE MANY "JENNYS" OUT THERE!

Seeing connective tissue deficiency as a visual representation really hit home for Jenny. She is still taking her oral contraceptive pills, but has incorporated more protein into her diet and takes some potent nutritional supplements. Even to her amazement, her energy level has improved and the mild aching she experienced in other parts of her body is going away. The Prolotherapy relieved her ankle pain and she is back to playing her various sports. Yes, there are many Jennys out there. People who want to completely heal their injuries also want to remain out of the doctor's office—permanently. In order to accomplish this, they should start eating an appropriate diet and taking supplements to enhance connective tissue regeneration.

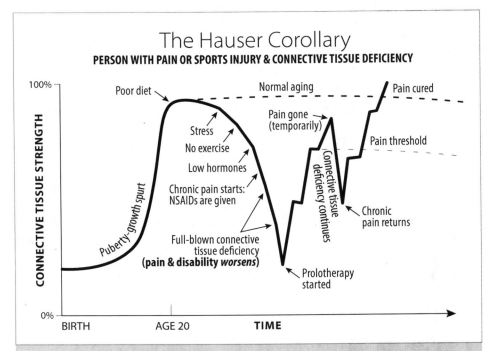

Figure 18-2: Connective tissue deficiency cured with Prolotherapy and Natural Medicine. For people with connective tissue deficiency (Hauser syndrome), Prolotherapy is utilized along with diet, stress reduction, exercise, nutriceuticals, anabolic hormones, and other natural remedies to cure the condition.

THE POSITIVE HAUSER COROLLARY

In the positive, The Hauser Corollary states that "If something changes, something changes." This sounds just too profound for words, but bear with us! An expanded, more thorough representation of The Hauser Corollary is: **"If nothing changes, nothing definitely changes. If something changes, generally something changes, but eventually something will change with enough changes."** How's that for a lot of words?

For the person with a chronic injury, one can be assured that if the same treatments continue to be used, then the same result will occur. For example, athletes jump around from athletic trainer to physical therapist, to massage therapist to chiropractor, back to athletic trainer to physical therapist, to acupuncturist to a different massage therapist or chiropractor, and the cycle continues to repeat. Obtaining some symptomatic relief with these types of therapies is fine for the general population, but for the athlete, time is of the essence. Every day an athlete is out with an injury, another two days of rehabilitation and training are necessary to return to the pre-injury level. Thus, it is vital for athletes and others in pain to take it upon themselves to **change the type of treatments they are receiving.**

By applying The Positive Hauser Corollary, patients receive treatments that stimulate connective tissue growth in the ligaments and tendons, namely Prolotherapy, in combination with various nutriceuticals and the MEAT protocol.

It does not eliminate the need for specific training regimens, post-workout massages, or occasional chiropractic visits, but should abolish such phrases as RICE, NSAIDs, anti-inflammatories, and cortisone shots from medicine's vocabulary. The net result of this is a significant decline in the use of such procedures as arthroscopy, surgery, and joint replacement.

It is our hope that everyone, including athletes and sports medicine practitioners, as well as pain patients and practitioners, will take this Positive Hauser Corollary to heart…"If something changes, something changes." The changes we would like to see in the care of chronic injuries, such as those to ligaments and tendons, include the following:

1. Application of heat to injured areas instead of ice.
2. Early use of some type of active exercise program as opposed to rest.
3. MEAT rather than RICE protocol.
4. Discontinuation of most wraps and braces.
5. Women, cease taking estradiol in the form of birth control pills or allopathic hormone replacement.
6. Eliminate NSAIDs.
7. Use of proteolytic enzymes to reduce swelling.
8. Widespread utilization of nutritional supplements to aid healing.
9. The removal of cortisone, and its derivatives, in syringes pointed toward athletes and injury victims.
10. My Reproducibility Instrument (the thumb) to replace mechanical MRI.
11. A dramatic decline in the "look and see" arthroscopy.
12. Prolotherapy promoted to a first-line therapy.
13. Surgery only as a measure for emergencies or as a last resort.
14. Sports medicine specialist becomes synonymous with Prolotherapist.

Only when the principles of this book are applied will people be truly healed. The body has, does, and always will heal by inflammation. This is why we can confidently say that you can cure your chronic pain, arthritis, and sports injuries with regenerative injection treatments such as Prolotherapy. There is a cure for injuries and a way to enhance health and strength, and that way is Prolotherapy.

FACTORS AFFECTING HEALING

Generally, by the time people are seen at one of our Caring Medical offices, they have seen 10 prior health care clinicians and often none of them have considered any of the potential causes as to why they don't heal.

By definition, pain means something is weak or injured, assuming a musculoskeletal cause for the pain. Most people can tell the date and time when their pain started. "I was in a car accident on…I fell down the stairs on…I was playing a lot of golf when…" Most people with pain know what started the pain— they just want to find out how to end it!

TOP TEN REASONS WHY YOU DON'T HEAL

1. Nutrition: Deficiencies and eating the wrong food.
2. Hormone deficiency or imbalance.
3. Medications such as anti-inflammatories or narcotics.
4. Over-manipulation by self or other practitioner.
5. Inadequate Prolotherapy.
6. Sleep and inadequate rest.
7. Food sensitivities.
8. Chronic infection.
9. Melancholy temperament or negative attitude.
10. God's will for your life and 7 deadly stresses.

EATING THE WRONG FOODS

To grow ligaments, tendons, or for that matter to heal any bodily structure, it is safe to say that the whole gamut of essential nutrients is needed—this means amino acids, fatty acids, vitamins, minerals, and trace elements that are supposed to be consumed in a healthy diet.

Nutritional testing is recommended for those pain patients who are not healing properly. Sometimes the sole reason for inadequate healing is because the patient does not eat correctly. We recommend that the diet consist primarily of vegetables, proteins, and some complex carbohydrates, in the form of fresh foods, organic and non-processed as much as possible. Leave the white flour, chips, snacks, sugary foods, and sodas on the store shelves. Consuming too many simple carbohydrates is one of the primary reasons people are overweight. The joints and ligaments are strained when they have to carry so much more weight. Weight loss is, therefore, a part of curing chronic pain. You may not realize that one sugar load hampers immune function for four hours! So the person who consumes a soda every few hours is suppressing the immune system all day. This is the same immune system that heals your connective tissues. If you want to heal, cut out the sugar and take control of your diet.

This can include a high-grade multi-vitamin in addition to specific herbs that help collagen growth and proteolytic enzymes for tissue recovery. While many herbal products and enzymes are referred to as "anti-inflammatory" in the media or even their own marketing materials, the mechanisms are actually more pro-healing. They tend to speed the body through reparative processes faster, but from clinical experience we have seen that these are much different than taking NSAIDs.

EATING WRONG

Do you know for sure that you are eating the right kinds of foods in the right amounts? Why do some people feel great as a vegetarian, while others do not, and many people who count calories continue to put on weight and feel lethargic? If you answered "no", you are not alone. To help patients answer these questions we developed Hauser Diet Typing®.

The goal of Diet Typing is to find the foods that will give you the maximum amount of energy. Your body functions the best when energy reserves are highest. Basically, more energy = more health.

In a nutshell if you eat the wrong types of foods you will not feel well. *(See Figure 18-3.)* To have optimum energy and reach your physical potential it is necessary that the body extract the maximum amount of energy from the food consumed. Some humans have vegetarian physiology and others have carnivorous physiology. The

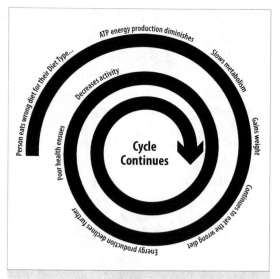

Figure 18-3: Eating wrong. Eating the wrong foods for your Diet Type can cause weight gain, diminished energy, and lead to further health problems.

majority of us are a combination. Thus we divided the various Hauser Diet Types according to the animals with a similar dietary breakdown that correspond to each Diet Type. These Diet Types are the Lion Diet Type®, Otter Diet Type®, Bear Diet Type®, Monkey Diet Type®, and Giraffe Diet Type®.

Realize however, it is not necessarily just learning your Diet Type that is important it is *actually eating right* once you are informed of your Hauser Diet Type!

HORMONE DEFICIENCY OR IMBALANCE

The engines driving your immune system are your hormones. Everything cannot be blamed on your chronic pain. The person who experiences thinning hair, loss of sex drive, decreased muscle tone, dry skin, menstrual cramping, irregular menses, chronic fatigue, decreased body temperature, and a feeling of coldness has a hormone deficiency until proven otherwise.

Like everything else in our bodies, hormone levels need to be balanced. The "correct balance" can change, based on our gender and age, but everyone needs their hormones balanced in order for their bodies to function the way they were meant to function. When your hormones are off balance, it is a sign that the body is not working correctly. When the body does not function optimally, it cannot heal the way it is supposed to heal. For instance, having high estradiol levels can decrease the ability of the body to make fibroblasts, the cells needed to make connective tissue. *(See Figure 18-4.)* This is a consideration for women who are on birth control, as it can hamper healing ability. Low hormone levels can most definitely alter your ability to heal, let alone make you feel sluggish and unhealthy. Fortunately, this can be fixed with Natural Hormone Replacement therapy regimens. We balance your hormones so that the levels are where they are supposed to be for your age and gender. After your hormones attain balance, your body is able to respond to Prolotherapy and heal your injury, so you are feeling your best!

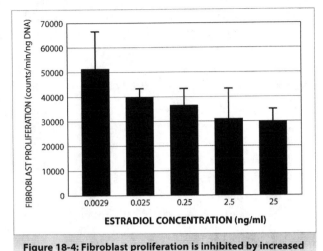

Figure 18-4: Fibroblast proliferation is inhibited by increased estradiol levels.
Adapted from *American Journal of Sports Medicine* Vol. 25, Page 707 © 1998.

We want to help you heal as fast as possible. Understanding your hormone levels may be the key to doing just that!

We commonly check the following hormone levels to optimize health, healing, and aging: thyroid, TSH, Growth Hormone, DHEA, pregnenolone, estrogen, progesterone, testosterone, melatonin, and cortisol at least to start. For the person in chronic pain, most assuredly, at least one of these levels will turn out to be suboptimal. Always keep in mind that certain hormones are anabolic, meaning they grow connective tissue, where others are catabolic and promote its breakdown. **(See Figures 18-5 & 18-6.)** When deficient, supplementing with natural hormones will generally enhance healing. More important is hormonal balancing, making sure that the hormonal milieu is anabolic and not catabolic.

MEDICATIONS: THE EFFECTS OF NARCOTICS AND ANTI-INFLAMMATORIES ON HEALING

Nothing pains us more than seeing a chronic pain patient addicted to narcotics. Hopefully, after reading thissection you will see why we feel that way. In regard to the anti-inflammatories, they have been covered adequately in this book but, in case you forgot, **nonsteroidal anti-inflammatory drugs (NSAIDs) stop the normal healing inflammatory reaction! In other words, they are anti-healing.** The body heals by

	Catabolic	Anabolic
Ability to train intensely	Poor	Excellent
Aging effects	Advanced	Diminished
Arthritis risk	High	Low
Connective tissue healing	Poor	Excellent
DHEA levels	Low	High
Estradiol levels	High	Low
Estriol levels	Low	High
Growth hormone levels	Low	High
Healing capacity	Poor	Excellent
Likelihood of injury	High	Low
Progesterone levels	Low	High
Recovery after workouts	Poor	Excellent
Testosterone levels	Low	High

Figure 18-5: Catabolic versus anabolic profiles. A person whose metabolism is anabolic has a much greater chance to heal an injury than if the metabolism is catabolic.

inflammation. The person with chronic pain has a choice—anti-inflame your way to terrible arthritis or Prolo your way to freedom from pain!

As detrimental to healing as NSAIDs are, they are no match for narcotics. Why don't we start with the known effects of narcotics and go from there?

THE KNOWN EFFECTS OF NARCOTICS ON THE IMMUNE SYSTEM

1. Suppression of the cytotoxic activity of natural killer cells.[1]
2. Enhanced growth of implanted tumors.[1]
3. Depressed T–lymphocyte responsiveness to stimulation.[2]
4. Ablate delayed hypersensitive skin response.[3]
5. Spleen atrophy.[4]
6. Thymus atrophy.[4,5]
7. Decreased T-lymphocyte numbers.[5]
8. Decreased T-cell function.[6]
9. Inhibition of antibody production.[7]
10. Inhibition of B-cell activity.[7]
11. Decreased levels of interferon.[8]
12. Increased incidence of infections.[9]
13. **Depressed function of all cells of the immune system.**[10]

Once patients take regular narcotics for longer than two months, it is doubtful they will ever stop taking them. This is a sad statement—but it is true. If a doctor offered a chronic pain patient chemotherapy, he would most likely decline, even if it gave some pain relief, because everyone knows that chemotherapy can be dangerous. Well, guess what? **Narcotics have the same depressive effects on the immune system as chemotherapy!**

If you do not believe us, then listen to what the premier neuroimmunology journal in the world says. Yes, the *Journal of Neuroimmunology*, in an article from Toby K. Eisenstein and Mary E. Hilburger, from the department of microbiology and immunology at Temple University School of Medicine, stated it plainly.[10] The article is entitled, "Opioid Modulation of Immune Responses: Effects on Phagocyte and Lymphoid Cell Populations." It is a review article on the information known to date as to narcotics effects on the immune system. Their conclusion of the whole matter is, "**In aggregate, the literature supports the existence of *in vivo* neural-immune circuits through which morphine acts to depress the function of *all cells* of the immune system.**" In other words, taking the medical literature as a whole, narcotics suppress *every* cell of the immune system.

The body needs an intact immune system to heal. It does not matter if it is after an accident, sports activity, or Prolotherapy, the body heals by inflammation, and inflammation **only** occurs if the body can mount an immune reaction. The person who is on narcotics needs to cease taking them if healing is to take place.

WHAT ARE NARCOTICS?

The term "narcotic" is derived from the Greek word for "stupor" and, at one time, applied to any drug that induced sleep, but most often refer to drugs that have morphine-like, strong analgesic properties.[11] Narcotics are to morphine as NSAIDs are to aspirin. There are numerous NSAIDs because each touts that it is safer and more efficacious than the other. So it is with the various narcotics— each tries to become an even stronger pain reliever with fewer side effects. By definition, narcotics, which act as morphine does, are immunosuppressive. This goes for Vicodin®, Darvocet®, Duragesic®, morphine, Oxycontin®, codeine, Percodan®, and any other such addictive substances.

It is not necessary to be completely off narcotics to begin Prolotherapy, though this is preferred;

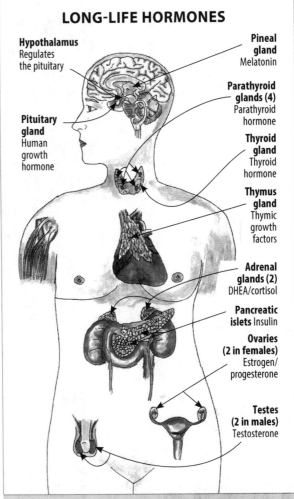

LONG-LIFE HORMONES

Hypothalamus
Regulates the pituitary

Pituitary gland
Human growth hormone

Pineal gland
Melatonin

Parathyroid glands (4)
Parathyroid hormone

Thyroid gland
Thyroid hormone

Thymus gland
Thymic growth factors

Adrenal glands (2)
DHEA/cortisol

Pancreatic islets Insulin

Ovaries (2 in females)
Estrogen/progesterone

Testes (2 in males)
Testosterone

Figure 18-6: The endocrine system. The endocrine glands secrete the hormones that help the body stay healthy. The hormones DHEA, testosterone, progesterone, and Growth Hormone stimulate the repair of the connective tissues, thus they are anabolic.

but there must be a willingness to begin weaning off of them. For people unable to do so, there is little hope of curing their pain. Typically, a person's dose of narcotics is weaned by 5 to 10 mg per week until he or she is completely off of narcotics. It is always helpful for a person on narcotics to have nutritional and hormonal assessments in order to determine appropriate treatments to enhance their immune function, which is depressed from the narcotics. By taking this approach, we have had success, even with heroin addicts, in not only curing their chronic pain—but also curing their addictions.

OVER-MANIPULATION

Self or chiropractic manipulation has the potential to loosen ligaments or make them lax, which then causes them to sublux even more, not less. *(See Figure 18-7.)* This leads to the joint becoming more and more unstable, a condition we termed over-manipulation syndrome (OMS). We published an extensive research article on this concept in the *Journal of Applied Research* in 2013.[12]

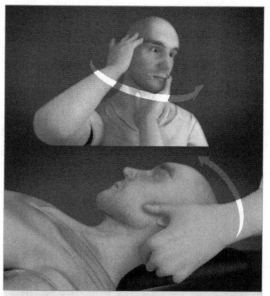

Figure 18-7: Over-manipulation negatively affects healing. Chiropractic high velocity adjustments and self-manipulation may correct subluxations temporarily, but they have a negative long-term effect because they worsen joint instability by continuously re-loosening and overstretching the ligaments.

SELF-MANIPULATION:

If you are voluntarily manipulating your back or neck repeatedly throughout the day, you are worsening the spinal instability. For some patients it develops into a chronic habit or addiction. We have seen patients come in for a consultation with neck or back pain and it is not uncommon for patients to tell us that they adjust their necks or backs many times per day. One of the record number of times reported was someone who said that he had been self manipulating his upper back for 25 years every 5-10 minutes! He was finally able to reduce it to 25 times per day. After his first Prolotherapy treatment he reduced it even further to 2 or 3 times per day. Obviously we urged him to completely stop, so that he could allow the Prolotherapy to do its job: strengthen and tighten loose ligaments and joints.

CHIROPRACTIC MANIPULATION

We have also seen many patients who have received hundreds of chiropractic high velocity manipulations over many years in order to manage their chronic pain. Patients who already have loose or lax ligaments should avoid these entirely because high velocity manipulations can put extra strain on ligament tissue, further causing it to become damaged or lax. This is especially true in those with congenital hypermobility. Those with this condition already have loose ligaments to begin with, so if they continue to receive high velocity adjustments on a regular basis they could potentially set themselves up for further pain and complications.

If you need to self manipulate or receive chiropractic manipulation repeatedly then you need to consider resolving the issue with Prolotherapy.

INADEQUATE PROLOTHERAPY

We are often asked the question, "Where can I get Prolotherapy the way you perform it at Caring Medical?" The answer to this question is "Caring Medical." Each practitioner has their own way of doing things. We feel our comprehensive approach at Caring Medical is highly effective and our study results prove that.

Prolotherapy's efficaciousness in curing chronic pain is completely dependent on the Prolotherapist's ability to **completely** treat the injured structures. This means that all of the injured structures are treated with a strong enough solution to heal the area in a reasonable period of time. We have heard of people getting 30 or 40 sessions of Prolotherapy without good results, or receiving three injections during a Prolotherapy session for the lower back. As this book discusses, most people are cured of their pain with 3-6 Prolotherapy sessions. If by the sixth Prolotherapy session, a patient has not experienced significant improvement, we search for an additional cause of his/her pain.

A general rule of thumb when receiving the Hackett-Hemwall-Hauser technique of Prolotherapy, is to receive 30 to 40 injections for an extremity (knee, ankle, or shoulder) and anywhere from 50 to 80 injections for the neck, back, or thoracic spine. *(See Figure 18-8.)* Someone getting three shots to the lower back during a session is probably not getting Prolotherapy, but most likely trigger point injections. Trigger point injections are given into the muscle to decrease muscle spasms. Sometimes you are being given Prolotherapy injections, but just very few of them. Some doctors who administer cellular forms of Prolotherapy, such as Platelet Rich Plasma or Stem Cell Prolotherapy, will only provide one injection into the joint. We find that the entire support structure of the joint needs to be treated in order to fully treat the painful area. This involves injecting at all of the attachments that support the joint versus just providing one injection into the joint.

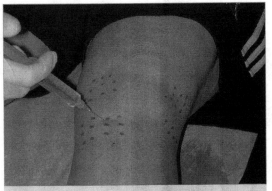

Figure 18-8: Typical injection sites for Hackett-Hemwall dextrose Prolotherapy of the knee. As you can see, it is a much more comprehensive treatment technique than only one or two injections.

Another reason for suboptimal results with Prolotherapy is due to inadequate inflammation with the Prolotherapy treatment. Remember, **the body heals only by inflammation.** In some people, stronger Prolotherapy solutions are needed to achieve an adequate inflammatory reaction after the treatment. Until the injured structures are completely treated with Prolotherapy—with a strong enough solution—Prolotherapy has not failed. It is important that the patient feel stiff for at least one to two days after a Prolotherapy session. If the stiffness after the treatment lasts only a few hours, then the immune reaction to the treatment, most likely, will not be enough to regenerate the connective tissue needed for healing. In such a situation, there are two options. First, figure out why you have a poor immune response by doing metabolic, nutritional, and hormonal testing, or, second, use a stronger Prolotherapy solution. Physicians who have a lot of experience doing Prolotherapy may have a dozen different solutions they can use, depending on the individual case.

SLEEP AND INADEQUATE REST

Inadequate or poor sleep is often an overlooked factor in health and healing. Do you get enough good quality sleep? If you do not feel rested in the morning or if you rely on an alarm clock to wake you up, you may not be getting enough sleep. If you aren't allowing enough time for sleep, it may be time to look at your schedule and get to bed earlier.

Sleeplessness has a cause. Find the cause and the insomnia typically goes away. Insomnia is a common cause of chronic fatigue, body pain, poor concentration, anxiety, depression, and poor athletic performance.

When did it start? What was going on in your life when the insomnia started? It started with being married. Was this due to the fact that your spouse likes the room warmer than you? The solution might be as simple as putting a fan on your side of the bed. It started with a new job. Figure out why this is causing sleeplessness. Talk about it. Figure out what bothers you about your job. Resolving the underlying cause of the insomnia can help resolve it.

Excessive thinking can keep people awake at night. Not just thinking, but excessive worry. *(See Figure 18-9.)* Edmund Jacobson, MD, a Chicagoland physician, the first person to measure electrical activity in muscles at rest in the early 1900s discovered that excessive thinking caused the muscles of the jaw to contract and keep people awake.[13] Someone who is worrying excessively and thinking all the time, has no capacity to go to sleep at night unless a sedative is taken (such as a sleeping pill). A better approach

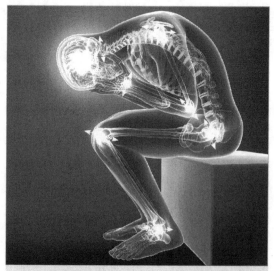

Figure 18-9: Excessive worry and negative thought patterns can cause sleeplessness, impair healing, and worsen pain. Obtaining enough rest and a good night's sleep is a very important part of the body's repair process.

is to be "in the moment." Concentrate on what you are doing moment to moment which will cause you to work more efficiently, to focus on people more who are talking to you (which is what you should be doing any way) and allow you to enjoy life more because you aren't worrying about all that is wrong with the world, your life, or the future!

Another weapon that you need to know about to feel rested and refreshed: the nap. Read the book by Sara Mednick, PhD, Harvard researched called *Take a Nap! Change Your Life.* (Workman publishing, New York, 2006). Most of us who enjoy naps, know that naps can give you instant energy. Dr. Mednick documents very well in this book how there are two periods of drowsiness one during the day but another one just after lunch. A nap from 20–90 minutes mid–day can have the same effects basically as a full–night's rest. We were designed by God to take naps in order to function optimally.

PAIN AND INSOMNIA

Many of our patients' insomnia issues are due to pain. Get rid of the pain and sleep is improved. If pain is keeping you awake, then Prolotherapy could be the key to a good night's sleep.

CORTISOL, STRESS, AND INSOMNIA

The stress hormone in your body that controls when you wake up and when you go to sleep is called cortisol. Blood cortisol levels are supposed to be high in the morning and low in the evening. The high levels in the morning help you wake up and the low levels in the evening help you feel tired in preparation for sleep.

Not eating may actually cause insomnia. If you don't eat at night because you aren't hungry or you are working late, then the body makes cortisol to keep your blood sugar up. The high cortisol could keep you up at night.

URINATING DURING THE NIGHT

Many people don't sleep because they are urinating throughout the night. This could be because of too much coffee or fluid consumption at night. So stop doing it! Excessive thirst or urination can, however, be related to a significant problem called diabetes insipidus.

Diabetes insipidus is caused by a deficiency in the hormone Vasopressin or Antidiuretic Hormone (ADH). This is one of the main hormones that helps the body retain the water it needs. Inadequate ADH may cause you to become chronically dehydrated. Diabetes insipidus can cause dehydration, joint pain, vertebral disc dehydration, cartilage problems, dizziness, and fatigue. It is documented by urine and blood tests.

Rhonda came to see us with a myriad of complaints, including fatigue, dizziness, body pains, and poor concentration. She thought she was a good candidate for Prolotherapy. Upon further questioning, she revealed that she was getting terrible sleep. Rhonda said that she needed to drink a gallon of water every day. Therefore, she would have to get up multiple times in the night to go to the bathroom. Blood and urine tests confirmed diabetes insipidus. Rhonda was placed on Antidiuretic Hormone, and her dose was carefully increased to the point where she could sleep through the night without having to get up to use the bathroom.

INADEQUATE REST

Many of our patients are very driven, accomplished people. They love to exercise, train, and stay physically fit. Thus, when injury hits, they are extremely upset, and rightly so. However, one of the factors that we find will contribute to non-healing is not allowing enough rest time between workouts, after long work days, or during stressful life events. When your body tells you that it needs rest, you should listen. Certain times in your life require more rest. If you stop doing what you are doing and listen to your body and take the time to rest, it will typically pay off in the long run. One day of added rest can lead to a healthier life and make you less likely to injure yourself.

CREEP

Creep is actually a medical condition that results from the elongation of ligaments stemming from long-term tension put on them. **(See Figure 18-10.)** This can be caused from improper form at the gym, standing too long with terrible posture, or even slouching in a chair too long. We are discussing this

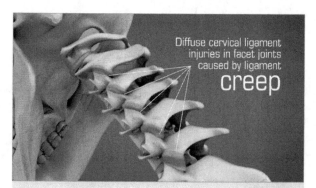

Diffuse cervical ligament injuries in facet joints caused by ligament **creep**

Figure 18-10: Ligament creep. Ligaments, when subjected to a constant stress, display Creep behavior—a time-dependent increase in strain or the fact that ligaments slowly "stretch out" over time.

in the healing chapter of the book because again, if you continue to perform the same tasks repeatedly, you will find it difficult to heal. One common example of this is related to those who use their smart phones for emailing and texting. These patients may be receiving Prolotherapy to their necks, upper backs, wrists, and even their thumbs, but because they have not rested the body, they have not allowed the body to heal itself as it should be able to do.

FOOD SENSITIVITIES

Part of knowing which foods to eat involves getting a blood food sensitivities profile in addition to Hauser Diet Typing. For example, if you typed out a Lion Diet Type®, milk would be allowed on that diet. But if you were severely allergic to the milk, drinking milk or eating cheese, in this instance, would not help you achieve maximum energy, it would actually take away energy.

Food sensitivities are tested by a blood sample. The laboratory checks for IgG antibodies against certain foods. When we eat foods to which we have sensitivities, our immune cells produce antibodies, which are like little torpedoes, made to destroy the invading substance. Yes, there are certain foods that people eat everyday that may actually be seen by the body as invaders. Instead of these foods giving you energy (the ultimate purpose of food), the foods actually take energy away from the body. *(See Figure 18-11.)*

For example, patients will report that certain joints hurt when they consume dairy products such as milk, pizza, ice cream and the like. This may not occur immediately after eating the dairy products, but can occur days later. Food sensitivities create a systemic inflammation in the body, noticeable by increased pain, an indication that there is something wrong when this food is consumed. Never underestimate the power of food!

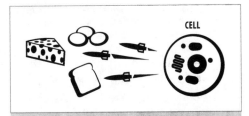

Figure 18-11: Cells send out antibodies to attack sensitive foods because these foods are detected as harmful.

CHRONIC INFECTIONS

For the person who has multiple areas of pain, especially chronic body aching, the cause may be "leaky gut syndrome." This condition is caused by a disorder of the tight junctions of the digestive tract no longer being "tight" and allowing particulates from food or infectious agents into the blood stream. If a person has an overgrowth of a bad organism in the digestive tract or food sensitivities, the tight junctions of the intestines are no longer tight and allow toxins into the body and these then get absorbed into the blood stream. One can easily document this for instance by doing a blood test for candida immune complexes, which shows that not only did candida come across the digestive tract but the body sent an antibody to "complex" with it. Do you think your body would be hurting all over, like you have the flu if this was occurring? *(See Figure 18-12.)*

To overcome leaky gut syndrome, nutritional status must be improved. A chronic infection in the digestive tract is called intestinal dysbiosis. The easy treatment for this is to clean up the diet and take a lot of probiotics (good bacteria) such as lactobacillus acidophilus and bifidobacterium bifidum. The probiotics crowd out the bad bacteria or fungus. The person who has been on a lot of antibiotics, most likely has destroyed the good bacteria and then allowed these bad bacteria, fungi and parasites to take over, which perpetuate the leaky gut syndrome. Sometimes a comprehensive stool digestive analysis needs to be done to see what the intestinal flora look like.

There are a host of other chronic infections that plague folks with chronic pain. "I don't have any fevers, so I don't have an infection." So the arguments go. All

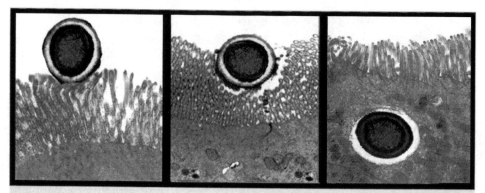

Figure 18-12: Yeast burrowing through the intestinal wall. Candida fungus infection is one of the causes of "leaky gut syndrome." Pictures courtesy of Great Smokies Diagnostic Laboratory, Asheville, North Carolina.

you have to do is point to the fact that people get cold sores. Most cold sores are a herpes viral infection, yet the people have no fevers. You can have an indolent, low-level, yet raging infection causing your chronic pain without knowing it. The most common ones that we test for in the office are Mycoplasma, Lyme, Babesiosis, and various fungal infections, including Candida. Research is mounting that all four of these are much more prevalent than most people think and all of them can cause chronic pain.

MYCOPLASMA INFECTIONS

Many people with chronic pain are also wracked with chronic fatigue. Often the pain is blamed as the cause for the chronic fatigue. Unfortunately, this is not the case in most instances, because Mycoplasma infection is the cause. Mycoplasma is the smallest, simplest known bacterium. These bacteria are invasive and burrow themselves deep within the body tissues, including the brain, central and peripheral nervous systems, muscles and joints, bone marrow, digestive tract, lungs and heart, and the immune system. They can virtually "hide" within the white blood cells of the human body, which makes them undetectable by the immune system and very difficult to treat.

It is now possible to diagnose Mycoplasma by a simple blood test. Researchers are finding that the incidence of Mycoplasma infection in disorders such as Gulf War syndrome, chronic fatigue syndrome, fibromyalgia, and rheumatoid arthritis is around 65%.[14,15] The most common symptoms found from Mycoplasma infection include fatigue, clouded thinking, depression, memory problems, balance disorders, joint stiffness, and various types of chronic pain.

The main treatment for Mycoplasma infection is long-term antibiotics. Because of the risk of a depletion of the normal flora bacteria in the intestines, probiotics are given along with an antifungal regimen or medication. If the infection is the cause of the patient's symptoms, generally a gradual decrease in pain and increase in energy is seen. Remarkable as it sounds, some who have rheumatoid arthritis and other autoimmune diseases, including lupus and scleroderma, have remissions of the disease while on the antibiotics. Anyone with these conditions should get checked for this organism because resolution of your pain or fatigue could depend on it.

MUSCULOSKELETAL MANIFESTATIONS OF LYME DISEASE

Most people have heard of Lyme disease but know very little about it. Lyme disease is caused by the spirochete *Borrelia burgdorferi*, which is carried by infected ticks. This disorder has a variable clinical course and involves multiple systems, affecting the skin, nervous system, heart, and eyes. Early in the illness, many patients experience migratory musculoskeletal pain in joints, bursae, tendons, muscle, or bone, in one or a few locations at a time, frequently lasting only hours or days in a given location. Weeks to months later, untreated patients often have intermittent or chronic arthritis, primarily involving the large joints, especially the knees, over a period of several years.[16,17] *(See Figure 18-13.)*

Since the clinical course of the disorder is so varied, from mild aches and pains to debilitating memory, neurologic and heart conditions, there is no one symptom that is diagnostic for Lyme disease. For this reason, it is important for those with chronic pain and/or fatigue to get the various blood and urine tests for the condition.

The treatment for this condition is similar to Mycoplasma infection, involving long courses of antibiotics. For the person desiring to avoid antibiotics, we prescribe various herbal programs and add connective tissue products for the patients with chronic musculoskeletal complaints.

BABESIOSIS

Babesiosis is an infection that may be spread by the same tick that carries borreliosis (Lyme disease). It is caused by *Babesia microti*, which is a protozoa—not bacteria, virus, fungus, or yeast. Other examples of protozoal infections are malaria and giardia.

Babesia infection can cause all of the same symptoms as

Joint	# of Patients Affected	Periarticular Site	# of Patients Affected
Knee	27	Back	9
Shoulder	14	Neck	6
Ankle	12	Bicipital	4
Elbow	11	Lateral epicondyle	2
Temporomandibular	11	Lateral collateral	2
Wrist	10	de Querva's disease	1
Hip	9	Prepatellar	4
Metacarpophalangeal	4	Subacromial	2
Proximal interphalangeal	4	Infraspinatus	2
Distal interphalangeal	4	Olecranon	2
Metatarsophalangeal	4	Sausage digits	2
Sternoclavicular	1	Heel pain	2

Figure 18-13: Joints and periarticular sites affected out of 28 patients with lyme arthritis.

Lyme disease, and in many ways, it masks the disease. Anyone who is suspected of having Lyme disease should also have Babesiosis testing. Like Lyme disease, the best test is a blood test. The treatment course of long-term antibiotics is also similar.

CANDIDA

Because of the indiscriminate use of antibiotics, cortisone shots, prednisone prescriptions, and the like, fungal infections are prevalent. Candida is a yeast that is the most common cause of systemic fungal infections and is common in people with pain throughout the whole body. There are various methods to document an internal fungus infection, most commonly a stool culture or blood antibody test. Once a fungal infection, such as candida, is found, antifungal herbal remedies or medications are needed for several months. In addition, patients are put on a strict diet, high in fresh, non-processed protein and vegetables. The diet also severely restricts carbohydrates from fruit, bread, sugar, juice, starches, alcohol, and fermented foods. The diet is designed to stop feeding the candida. It is also advised to supplement with high amounts of probiotics to restore the balance of gut flora overtaken by gastrointestinal candida overgrowth.

MELANCHOLY TEMPERAMENT

"Negative thoughts have a negative effect on the body and positive thoughts have a positive effect on the body." —Ross A. Hauser, MD

The next two sections of this chapter focus on the emotional side of pain. We put these toward the back of the book to focus the attention on the true cause of most structural chronic pain, which is joint instability, and its treatment with Prolotherapy. But make no mistake, all pain has an emotional component. In some instances, it is the central piece that has to be resolved in order to cure the chronic pain!

> *"Do not judge, or you too will be judged. For in the same way you judge others, you will be judged, and with the measure you use, it will be measured to you. Why do you look at the speck of sawdust in your brother's eye and pay no attention to the plank in your own eye? How can you say to your brother, 'Let me take the speck out of your eye,' when all the time there is a plank in your own eye? You hypocrite, first take the plank out of your own eye, and then you will see clearly to remove the speck from your brother's eye."*

These words were spoken by Jesus Christ, as recorded in the Bible in Matthew 7:1-5. No matter if you are a Christian or not, the principle of "be careful of judging or drawing conclusions" still applies. As it turns out, some people are more apt to judge, be critical, and/or look at the negative side of events. Unfortunately for these people, they are more prone to developing chronic illness and pain. Perhaps the simplest explanation for this is that negative thoughts have a negative impact on the body and positive thoughts have a positive impact on the body.

Too often people want to blame the circumstances of their lives as the reasons why they act certain ways. The fact is, circumstances reveal what is deep down inside of a person. The person who has strong self-esteem and a strong faith can face even the most difficult of situations with grace, peace, and calmness; whereas the person who struggles without these virtues reacts to the same stimulus with bitterness, anger, and resentment. Much of the difference in the way people react to illness and life circumstances, as well as to each other, can be found in the different temperaments people possess.

Temperament is defined as "constitution of a substance, body, or organism with respect to the mixture or balance of its elements, qualities or parts; makeup; characteristic or habitual inclination; or mode of emotional response."[18] There are four basic temperaments: choleric, sanguine, phlegmatic, and melancholy; each of which has strengths and weaknesses. Believe it or not, the person to first describe these four temperaments was Hippocrates, who lived from 460 to 370 B.C. The basic characteristics of the four temperaments are found in *Figure 18-14*.

Learning about their own temperament helps people see themselves as others see them. Often these two viewpoints are completely opposite. A complete description of the temperaments, as well as personality profile tests people can take to determine their temperament, are available. We encourage everyone with chronic pain to explore this.[19-22]

After treating many thousands of chronically ill people, it is our contention that a good percentage of them have melancholy temperaments. The strengths of the melancholic are that they are the most sensitive and the "deepest thinkers" of all the temperaments, and are thus the playwrights, authors, artists, and those in the creative arts. The melancholic is often thinking, and often thinking too much. "What did he or she mean by that, why did they look at me that way, did the doctor mean such and such?" The melancholy temperament has a strong perfectionist tendency, with standards of excellence that exceed those of others and requirements of acceptability—in any field—that are often higher than anyone can maintain. This is a great set-up for disappointment and, thus, the melancholy tendencies.

Temperament	Strengths	Weaknesses
Sanguine	Enjoying	Restless
	Optimistic	Weak-willed
	Friendly	Egotistical
	Compassionate	Emotionally unstable
Choleric	Strong willpower	Hot-tempered
	Practical	Cruel
	Leader	Impetuous
	Optimistic	Self-sufficient
Phlegmatic	Witty	Slow and lazy
	Dependable	Teasing
	Practical	Stubborn
	Efficient	Indecisive
Melancholy	Sensitive	Self-centered
	Perfectionist	Pessimistic
	Analytical	Moody
	Faithful friend	Revengeful

Figure 18-14: Characteristics of the four temperaments.

The melancholic is very analytical, but in relation to getting ill, this can be a bad thing. "Why did this happen to me?" Because illness doesn't fit into the perfectionist imaginary world in which the melancholic lives, pessimism, bitterness, and self-centeredness results, especially relating to the aches and pains the person experiences.

A good description of the melancholic is as follows: "He is surely more self-centered than any of the other temperaments. He is inclined to that kind of self-examination, that kind of self-contemplation which paralyzes his will and energy. He is always dissecting himself and his own mental conditions, taking off layer after layer as an onion is peeled, until there is nothing direct and artless left in his life; there is only his everlasting self-examination. This self-examination is not only unfortunate, it is harmful. Melancholies usually drift into morbid mental conditions. They are concerned not only about their spiritual state; they are also **unduly concerned about their physical condition.** Everything that touches a melancholic is of prime importance to him, hence no other type can so easily become a hypochondriac."[19]

Good examples of this are people who want to tell you about every single ache or pain, and as soon as one pain goes away, another starts. A melancholic would describe pains in great detail even if they just lasted a few minutes. "My rib started hurting after dinner a few days ago, then it was gone. I wonder what that was?" "Doctor, I got a sharp pain in my foot only upon rising out of bed the other day. What do you think that was?" Most people would ignore a "one-time" pain, but not melancholics. For the melancholics to be truly free of pain, they are going to have to realize they are melancholy and work on minimizing the weaknesses of this personality trait.

A person with a melancholy temperament who has difficulties in life, such as marital problems, strained relationships with family or children, a bad job, or money issues, will often **develop physical complaints to cope with these life disappointments.** It is much more difficult for melancholy temperaments to take responsibility for these disappointments and to admit to themselves that life is not all that great and it is partly their fault. If melancholics do get legitimate musculoskeletal pain, the emotional reaction to it can often be blown out of proportion to the actual structural injury. For such people, Prolotherapy may help them, but they won't admit that they are totally better. They need some of the pain to remain so they have an excuse for not working on the emotional, spiritual, or relational problems they are having.

Once patients admit to themselves that they are melancholy, they experience fewer emotional swings. Confidence level is much improved, and they are better able to step back to analyze perceived criticism for what it really is. More often than not, people are just stating facts, not judging. Knowing your temperament can change your life for the better. If it is melancholy, properly thinking about your life in a true and honest sense will help you solve your problems and your temperament will not be one of them.

GOD'S WILL FOR YOUR LIFE AND 7 DEADLY STRESSES

For the person who really desires to delve into the subject of the spiritual reasons for illness, besides studying the Bible, we would encourage you to read the book *A More Excellent Way* by Pastor Henry Wright.[23] In the book, he says that the **beginning of all healing of spiritually related diseases begins with:**

1. Your coming back in alignment with God, His Word, His person, His nature, His precepts and what He planned for this planet for you from the beginning. The solution is restoration.
2. Accepting YOURSELF in your relationship with God; getting rid of your self-hatred, getting rid of your self-bitterness, getting rid of your guilt and coming back in line with who you are in the Father through Jesus Christ.
3. Making peace with your brother, your sister, and all others, if at all possible.

There are many causes of pain and illness and one should not overlook the possible "big picture" reason for pain. It could be God's purpose for your life at this particular moment to have pain because He wants you first and foremost to acknowledge Him in your life.

> *"Jesus replied: 'Love the Lord your God with all your heart and with all your soul and with all your mind. This is the first and greatest commandment. And the second is like it: Love your neighbor as yourself. All the Law and the Prophets hang on these two commandments.'"* Matthew 22:37-40

It could be that *your* healing will start the moment you restore the relationship that God desires to have with you by loving the Lord your God with all your heart, soul, mind, and strength. The second relationship that must be restored is loving your neighbor. Notice from the above verses that you cannot love your neighbor if you do not love yourself. It is not possible. For the person who is filled with God's love, it is easy to love yourself and, thus, love your neighbors.

> *"I pray that out of His glorious riches He may strengthen you with power through His Spirit in your inner being, so that Christ may dwell in your hearts through faith. And I pray that you, being rooted and established in love, may have power, together with all the saints, to grasp how wide and long and high and deep is the love of Christ, and to know this love that surpasses knowledge—that you may be filled to the measure of all the fullness of God."* Ephesians 3:16-19

For the person who has experienced the love and forgiveness of God through Jesus Christ, anything is bearable, even horrible, unrelenting pain. For the person who has no belief in God and does not see the higher purpose for everything in life, it is easy to see why depression and hopelessness prevail. God has a purpose for everything and, when one takes an eternal perspective, it is easy to see the many reasons it may not be God's will for your life to free you of the pain.

CHRONIC PAIN CAN HELP YOU REALIZE:

1. The need for God in your life.
2. The need for forgiveness of your sins through Jesus Christ.
3. The need to start going to church again.
4. The need to work on family and other strained relationships.
5. The need to be more thankful for what you have in life.
6. The need for more humility.
7. The need to free yourself from all bitterness and anger.
8. The need to love and serve others more than yourself.
9. The need to realize that every day is a gift from God.
10. The need to accept that there are no promises for tomorrow, so live each day to its fullest!

A HEALING JOURNEY

By the time someone seeks out a Prolotherapist, especially one across the globe, he/she has often been through the wringer, physically, emotionally, mentally and spiritually. Sadly, Lea was one of these patients. Lea started flying in to see us from her home country of Australia because chronic pain was beginning to prevent her from performing as a singer, her chosen profession. Her most debilitating condition was migraine headaches that were always preceded by neck pain. These would incapacitate her for eight or more hours at a time. She also suffered from accompanying nausea and vomiting. Physical exam showed cervical and thoracic spine instability. Her history involved some physical traumas, including a first-floor fall onto her head and emotional abuse as a child, and then being in a physically abusive relationship as an adult. These traumas mixed with the professional demands of being a traveling musician with long, late hours took a great toll on her overall health.

If all of these aspects of the human condition are not addressed, what are the chances of making significant progress in reversing such debilitating chronic pain, no matter how sophisticated and advanced the treatment? Not very good. We knew that Lea was determined to address all the necessary aspects of her life to get better. We discussed the need to find peace and closure on the things she could control, including past relationships and personality conflicts with family. Often, this peace comes when a person chooses an attitude of gratitude for all things in life: aspects of life that are working well (even little, often overlooked things), the good in current relationships, and even the lessons learned in previous relationships. Lea is a Christian and we encouraged her to continue to work on her faith and relationship with God that through the challenges of mending extremely hurtful relationships, she would feel His peace and reassurance. She began spiritual counseling outside of our office, and with our team, she began Prolotherapy for her spine.

As Lea made several trips to our office, her healing took two steps forward and one step back. She reported being able to move better and that her migraines became fewer and less intense. Physical improvement occurred with Prolotherapy treatments, but then she would get mentally and spiritually bombarded with family drama and emotional setbacks. It is without a doubt that emotion and mental strain has a direct correlation with chronic pain. The body, mind, and spirit are interconnected. The physical relief that Lea experienced from Prolotherapy helped give her some physical relief and renew her hope that she could also find the strength to deal with emotional pain that often takes much longer to mend than ligaments with Prolotherapy. Her relationships with God and her current husband continue to strengthen. We continue to encourage Lea in her journey and see her occasionally when she experiences recurrence of her spine pain.

7 DEADLY STRESSES

"Stress begins when we fail to recognize that difficult situations are designed by God for our benefit."[24]

Most people want not only to cure their painful conditions, but lead healthy active lives, without having to face diseases that limit their function. Most diseases are preventable when people make healthy changes to their lifestyles. Over the years, we have come to realize that disease and illness can also be associated with five factors that traditional medicine may overlook:

1. What we think.
2. What we say.
3. What we do.
4. What we eat.
5. What we inherit.

We all face a wide array of stresses in our lives related to things such as trying to juggle work and personal lives, provide adequately for ourselves and/or our families, relationship issues, illnesses of loved ones, and the list goes on. Some aspects of stress that may not normally be addressed by your medical practitioner are stresses that result from attitudes of anger, guilt, lust, bitterness, greed, fear, and envy. These stresses can destroy the immune system and therefore inhibit the body from fully healing. There is growing research documenting that psychological and social stress affect cardiovascular, nervous system, endocrine system, digestive system, and immune system function. *(See Figure 18-15.)*

Recognizing the possible connection between stresses and physical symptoms has been helpful for some of our patients to discover the underlying cause of their diseases and them resolve these underlying stressors which in turn leads to better health and healing.

SUMMARY

There are many reasons why a person develops chronic pain. Generally, chronic pain is due to inadequate ligament and tendon healing, which may stem from nutritional and/or hormonal deficiencies, along with the ingestion of anti-inflammatory medications and receiving steroid shots. There are additional factors that hamper healing, including musculoskeletal asymmetries, such as leg-length discrepancies, along with chronic infections and food sensitivities. The latter two, in and of themselves, can lead to chronic pain. The most common infections that are found in people with chronic pain are *Borrelia* (Lyme disease), Mycoplasma, *Babesia*, and fungal infections.

Stresses in relationship to the seven primary systems in our body

 Anger - including frustration and irritation, affects the **cardiovascular system**

 Guilt - reflected in blame and anxiety, affects the **nervous system**

 Lust - unrestrained passions and addictions, affects the **endocrine system**

 Bitterness - involving hatred and revenge, affects the **digestive system**

 Greed - for money, possessions, or power, affects the **immune system**

 Fear - of rejection, failure, and the future, affects the **respiratory system**

Envy - expressed in desiring what others have, affects the **musculoskeletal system**

Figure 18-15: Stresses and their relationship to bodily systems.

There is a greater tendency for people who suffer from chronic pain to have a melancholy temperament. People with this temperament are very pessimistic and are often considered "negative" or classified as "having a bad attitude" because they live in an idealistic world in their minds and, when events or relationships do not develop as they had hoped, the melancholy nature sets in. Sometimes the chronic pain they are suffering from is a direct result of this melancholy attitude.

Pain always has a cause and, for some, the cause is spiritual. There are many reasons why, for some, it is not God's will yet that they be freed from their pain. Pain can help a person realize his or her need for God, change an attitude, or restore relationships. Addressing stresses in your life can help you achieve resolution of past issues and achieve better health and healing. Yes, chronic pain can be life-changing and, for many, it changes their lives for the better. ∎

RESOURCES

To learn more about Christianity, the Bible, and health we have found the following books very helpful:

The Word on Health
By Dr. Michael D. Jacobson
Moody Press, Chicago, Illinois

What a Christian Believes
By Dr. Ray Pritchard
Crossway Books, Wheaton, Illinois

Anchor for the Soul
By Dr. Ray Pritchard
Moody Press, Chicago, Illinois

Stealth Attack
By Dr. Ray Pritchard
Moody Press, Chicago, Illinois

The Purpose Driven Life:
What on Earth am I here for
By Rick Warren
Zondervan, Grand Rapids, MI

How to Resolve Seven Deadly Stresses
A Health Manual for All Nations
By Institute in Basic Life Principles, Inc.

Lies We Believe that cause Stress and Disease
By Dr. Bill Gothard
IBLP Publications

Why Did God Let It Happen
By Institute in Basic Life Principles, Inc.

Why Do We Get Weary?
By Dr. Bill Gothard
IBLP Publications

The Missing Commandment:
Love Yourself: How Loving Yourself
the Way God Does Can Bring Healing
and Freedom to Your Life
By Jerry and Denise Basel
Heart and Life Publishers

19

PROLOTHERAPY VS. SURGERY

Chances are that if you are reading this book, you have already had joint surgery which failed to relieve your pain, or you are hoping to avoid surgery. Prolotherapy is an excellent alternative to surgery, and a powerful treatment to help with post-surgical pain. Unlike surgery, Prolotherapy is a regenerative treatment that addresses the actual cause of the pain. *(See Figure 19-1.)* It is not surprising that more people do not know of Prolotherapy when we consider what most people consider "normal" or even

Pain Complaint	Body Part Operated On	Surgery	Actual Cause of Pain
Low back pain	Bone/disc	Laminectomy/ discectomy	Sacroiliac joint
Medial knee pain	Meniscus	Meniscectomy	Pes anserinus tendon
Neck pain	Bone/disc	Laminectomy/ discectomy	Cervical ligaments/facets
Diffuse knee pain	Whole knee	Debridement/ lavage	Knee ligaments
Shoulder pain	Labrum	Resection	Shoulder ligaments
Hip pain	Labrum	Refixation	Hip ligaments
Shoulder pain	Bone/cartilage	Debridement/ lavage	Shoulder labrum/ ligaments

Figure 19-1: Common painful conditions not addressed by surgical procedures.

"good" medical care. Most people believe that if they have pain, the first course of action is to get an MRI and see an orthopedic surgeon. Why would there be any surprise if the next step is surgery if the first doctor you see is a surgeon? Since joint instability is the cause of most chronic pain, and surgery typically involves cutting, shaving, or removing tissue, it tends to make the joint more unstable. *(See Figure 19-2.)* Thus, leading to additional surgeries, revisions, and fusions. We are living in a time of runaway medical supply and insurance costs, and also in the midst of an opiod addiction crisis, because the standard of care has been to prescribe drugs and surgery for patients with chronic pain. There is mounting evidence that this should not be considered the standard of care, and that more conservative, regenerative models should be the standard. This has been our crusade since the early 90's, because patients certainly deserve better.

Surgeries that Potentially Worsen Joint Instability

- ACL reconstruction
- Arthrodesis
- Arthroscopic debridement
- Arthroscopy
- Autologous chondrocyte implantation
- Capsulotomy
- Chondroplasty
- Debridement and lavage
- Disc replacement
- Discectomy
- Facetectomy
- Foraminotomy
- Fusion
- Joint replacement
- Joint resurfacing
- Labral debridement
- Labral refixation
- Labral repair
- Labral resection
- Laminectomy
- Laminoplasty
- Laminotomy
- Meniscal repair
- Meniscectomy
- Microdiscectomy
- Osteochondral autograph transplantation
- Osteochondral allograft transplantation
- Osteoplasty
- Rotator cuff repair
- Tommy John surgery

Figure 19-2: Orthopedic surgeries that potentially worsen joint instability. All of these surgeries can cause or worsen long-term joint instability and chronic pain.

CT, MRI, AND X-RAYS ARRIVE ON THE SCENE

The CT scan became widely available in the early 1970s and was used, among other things, to view the intervertebral discs. Chronic pain physicians in the early 1970s found abnormalities in this area and concluded that the disc problems caused chronic pain. Millions of people underwent surgical procedures to correct some "abnormality" of the disc, as seen on the CT scan, only to experience minimal pain relief.

Not until the early 1980s were the CT scans of people without pain examined.[1] A study published in 1984 by Sam W. Wiesel, MD, found that 35% of the population, irrespective of age, had abnormal findings on CT scans of their lower backs even though they had no pain complaints. In CT scans of people over 40 years of age, 50% had abnormal findings. Twenty-nine percent showed evidence of herniated discs, 81% facet degeneration (arthritis), and 48% lumbar stenosis (another form of arthritis). This meant that for people over 40 years of age who do not have symptoms of pain, a 50% chance of abnormality on their CT scans existed, including a herniated disc.

WHY IS A CORRECT PATIENT HISTORY BETTER THAN AN MRI?

The difference between a patient history and an MRI is that the MRI can be interpreted subjectively, open to interpretation, and often be a "roadblock," in helping the patient heal. Our patients are incredibly well educated when it comes to pain. Good patient histories are more important than looking at films.[2] Some of the most common surgeries, such as arthroscopy for meniscal tears, are based on MRI findings, which have an increasingly high percentage of false-positive rates as we age. *(See Figure 19-3.)*

In one study that looked at the widespread use of MRI to identify joint disease, the study says that semiquantitative assessment (which is a non precise – subject to interpretation reading) of the joints by expert interpreters of MRI data is a powerful tool that can increase understanding of joint disease in osteoarthritis. Using a scoring system for different joint diseases, doctors can precisely diagnose problems of the joint as seen on the MRI. BUT, the researchers warn – it is still not accurate!

"Although these new scoring systems offer theoretical advantages over pre-existing systems, whether they offer actual superiority with regard to reliability, responsiveness and validity remains to be seen."

The entire study points to the use of MRI as a valuable tool until the end, which states in theory this should work, but that remains to be seen. In other words — there is a doubt that the latest in MRI enhancements help the patient's situation.[3]

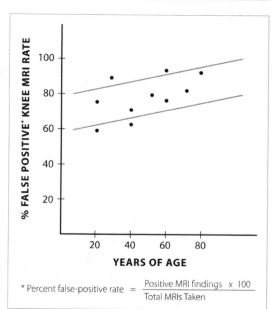

* Percent false-positive rate $= \dfrac{\text{Positive MRI findings} \times 100}{\text{Total MRIs Taken}}$

Figure 19-3: Graph of the percent of false-positive knee MRIs of the medial meniscus, findings in asymptomatic people relative to age. Studies show that even by age 20, the number of abnormal MRIs of the knee, in people without any symptoms, is quite substantial. So patients, beware of arthroscopies that are recommended based primarily on MRI scans.

Data from: Kornick J. Meniscal abnormalities in the asymptomatic population at MR imaging. *Radiology.* 1990;177:463-465.

AN ACCURATE MRI – LACK OF CONSENSUS

No consensus yet exists regarding how to perform a proper consultation that best helps the patient. Here is what these researchers came up with: The model osteoarthritis consultation included 25 tasks to be undertaken during the initial consultation between the doctor and the patient presenting with peripheral joint pain. The 25 tasks provide detailed advice on how the following elements of the consultation should be addressed:

1. Assessment of chronic joint pain.
2. Patient's ideas and concerns.
3. Exclusion of red flags.
4. Examination.
5. Provision of the diagnosis and written information.
6. Promotion of exercise and weight loss.
7. Initial pain management.
8. Arranging a follow-up appointment.

This study has enabled the priorities of the doctors and patients to be identified for a model osteoarthritis consultation.[4] The study did not say — look at film and treat.

Hopefully technologies of the future will assist in making a determination of the patient's true cause of pain, but for today, in our opinion and that of certain researchers – physical examination and patient history is superior to the current technology.

In regard to pain management, diagnostic tests, such as x-rays, magnetic resonance imaging (MRI), or CT scans, should never take the place of a listening ear and a strong thumb to diagnose the cause of chronic pain. It is necessary for the clinician to understand where the pain originates and radiates. They must fully understand the referral pain patterns. In summary, it should be obvious that a scan should not be used solely as the criterion for determining the cause of a person's pain.

To properly diagnose the cause of a person's pain it is important for the physician to touch the patient. Medical doctors are too quick to prescribe an anti-inflammatory medication or order an MRI. The best MRI is a physician's thumb, which we call My Reproducibility Instrument, used to palpate the ligament or tendon suspected to be the problem. *(See Figure 19-4.)* If the diagnosis is correct, a positive "jump sign" will occur because the weakened ligament or tendon will be very tender to palpation. If the physician does not reproduce a person's pain during an examination, the likelihood of eliminating the pain is slim. How can a physician make a correct diagnosis without reproducing the pain? Our patients often say that this initial examination was the first real examination performed since experiencing the pain.

BACK SURGERY

In this section, we will detail some of the most common surgical procedures that are recommended for patients with chronic pain. Post-surgical pain, including failed

MRI Versus the Thumb

		MRI	THUMB
False-positive rate of static MRI positive in asymptomatic middle-aged persons (conservative estimate)	Lower back	64%	0
	Neck	50%	0
	Shoulder	54%	0
	Knee	62%	0
Cost		Thousands	Free (Included in office visit)
Ability to reproduce pain		None	100%
Likelihood of progression to surgery		High	Low

Figure 19-4: MRI versus the thumb.
Which do you want diagnosing your injury?

back surgery syndrome (yes, a condition so prevalent that it has an official diagnosis) is one of the top reasons that patients take matters into their own hands and end up in our office seeking to relieve their pain once and for all.

LAMINECTOMY

The laminectomy procedure involves removing some of the bone, called lamina, from the supporting structure of the back. Its removal creates stress on other areas of the lumbar spine. *(See Figure 19-5.)*

Because some of the lamina are removed, the discs, ligaments, and muscles have to do more work. As a result, the vertebral discs degenerate. The vertebral segments then move closer together and eventually become hypermobile. Back muscles tense to stabilize the segment. When they cannot stabilize the segments, the vertebral ligaments are then

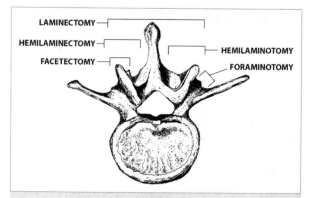

Figure 19-5: The areas of vertebral bone removed with the various types of surgery. The weakness caused by bone removal from back operations often leads to vertebral instability resulting in long-term low back pain.

forced to do this alone. They eventually become lax and subsequently cause pain. This is probably why back pain so commonly occurs several years after this operation. If the muscles and ligaments cannot stabilize the joints in the lower back, the vertebrae loosen and eventually rub together and crack, causing excessive bone growth in order to stabilize the joint. The stabilization results in spondylosis, or arthritis of the lumbar spine. Often the person then succumbs to another operation for the arthritis that formed as a result of the first operation. Unfortunately for the patient, the second operation is not a panacea of pain relief either. A simpler approach is for Prolotherapy to correct the underlying ligament laxity that was causing the pain in the first place. This sequence of events is also applicable to other areas of the body. *(See Figure 19-6.)*

DISCECTOMY

Discectomy, another common back surgery, follows the same degenerative sequence as a laminectomy. Once the disc material is surgically removed, stress is added to the segments above and below the removed disc segment. These segments may eventually degenerate and become a cause of chronic pain.

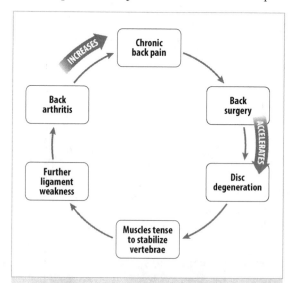

Figure 19-6: How back surgery leads to the perpetuation of chronic pain. Back surgery, by removing important tissue, puts greater strain on remaining tissues, which eventually weaken and become a source of chronic pain.

In a study by John Maynard, MD, 10% of people after disc operation re-herniated the same disc at a later date. Four years after surgery, 38% of the patients still had persistent pain in the back and 23% had persistent pain in the lower limbs.[5]

LUMBAR SPINAL FUSION

Lumbar spinal fusion operations fuse together several segments of the vertebrae. Such an operation is commonly performed for spondylolisthesis, a condition where one vertebral segment slips forward on another. This causes back pain, especially when bending. By definition, spinal fusion causes permanent bonding or fusing of several vertebral segments. Mobility is decreased, causing increased stress on the areas above and below the fused segment. While fusion is sometimes a necessary surgery, the long-term consequences should be known and all conservative efforts tried, including Prolotherapy. Even in the beginning when surgical fusions were just gaining momentum as a surgical procedure, Dr. Ehni asserted that, "fusion generates a conflict between immediate benefit and late consequences."[6] Studies have shown that some of the biomechanical changes that occur in adjacent segments after fusion include increased intradiscal pressure, increased facet loading, and increased mobility in the facet joints. All of these ultimately lead to adjacent segment disc and facet degeneration.[7,8] Adjacent segment disease (ASD) after a single-level cervical or lumbar fusion occurs at an annual incidence of around 2.5-3%.[9] This means that every year there is about a 3% chance that the segments next to the fusion will shows signs of instability and degeneration. A laminectomy adjacent to a fusion increases the relative risk of ASD by 2.4 times, as does fusions that involve two or more segments.[9] The additional stress creates instability and degeneration in adjacent spinal segments. Over two-thirds of patients who get symptomatic ASD fail traditional therapies and end up with more surgery.[10] *(See Figure 19-7.)*

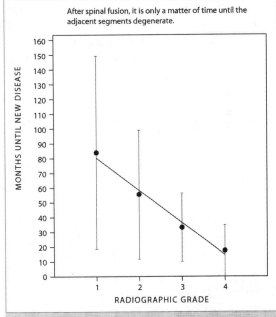

Figure 19-7: Graph showing when the neck or back will hurt after a fusion operation. This graph shows the durations until symptomatic adjacent-segment disease developed according to the radiographic grade for the forty-nine patients (fifty procedures) for whom radiographs were available.

Adapted from Figure 3. Hilibrand AS, et al. Radiculopathy and myelopathy at segments adjacent to the site of a previous anterior cervical arthrodesis. *The Journal of Bone and Joint Surgery.* 1999;81-A(4):519-528.

In her article, published in the *Journal of the American Medical Association* in 1992, entitled, "Patient outcomes after lumbar spinal fusions," Judith A. Turner, PhD, noted that there has never been a randomized or double-blind study comparing lumbar spinal fusion with any other technique. In some cases, only 16% of the people experience satisfactory results after the operation. On average, 14% of the people experience

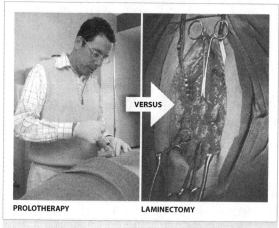

Figure 19-8: Back Prolotherapy versus laminectomy surgery. Which would you rather have?

incomplete healing of the surgical site. The most frequent symptom persisting after the operation is low back pain, which is often the reason for the operation in the first place. Turner concluded her article by saying that the wide variability in reported success rates is bothersome and should be carefully considered by patients and their physicians when contemplating this procedure.[11]

Prolotherapy is a much safer and effective alternative to a laminectomy, a discectomy, or a lumbar spinal fusion. *(See Figure 19-8.)* Prolotherapy initiates the repair process of the loose ligaments in spondylolisthesis and degenerated and herniated discs.

ARTHROSCOPY: THE QUICKEST WAY TO ARTHRITIS

There is a high likelihood that you will develop aggressive arthritis in the future if an arthroscope enters your joints. This does not apply to complete ligament tears. These may actually need surgical repair to regain function. Prolotherapy cannot reattach two loose ends. For all the other conditions, any tissue removal inside the knee will most likely give you an increased chance of a future filled with arthritis and the accompanying pain and a lessened ability to play sports or perform daily activities. A well-accepted schemata on the development of arthritis is shown in *Figure 19-9.*

Arthritis begins immediately after chondrocyte function is altered. This leads to altered production of ground substance, or proteoglycans. Because the articular cartilage is now in a weakened state, breakdown begins. Orthopedists have fancy terms for this breakdown such as fibrillation, fissures, flaking, and vascularization. *(See Figure 19-10.)* When they use these terms it just means your cartilage is degenerating. Thinning articular cartilage shows on x-ray as a loss of joint space. This causes a transmission of pressures that are too high for the bones to handle. The tibial bone in the knee, for example, will attempt to harden by sclerosis,

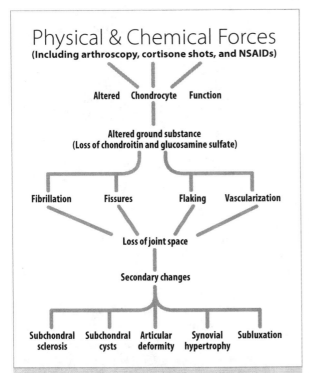

Physical & Chemical Forces
(Including arthroscopy, cortisone shots, and NSAIDs)

Altered   Chondrocyte   Function

Altered ground substance
(Loss of chondroitin and glucosamine sulfate)

Fibrillation   Fissures   Flaking   Vascularization

Loss of joint space

Secondary changes

Subchondral   Subchondral   Articular   Synovial   Subluxation
sclerosis   cysts   deformity   hypertrophy

Figure 19-9: The development of degenerative joint disease. The process can be accelerated by arthroscopy, cortisone shots, and NSAIDs, the primary "tools" of most traditional pain doctors. Adapted from: *Essentials of Skeletal Etiology*, Vol. 2. by Yochum, T. Page 547, 1987, Williams and Wilkins, Baltimore, MD.

forming cysts. The bone itself will actually overgrow to stabilize the area. This is why arthritic joints are called articular deformities, which is actually bone overgrowth.

A patient who undergoes arthroscopy receives a direct assault to the surrounding tissues. It is very rare for an orthopedist to just look into a joint. Tissue is shaved and cut because the physician truly believes that this helps the person. Even if the area is fibrillated or has frayed edges, how could removing the tissue possibly help the individual? It does nothing to help repair the area. Arthroscopic shaving or abrasion of fibrillated and irregular cartilage may relieve symptoms temporarily, but long–term it aids in the destabilization and degenerative process of the joint. Many times the argument is made that the cartilage was smoothed by arthroscopy. This now smoother cartilage (because the fibrillations and frayed edges were shaved) will allow a more normal glide of the bones. The research does not support this. Schmid and Schmid reported that shaving did not restore a smooth congruent articular surface and may have caused increased fibrillation and cell necrosis in and adjacent to the original defect.[12]

PROLOTHERAPY VERSUS ARTHROSCOPY

Prolotherapy has many advantages over arthroscopy. It is, first of all, a much safer and conservative treatment.

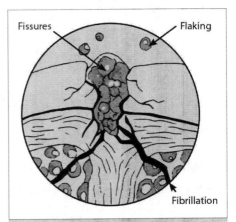

Figure 19-10: Articular cartilage deterioration as evidenced by fibrillation, fissures, and flaking.

	Prolotherapy	Arthroscopy
Stimulates repair	Yes	No
Increases collagen strength	Yes	No
Arthritis risk	Decreased	Increased
Return to normal activities	Quick	Slow
Rehabilitation time	Short	Long
Exercise	Encouraged	Cautious
Cost	Hundreds	Thousands
Time involved in procedure	Minutes	Hours
Instrument used	Thin needle	Massive scopes

Figure 19-11: Prolotherapy versus arthroscopy.
Which would you rather have—Prolotherapy OR Arthroscopy?

It works faster. *(See Figure 19-11.)* The procedure does not take long to administer to the patient. Prolotherapy stimulates the body to heal the painful area. The new collagen tissue formed is actually stronger. It reduces the chance of long-term arthritis, whereas arthroscopy increases the chances for it.[13-19]

Furthermore, arthroscopic surgery has also been proven to have equal results to that of a sham surgery for osteoarthritis in highly regarded randomized studies published in the *New England Journal of Medicine*.[20-21] Prolotherapy also increases the chances of athletes being able to play their sports and regular people staying active, whereas arthroscopy decreases those chances.[22-25] Most people may return to activity almost immediately after Prolotherapy. They are encouraged to exercise while getting Prolotherapy, whereas after arthroscopy, patients must often be very cautious and undergo extensive rehabilitation programs.

PROLOTHERAPY VERSUS MENISCECTOMY

One of the most common calls our office receives involves patients who have had part or all of their meniscus removed and are suffering with continued pain or arthritis that was accelerated due to the surgery. Meniscectomies worsen knee joint instability by negatively influencing other supporting knee structures, increasing contact stress, and leading to arthritis.[26-31] For those who are considering meniscectomy surgery, we strongly suggest at least a consultation with a Prolotherapist who does Comprehensive Prolotherapy. The success with being able to keep patients out of surgery with Prolotherapy is excellent.[32,33] Keep and repair the tissue with regenerative treatments versus surgery to improve longevity of the knee. *(See Figure 19-12.)*

PROLOTHERAPY VERSUS TOTAL KNEE ARTHROPLASTY

One of the top reasons people seek Prolotherapy is to avoid a knee replacement, whether it has already been recommended or because they know that is the inevitable recommendation if something is not done to halt the degenerative process. *(See Figure 19-13.)* In an article published by the journal *Orthopedics*, 273 patients who

Effects of treatment	Meniscal removal	Meniscal repair	Meniscal transplant	Untreated injury	Prolotherapy
Articular cartilage deterioration	YES	YES	YES	YES	**NO**
Bone deformity	YES	YES	YES	YES	**NO**
Chronic pain	YES	YES	YES	YES	**NO**
Continuing instability	YES	YES	YES	YES	**NO**
Joint space narrowing on MRI	YES	YES	YES	YES	**NO**
Likely to be re-injured	YES	YES	YES	YES	**NO**
Long-term osteoarthritis	YES	YES	YES	YES	**NO**
Restricted motion	YES	YES	YES	YES	**NO**
Weakened ligaments	YES	YES	YES	YES	**NO**
Stimulates meniscus repair	NO	NO	NO	NO	**YES**

Figure 19-12: Effects of treatments for meniscal tears. Only Prolotherapy stimulates the repair of injured meniscal tissue.

underwent primary knee arthrotplasty were studied a minimum of one year after surgery. Thirty-nine percent of patients reported persistent pain after the procedure, with an average median pain score of 3 out of 10, and worst pain score of 5 out of 10.[34] Think about it this way, if your surgeon told you that if he or she performs a drastic, irreversible surgery in which there is more than a 1 in 3 chance that you will continue to have a significant level of pain, would you consider it a successful procedure? Probably not. Yet, surgery continues to grow by leaps and bounds. Go to any cocktail party with people 50 and older who suffer from joint pain and you will find that most of them have a glorified idea of surgery, and some seem downright giddy about their future joint replacement. We've got a suggestion for you... Make sure that after the Orthopedic visit, you go talk to the people in the rehab center and do your own patient satisfaction survey. Then call a Prolotherapist for a second opinion! For those of you who already had the surgery and are experiencing this pain first-hand, Prolotherapy can still work well for post-surgical pain.

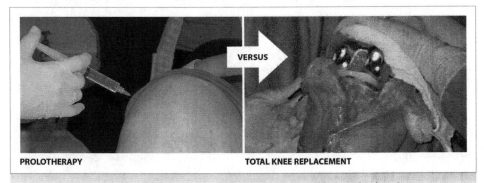

VERSUS

PROLOTHERAPY

TOTAL KNEE REPLACEMENT

Figure 19-13: Knee Prolotherapy versus knee surgery. Which would you rather have?

ANTERIOR CRUCIATE LIGAMENT TEARS

Surgical outcomes for ACL tears have their own fair share of disappointing results, including as high as a 25% failure rate, that can be especially devastating for young athletes.[35] Using tissue from cadavers (allograft) or from a patient's own tissue (autograft) is used for ACL reconstruction, as well as for many other areas of the body, because it sounds promising to a patient in pain who is looking for repair, and is necessary in the instance of grade III (complete) tears. *(See Figure 19-14.)* The long-term results, however, demonstrate that untreated joint instability remains. In one study, of the over 23,000 pediatric patients who underwent ACL reconstruction, 8.2% had a subsequent ACL reconstruction and 14% had subsequent non-ACL knee surgery. The median time lapse between the first and second surgeries were 1.4 and 1.6 years, respectively. It was noted that this may be a conservative number of patients who had repeat tears, as the data only included those who underwent a second surgery, and not those who decided not to have the additional surgery.[36] This time line can kill a young athlete's career. Athletes have a low rate of returning to sports, and a high rate of developing new injuries, including to that of the other knee![37-39] Yes, a ligament injury in one limb can affect the ligaments of the contralateral limb.[40] This cycle can lead to surgery after surgery if it is not stopped.

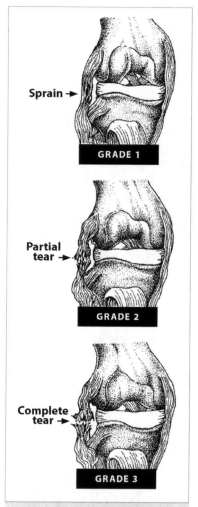

Figure 19-14: Grading of ligament severity. Grade 1 and 2 ligament injuries are successfully treated with Prolotherapy. Grade 3 injuries (complete ligament tears), however, often need surgery.

It makes no sense that a person is subjected to multiple surgeries when it is obvious that joint instability is the cause of the problem. There is often instability of other ligaments of the knee that can contribute to the failure of the ACL surgery, as often seen when revision surgery is done.[41,42] We know that surgery makes joint instability worse, not better. Joint instability is the missing diagnosis for athletes with ACL tears, and additional surgeries, no matter how sophisticated, are not the answer to the problem of joint instability. Pain, swelling, weakness, popping, grinding, and other symptoms associated with ACL tears can be addressed not with surgery, but with Prolotherapy. There is no comparison.

SURGERY DECREASES TISSUE PLIABILITY

Many surgeries such as labral repair and ACL reconstruction provide remarkable short-term pain relief. Temporarily they provide more stability to the joint. Unfortunately, the stability doesn't last because no matter how hard they try, they can not simulate exactly the same biology of what God gave the human body. If someone has a complete, grade 3 ligament tear, surgery is indicated. The cadaver or tendon graft that is replacing the torn ligament, however, will not function long-term like the original ACL. Once it starts becoming lax or weak, get Prolotherapy! We have patients that do not want to take chances and get Prolotherapy once they are cleared by the surgeon to start doing aggressive rehabilitation.

ACL grafts, as well as titanium tacked labral repairs do not have the same pliability as nascent tissue. In other words, ligaments, labrum, menisci are pliable, they can stretch. Surgerized ACLs, menisci and labrum no longer have the pliability and for the active person will cause long-term problems.[43-45] Thus, when the surgeon performs a hip labrum "repair," the repair does not restore the normal histologic structure, tissue permeability, hip hydrodynamics, load transfer, and normal kinematics.[45-47] So if a patient lives an active lifestyle, there is no way that two titanium staples inside the hip are not going to cause problems. It is physically impossible! The part of the labrum containing the titanium staples is surely not going to have the same stretch ability as the rest of the labrum. That part of the labrum will sustain increased forces on it with movement of the hip, especially external and internal rotation. **(See Figure 19-15.)** Long-term this will either cause another hip labrum tear or excessive pressures to be transmitted to the articular cartilage, causing femoroactacular impingment and/or accelerating the degenerative process.

If a person drastically reduces the stressors on the knee, hip or shoulder after surgery it is possible not to have any long-term problems, but let's not kid ourselves to think surgery cured the problem. All one can say is surgery helped stabilize the joint enough so that the person can walk around.

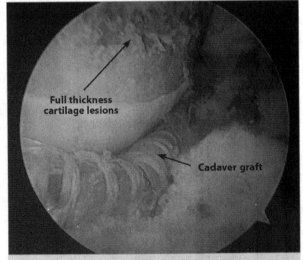

Figure 19-15: Arthroscopic picture showing the aftermath of a hip labrum repair with cadaver graft. Full thickness cartilage lesions are seen, even after hip surgery. It was these and other mechanical problems, including joint instability, which continued to cause enough pain that this patient sought Prolotherapy for pain relief.

PROSPECTIVE PILOT STUDY

In 2010, we published a prospective pilot study of 34 patients who were previously told that surgery was necessary for their condition, and 91% of the patients were told surgery was their only option.[48] The patients represented 21 knees, 5 hips, 2 wrists, 2 ankles, 2 feet, 1 shoulder, and 1 lower back. The operations the patients were trying to avoid were 20 joint replacements, nine arthroscopic procedures, three fusions, and four tendon/ligament repairs. The reasons the patients chose not to have surgery varied: 34% Natural Medicine minded, 18% personal choice, 18% risks, 9% family decision, 3% expense, and 3% fear. *(See Figure 19-16.)*

Prolotherapy vs. Surgery Study Patients

Total number of patients treated	34
Percent told surgery was needed	100%
Percent told surgery was only option	91%
Average age of the patients	57
Average number of prior physicians seen	2.5
Average length of pain (in months)	27

Figure 19-16: Patient characteristics at baseline.

TREATMENT OUTCOMES

Patients received an average of 4.5 Prolotherapy treatment sessions. The average time of follow-up after their last Prolotherapy session was 10 months. Prior to Prolotherapy the average patient was taking 1.1 medications for pain, but this decreased to 0.2 after Prolotherapy. Thirteen patients were able to stop taking medications or decrease them because of Prolotherapy. One of the 26 patients not on pain medications following Prolotherapy had to resume since stopping Prolotherapy.

Patients were asked to rate their levels of crunching, stiffness, and pain on a scale of 0 to 10, with 0 being no crunching/stiffness/pain and 10 being severe/crippling crunching/stiffness/pain. The average starting crunching level was 5.2, the average starting stiffness level was 7.2, and the average starting pain level was 7.6. Following Prolotherapy, patients reported an average ending crunching level of 1.5, an ending stiffness level of 2.5, and an average pain level of 1.3. *(See Figures 19-17 & 19-18.)*

When patients were asked if Prolotherapy had changed their life for the better, 91% answered "yes." Only one out of the 34 patients said Prolotherapy did not help the pain. Three out of 34 (9%) received less than 25% pain relief with Prolotherapy. Seventy-nine percent of the patients answered "yes" to having enough relief after their Prolotherapy treatment that they felt they will never need surgery. For the seven patients (21%) who answered "no" to that question, three felt they will need surgery. The four remaining patients noted greater than 50% pain relief, but plan to receive additional Prolotherapy treatment in the future. Of interest, is 100% of the patients treated stated that they have recommended Prolotherapy to someone else.

In regard to the three participants who ended up needing surgery; one had terrible shoulder pain especially with playing sports. He had failed physical therapy, cortisone injections, and medications for an intrasubstance tear of the supraspinatus tendon and impingement syndrome. He stated the two Prolotherapy treatments helped him 15%, but he was and is an active cricket player and decided on surgery. He is back to playing. Of interest is this participant at various times had five other body areas treated with Prolotherapy and responded 100%. The second patient who ended up needing surgery had osteoarthritis of the hip. He had six Prolotherapy treatments and felt he was 90% better in regard to pain from the Prolotherapy. He noted that he was

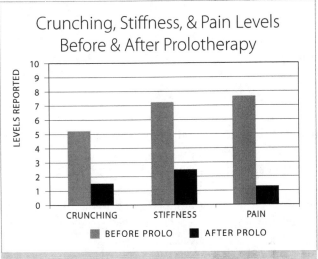

Figure 19-17: Starting and ending crunching, stiffness, and pain levels in 34 patients who underwent Prolotherapy treatments as an alternative to surgery.

sleeping and walking better since receiving Prolotherapy. Objectively, he had more range of motion with the Prolotherapy, but not enough for his activity level. He had a successful hip replacement. The third participant received two Prolotherapy treatments to her degenerated knee. She stated the Prolotherapy helped 50% with the pain but she was anxious to get back to dancing (her passion), and decided to get a total knee replacement. She is back to dancing.

While these three participants would be considered "failures" of Prolotherapy because they needed surgery, on closer examination it is clear that two of the patients did not receive the recommended number of treatments before stopping Prolotherapy. In our experience, patients who have been told by surgeons that surgery is their only option can often require at least six visits of Prolotherapy, especially if they have joint degeneration to the point of "bone on bone." These three patients do demonstrate the challenge that Regenerative Medicine doctors face daily in active patients, that they

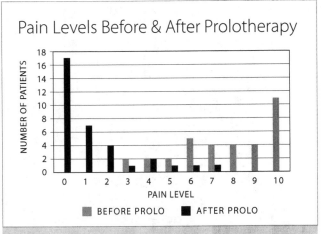

Figure 19-18: Starting and ending pain levels in 34 patients who underwent Prolotherapy treatments as an alternative to surgery.

want to get better quickly. Prolotherapy does require a patient to go to a doctor's office and receive the treatment every month, sometimes for six months to a year. While this can be a stumbling block to some patients, for the patient who does not want to have surgery, surely this is a small inconvenience for a lifetime of pain relief.

SURGERY IS YOUR ONLY OPTION

In a number of our studies, we looked at sub-groups of patients who were previously told that surgeries were their only treatment options. These cases tended to be more advanced and had exhausted all other efforts, such as the typical recommendations of exercise, rest, ice, pain medications, physical therapy, and cortisone injections. Typically, they had also seen a number of practitioners prior to trying Prolotherapy, and this was their last ditch effort to avoid joint surgery. Even in these tough cases, Prolotherapy had noticeable benefits. *(See Figure 19-19.)* We only wish that these

Study	Total patients in study	Subgroup of "surgery only" patients	Average pain level before Prolotherapy	Average pain level after Prolotherapy
Low back pain[1]	145	26	6.0	2.1
Shoulder pain[2]	61	20	7.0	2.6
Wrist pain[3]	31	5	4.8	1.2
Hip pain[4]	94	8	8.4	2.4
Neck pain[5]	98	21	6.6	2.1
Knee pain[7]	80	10	6.5	2.3
Chondromalacia patella[8]	69	16	4.9	0.8
Direct bone marrow aspirate[9]	24	18	5.8	0.4
Hip labrum lesions[10]	19	12	6.8	2.3

1. Hauser R, et al. Dextrose Prolotherapy for unresolved low back pain: a retrospective case series study. *Journal of Prolotherapy.* 2009;1(3):145-155.
2. Hauser R, et al. Retrospective study on Hackett-Hemwall dextrose Prolotherapy for chronic shoulder pain at an outpatient charity clinic in rural Illinois. *Journal of Prolotherapy.* 2009;4:205-216.
3. Hauser R, et al. Dextrose Prolotherapy for unresolved wrist pain. *Practical Pain Management.* 2009;Nov/Dec:72-79.
4. Hauser R, et al. A retrospective study on Hackett-Hemwall dextrose Prolotherapy for chronic hip pain. *Journal of Prolotherapy.* 2009;2:76-88.
5. Hauser R, et al. Neck pain. *Practical Pain Management.* 2007;7(8):58-69.
6. Hauser R, et al. Dextrose Prolotherapy with human growth hormone to treat chronic first metatarsophalangeal joint pain. *The Foot and Ankle Online Journal.* 5 (9):1. doi: 10.3827/faoj.2012.0509.0001.
7. Hauser R, et al. A retrospective study on dextrose Prolotherapy for unresolved knee pain at an outpatient charity clinic in rural Illinois. *Journal of Prolotherapy.* 2009;1:11-21.
8. Hauser R, et al. Outcomes of Prolotherapy in chondromalacia patella patients: improvements in pain level and function. *Clinical Medicine Insights: Arthritis and Musculoskeletal Disorders.* 2014;7:13-20.
9. Hauser R, et al. Treating osteoarthritic joints using dextrose Prolotherapy and direct bone marrow aspirate injection therapy. *The Open Arthritis Journal.* 2014;7:1-9.
10. Hauser R, et al. Regenerative injection therapy (Prolotherapy) for hip labrum lesions: rationale and retrospective study. *The Open Rehabilitation Journal.* 2013;6:59-68.

Figure 19-19: Surgery is not the only option. In many of the Hauser R, et al. studies, a subgroup of patients were told by another doctor that surgery was their only option. Those patients chose to receive Prolotherapy instead. The overwhelming majority of patients reported improvement in their pain and overall quality of life indicators after Prolotherapy, and most reported recommending Prolotherapy to others.

patients would have tried Prolotherapy sooner! In our experience, the sooner the patient begins a regenerative treatment course of Prolotherapy, the sooner they begin feeling better and can avoid years of continued medical care for their ailment.

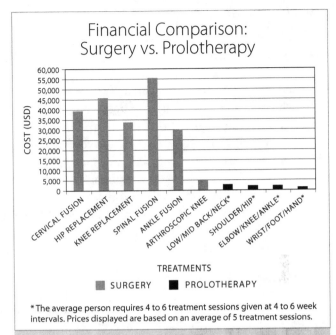

Figure 19-20: The cost of Prolotherapy is significantly lower as compared to surgical procedures.

As a whole, Prolotherapy can save patients and medical institutions millions in surgery fees, as the price for Prolotherapy is often in the hundreds or few thousands, versus tens of thousands with surgery. *(See Figure 19-20.)*

COMPLEX REGIONAL PAIN SYNDROME (CRPS)

One of the most painful, disabling, and even "bizarre" medical pain conditions is known as complex regional pain syndrome (CRPS), previously known as reflex sympathetic dystrophy (RSD). It is characterized by a variety of autonomic and vasomotor disturbances, of which diffuse pain, spreading edema, temperature disturbances, and functional impairment are most prominent.[49] *(See Figure 19-21.)*

CRPS generally appears in the extremities following a physical injury, is disproportionate to the precipitating event or level of tissue damage, progresses inconsistently over time, and is associated with nonspecific signs and symptoms.[50] It is a disease with an unpredictable and uncontrollable nature, and is a syndrome covered in confusion.[51,52] Spreading like wild fire, it may start in the foot, move its way up to the knee, back, down the other leg, and up into the arms.

Signs and Symptoms of CRPS

- Abnormal swelling/edema
- Allodynia
- Change in skin color
- Change in skin temperature
- Changes in skin, hair, and nail growth
- Decreased ability to exercise
- Feeling of limb disconnect
- Hyperalgesia
- Hyperesthesia
- Hyperpathy
- Inability to move extremity
- Incoordination
- Involuntary movements
- Limited range of motion/movement
- Muscle and skin atrophy
- Muscle spasms
- Osteoporosis
- Paraesthesias
- Paresis
- Pseudoparalysis
- Severe pain
- Sweating asymmetry
- Tremor

Figure 19-21: The signs and symptoms of complex regional pain syndrome (CRPS).

CAUSES OF CRPS

The majority of CRPS cases occur after orthopedic procedures.[50] *(See Figure 19-22.)* A chart review by Birklein et al. of 145 patients in 2000 suggested 41.3% of cases were due to fractures, 32% from soft tissue injuries, 9% due to surgeries, and 17.7% from minor traumas and lesions.[53-55] In the Duman study from 2006 which included 168 patients from two hospitals the percentage of CRPS from fractures was 55.3%, from soft tissue trauma 28%, and 16.7% from incisive injuries.[56] A review of 140 cases at the Mayo Clinic over a 2 year period also noted 65% from external trauma including 28.6% after soft tissue trauma, 20% after fractures, and 16.4% of the those cases were a result of surgery.[57] In the majority of pediatric cases, CRPS follows a soft tissue or joint injury.[58] It is perceivable that the aforementioned trauma cases including sprains, fractures and surgery also involved damage to the soft tissue. If we were to imagine the force required to break a bone, we could also appreciate that the ligaments supporting the joints were injured.

CRPS AFTER SURGERY

To further delineate the frequency of CRPS as far as surgery, the estimates include 2.3-4% after arthroscopic knee surgery, 2.1-5% after carpal tunnel surgery, 13.6% after ankle surgery, 0.8-13% after total knee arthroplasty, and 7-37% after wrist fractures.[50] Reuben noted that the development of CRPS is a common complication after fasciectomy for Dupuytreen contracture giving an estimate of 4.5-40%.[50,59]

Fractures and surgeries cause soft tissue damage involving the ligaments. Blood supply to bone is excellent, whereas blood supply to ligament tissue is poor. If the blood vessels supplying blood to the ligaments are sheered by fracture or surgery, this further impedes the ability of the ligaments to heal. Unfortunately, patients are recommended other non-healing therapies such as immobility, corticosteroid injections and NSAIDs, which all tremendously inhibit ligament healing!

Study name	Duman	Mayo Clinic	Birklein	de Mos 2006	de Mos 2008
Patient #'s in study	168	140	145	238	186
Fracture	55.3%	20.0%	41.3%	43.5%	49.0%
Soft tissue injury	28.0%	28.6%	32.0%	22.6%	26.0%
Surgery	16.7%	16.4%	9.0%	13.6%	11.0%
Spontaneous		15.0%		10.6%	8.0%
Other events, lesions, minor trauma, injections		19.0%	17.7%	9.6%	6.0%

Figure 19-22: CRPS precipitating events. Fracture and soft tissue injury are the most common precipitating events leading to CRPS.

Duman I, et al. Reflex sympathetic dystrophy: a retrospective epidemiological study of 168 patients. *Clin Rheumatol.* 2008;26:1433-1437.

Pak TJ, et al. Reflex sympathetic dystrophy: Review of 140 cases. *Minn Med.* 1970;53:507-512.

Birklein F, et al. Neurological findings in complex regional pain syndromes-analysis of 145 cases. *Acta Neurologica Scandinavica.* 2000;101:262-269.

de Mos M, et al. The incidence of complex regional pain syndrome: A population based study, *Pain* (2006), doi:10.1016/j.pain.2006.09.008.

de Mos M, et al. Medical history and the onset of complex regional pain. *Pain* (2008), doi:10.1016/j.pain.2008.07.002.

COMPREHENSIVE PROLOTHERAPY FOR CRPS

The same principles apply to resolving bizarre neurological conditions or symptoms, as it does to more traditional osteoarthritis pain complaints. **Find the ligament injury to resolve the condition!** When someone has local autonomic hyperactivity symptoms of the foot (i.e. the patient has a very cold foot compared the other foot) we determine which ligaments are injured in that foot and then treat them with Prolotherapy. Generally after 3-6 Prolotherapy sessions, the pain and the sympathetic symptoms are resolved.

If the condition has persisted for a long time and spread out to involve the other limb, a more comprehensive Natural Medicine approach to resolve the conditions is needed. By this time, there will be many "stressors" the person has to overcome including hopelessness, financial burdens, relationship issues and, of course, the devastating effect of CRPS on the body. In this instance, realistically the person probably needs therapy directed at their whole person; body, soul and spirit. As much as they allow us to, we will help.

A TOUGH CASE OF CRPS DEMONSTRATES WHY TO THINK TWICE BEFORE SURGERY

Jay had a long history of knee trouble, starting from two basketball injuries. At age nine, he tore cartilage in his right knee, and had it surgically repaired. Then at age 12, he tore his right ACL and also had it surgically repaired. For 20 years he had on and off knee pain, and at the age of 32 he sought care because he wanted to be active with his growing family and be able to maintain his job as a pharmacist. He was told he had meniscal tear, and he was advised to have it surgically repaired. During surgery, evidence was found that the ACL was torn again, so his surgeon tried to repair it with a graft. However, his pain continued, and later that year it was determined that the new graft had torn again, and he went in for yet another reconstruction surgery.

After the last surgery, Jay's pain level dramatically increased, and he was diagnosed with reflex sympathetic dystrophy (RSD), and later complex regional pain syndrome (CRPS). An external spinal cord stimulator seemed to help, but it was never implanted. He was referred for "pain management" which consisted of taking 8 Norco® pills per day. He gained 60 pounds and was tired all the time.

Jay's symptoms included constant numbness in the lateral knee, excruciating pain in the medial knee to lightest touch, and general constant ache in his whole knee. His right knee and right leg were colder to touch than the left. He also experienced numbness in both legs from thighs to feet, with numbness in the right 4th and 5th toes, cramping in right great toe, and coldness in all right toes.

When Jay came to Caring Medical, Dr. Hauser concurred with the RSD/CRPS diagnosis and told Jay that Caring Medical could most likely help him, but it would take a lot of work. The plan was to optimize his healing ability by weaning off narcotics, raising hormone levels, and improving his diet. These are ways to get the body into an anabolic state from a catabolic state. This would ensure that Jay would get the maximum benefit from Comprehensive Prolotherapy, the treatment that would repair the underlying tissue damage that was impacting the autonomic nervous system.

As expected, his labs showed low levels of testosterone, cortisol, and DHEA, and therefore, natural hormone replacement therapy was started. Jay was advised on a diet that would give his body the best foods to help him heal, in addition to a comprehensive multi vitamin and mineral regimen. A low-impact exercise program was also recommended. As a Christian, Jay understood the mind, body, spirit connection as it related to his health and he worked on his faith as well as his body. As is common in chronic pain, Jay also had problems sleeping which were addressed with a prescription medication which allowed him to have restful sleep.

Over the course of 18 months, Jay received 13 treatments which included, traditional Hackett-Hemwall, Stem Cell, and Neurofascial Prolotherapy. These treatments comprehensively treated the ligament weakness and damage inside and around the joint capsule, as well as the small sensory nerves that had been on high alert from all the injuries and surgeries.

It took several treatments for Jay to feel incremental improvement in his knee, but almost immediately he reported feeling much better on lower doses of pain meds, having higher levels of hormones and seeing the weight steadily fall off. Toward the end of his course of treatment, he was able to walk for hours with his family at the zoo and even go sledding, something he could not have imagined before starting Prolotherapy. Yes, Jay had more than the average number of necessary treatments, but he had an extraordinarily tough case of chronic pain. In addition, he had some setbacks over the course of treatment, including when a screw from one of his many procedures started to pop through his skin and exacerbated his symptoms. Still, in cases of chronic pain after numerous surgeries and rounds of narcotic pain medications, Prolotherapy and a Natural Medicine program can allow a person to heal beyond what they thought possible in the "pain management" system. This is an amazing example of a life changed by the power of Prolotherapy! It is also an important reminder that surgery has very real and long-term risks. Had Jay received Prolotherapy as a young athlete, who knows how much pain could have been avoided down the road.

WHAT TO DO IF SURGERY IS RECOMMENDED

It is inevitable that some people will need surgery for chronic pain. Based on our experience, however, most people who enter into a surgery have not fully explored their options or the potential long-term results of the surgery. This is particularly true of surgeries that involve the removal of the tissue.

OUR TOP CONSIDERATIONS IF SURGERY IS RECOMMENDED:

1. Did the surgeon take a thorough physical exam and history, or did he or she primarily rely on an MRI reading? Remember, the bias of the surgeon is to rely on tests such as MRI to see if there is something that can be surgically addressed. To make the right diagnoses you must start with the history. The diagnosis should make sense to you, and so should the reason for the recommended surgery.

2. Is the proposed surgery going to make the joint more stable in both the short and long-term? Often, when a surgeon plans to "repair" the joint, the real procedure may involve removing tissue, and making the joint less stable in the long-term. This is especially true if the surgeon drops a hint that a more drastic surgery, such as a replacement or revision surgery, will likely be needed within 5-10 years! You think you are signing up for one surgery, but it will lead to numerous over a lifetime.

3. Does the surgeon think you should exhaust all conservative measures before the surgery? Sometimes this is on the surgical consent form saying "Surgery is recommended after conservative measures failed." If so, then you have one more conservative therapy to try, and that is Prolotherapy.

4. Get an explanation, prior to surgery, that details all the vital soft tissue and bony structures that will be altered by the surgery. Then ask the surgeon how this will affect joint mechanics in both the short and long-term.

5. Ask the surgeon if you can run marathons (or whatever your activity of choice is) after the surgery rehabilitation is over. If he or she says "probably not," or "no," ask why? If he or she does not necessarily care if you get back to running, or you do not get a feeling that he/she are concerned about your long-term joint stability, politely decline the offer to slice up your joint, and call a Prolotherapist instead.

SUMMARY

Surgery is recommended based on MRI findings which may or may not be the sole cause of a person's chronic pain. This, along with the structural changes caused by the surgery, contributes to the growing number of patients whose chronic pain is not relieved by surgery. While surgery is necessary in a small percentage of patients, specifically for full thickness tears, it can accelerate the degenerative process leading to osteoarthritis.

Prolotherapy should be a first-line, conservative treatment tried prior to surgery based on its high success rate at relieving pain and allowing patients to quickly return to sports, work, and activities. It is also an excellent choice for cases of post-surgical pain and joint instability. Additionally, Prolotherapy can be done faster, more safely, and at a dramatically lower cost than surgery. ∎

CHAPTER

20

PROLOTHERAPY VS. OTHER POPULAR TREATMENTS

COMMONLY ASKED QUESTIONS

Dear Dr. Hauser: For the last 3 years I've been doing physical therapy and chiropractic adjustments regularly for my recurring sciatica pain. I thought I should be better by now. I researched other options and found your videos. Is it too late to try Prolotherapy? Please help. Jaime

Dear Dr. Hauser: I saw your website with the Prolotherapy shots. They appear to just be trigger point injections. I am a runner with a bad Achilles tendon problem. Trigger points helped for a few days—that was it. Are they the same? Thanks for your help. Pete

Dear Marion Hauser: I've read about a treatment I can receive in Europe that turns your blood to become an anti-inflammatory agent that is then injected into knees. I'm wondering if it's the same as Prolotherapy. I'm a basketball player and hoping to keep my scholarship and go professional after college. Thanks, Aaron

Dear Marion Hauser: I follow you on Facebook. My mom has been receiving viscosupplementation (chicken juice shots, as we call them- ha!). Her doctor told her she's still going to need a knee replacement. What do you guys think about these shots? Why aren't they helping her? She's uneasy about the thought of surgery. Best, Sandi

PS- thanks for the great recipes you post!

We could easily fill up several pages with the e-mail messages that we receive at CaringMedical.com or on social media. It's great that people have thought highly enough of us over the years to reach out with their most troubling health concerns. What is often more troubling is the treatments that have been recommended for them by well-meaning practitioners.

ACUTE PAIN IS DIFFERENT THAN CHRONIC PAIN

It is important to understand that chronic pain and acute pain are completely different diseases. They cannot be treated the same way. Consider the comparison of the two:

1. Acute pain is easy to treat and often goes away on its own.
2. Acute pain is typically from an injury that is very easily identifiable and localized.
3. Chronic pain (greater than 3-6 months of pain) is difficult to treat and by definition is not going away by itself.
4. Almost all therapies, help reduce chronic pain temporarily, so they all appear to be "successful" at first, but have no lasting effect.
5. Chronic pain spreads and is not an easily identifiable and localized problem. Thus, therapies toward them must be more comprehensive.
6. Chronic pain always has an emotional or stress component for the fact that it has been negatively affecting someone's life for a long time.

While this may the first time you heard a discussion on pain like this…acute pain is different than chronic pain, consider this quote from The American Academy of Pain Medicine who is the largest pain society in the United States:

> What is chronic pain?
> *While acute pain is a normal sensation triggered in the nervous system to alert you to possible injury and the need to take care of yourself, chronic pain is different. Chronic pain persists. Pain signals keep firing in the nervous system for weeks, months, even years.*[1]

Part of the problem with treating chronic pain with the same modalities as acute pain is that it results in "pain management" versus "pain cure." Treatments that work to temporarily relieve pain are not, however, correcting the underlying problem, so the pain returns.

WHY PHYSICAL THERAPY, MASSAGE, AND CHIROPRACTIC MANIPULATION MAY PROVIDE ONLY TEMPORARY RELIEF

We should first qualify this by saying there are some really awesome Natural Medicine practitioners who we love and use ourselves: massage therapists, reflexologists, chiropractors, and others. We use them for a variety of wellness treatments. What we want to cover in this chapter is how the most common treatments, both natural and traditional, compare to Prolotherapy for chronic pain.

For the chronic pain patient, the source of the pain is most commonly due to ligament laxity. These therapies usually treat the symptoms and not the underlying cause. Physical therapy modalities, such as TENS units, electrical stimulation units, massage, and ultrasound, will decrease muscle spasm and permanently relieve pain if muscles are the source of the problem. The chronic pain patients' muscles are in spasm or are tense usually because the underlying joint is hypermobile, or loose, and the muscles contract in order to stabilize the joint. Chronic muscle tension and spasm is a sign that the underlying joints have ligament injury.

Manual manipulation is a very effective treatment for eliminating acute pain by realigning vertebral and bony structures. Temporary benefit after years of manipulation treatment is an indication that vertebral segments are weak because of lax ligaments. Continued manipulation will not strengthen vertebral segments, and will more likely make the condition worse. Review the section in **Chapter 17** on over-manipulation syndrome where this concept is discussed more.

However, any treatment that improves blood flow while undergoing Prolotherapy, such as massage, myofascial release, ultrasound, and heat will enhance the body's response to Prolotherapy.

PROLOTHERAPY-SCREWDRIVER ANALOGY

Ligament injury and resultant joint instability account for the lack of long-term benefit from traditional and nontraditional approaches to chronic pain management, whereas Prolotherapy offers curative effects because it addresses the primary cause of chronic musculoskeletal pain: joint instability. Prolotherapy is used to tighten loose ligaments that cause joint instability the same way a screwdriver can tighten a screw in a loose hinge. **(See Figure 20-1.)** Ligaments are the most frequently injured tissues within a joint. About 150,000 ACL injuries occur each year and it isn't even close to the most common ligament injury![2] That title could go to the anterior talofibular ligament (ankle sprain) which occur in about 20,000 people per day! Ligaments, once stretched out, typically stay stretched out or injured because they have a terrible blood supply. Ligaments are white and heal poorly as do other "white" structures such as cartilage, menisci, tendons and labrum.

Traditional treatments such as physiotherapy, anti-inflammatories, bracing, manipulation, massage and others would perhaps help with the muscle spasm or joint swelling that can occur with ligament injury and resultant muscle spasm but do nothing to stimulate chronically-injured ligaments to heal. Since remodeled ligament tissue is morphologically and biomechanically inferior to normal ligament tissue, ligament laxity results, causing functional disability of the affected joint and predisposing other soft tissues in and around the joint to further damage.[3,4] When a ligament is injured and the joint unstable, excessive forces get transmitted to the joint. This causes a hardening of the bone underneath the cartilage. When extra pressure is put on a bone it hardens, plain and simple. The same thing happens to your hands and feet. Where there is extra pressure you get a callous right? Is a callous softer or harder than your normal skin? Harder. When the bone underneath the cartilage gets too hard, it has no cushioning effect. Guess what this does to the cartilage? This increases the forces on the cartilage so it starts to break. The cartilage develops fibrillations and when the fibrillations connect to each other a piece of cartilage breaks off and then the person is said to have an osteochondral defect. This free-floating cartilage fragment in the joint is called a "loose body." The accelerated degeneration leads to further joint deterioration, cartilage thinning and bone spur formation. Eventually the person has an extremely stiff and immobile joint and requires joint

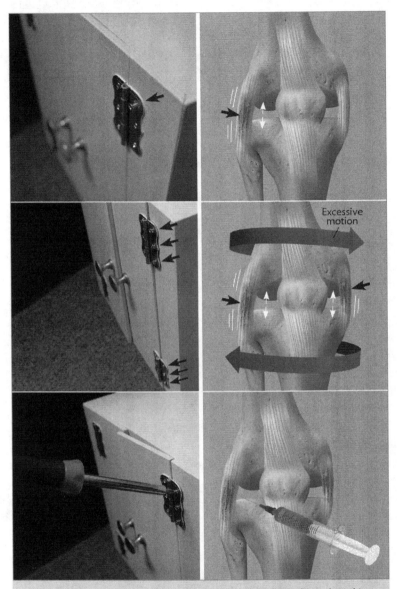

Figure 20-1: The Prolotherapy-Screwdriver Analogy. When cabinet doors hit each other it is because one or more of the hinges is loose. The weak link on a cabinet is the hinge (black arrows). Once a hinge is loose, it has the potential to make all the other hinges loose. The only curative treatment is to tighten the loose screws with a Phillips screwdriver. In the human body, the hinge is the joint. Around the joint are ligaments (not screws) to hold the bones of the joint together. For a loose joint (white arrows), the only curative treatment is to tighten the ligaments with Prolotherapy.

replacement surgery. Yes, nonhealing ligament injury and resultant joint instability explains the degenerative process in the peripheral joints and spine and the rising number of joint replacements.

DISAPPOINTING RESULTS WITH TRADITIONAL CHRONIC PAIN TREATMENTS

The traditional medicine approaches to chronic musculoskeletal pain include narcotic medications, NSAIDs (nonsteroidal anti-inflammatory medications), tricyclic antidepressants, GABA derivatives and medicinal injections including corticosteroids, anesthetics, and neuromuscular paralytic agents (botulinum toxins). Three major reviews by researchers from McMaster University in Canada noted "insufficient evidence" for use of all pharmacological agents including analgesics (including narcotics), anti-inflammatories, psychotropic agents, and medicinal injectable agents including corticosteroids, anesthetics and botulinum toxins.[5-7] In summary, they found no high or moderate quality studies with evidence of benefit of the therapy for chronic neck pain over control. Moderate quality evidence suggested little or no difference in pain or function/disability between nerve block injection of steroid and bupivacaine vs bupivacaine alone at short, intermediate and long-term for chronic neck pain.

Similarly with back pain, traditional pain management therapies including epidural steroid injections, facet joint injections or other nerve blocks cost thousands of dollars per procedure. The sad news is, patients are heading in droves to doctors to receive them. An analysis published in 2012 of the Medicare population documents an increase in interventional procedures for low back from 1,460,495 to 4,815,673 in only 11 years! Epidural injections increased in that time period from 832,000 to 2.3 million![8]

The most common reason given by physicians for the use of epidural or other steroid injections is to treat a pinched nerve. This condition in the spine is called radiculopathy; for the low back, lumbar radiculopathy and for the neck, cervical radiculopathy. Let's think about it. Would injecting a steroid shot into or around a pinched nerve have a beneficial effect on pain relief? Yes, of course! Remember, though, we are talking about chronic pain. To cure chronic pain you have to treat the cause of the nerve irritation. Without treating the cause, the beneficial effects will only be temporary and the person will be left with the same symptoms once the steroid shot wears off. That is exactly what the scientific literature shows.

Consider these conclusions by the American Academy of Neurology: "Based on the available evidence, the Therapeutics and Technology Assessment subcommittee concluded that 1) epidural steroid injections may result in some improvement in radicular lumbosacral pain when assessed between 2 and 6 weeks following the injection, compared to control treatments; 2) In general, epidural steroid injection for radicular lumbosacral pain does not impact average impairment of function, need for surgery, or provide long-term pain relief beyond 3 months. Their routine use for these indications is not recommended; 3) there is insufficient evidence to make any recommendation for the use of epidural steroid injections to treat radicular cervical pain."[9] Even with a pinched nerve in the neck or lower back, no evidence that exists supporting injections of steroids into and around the nerve for long-term benefit.

ACCEPT NO IMITATIONS

Prolotherapy is an injection technique that stimulates the body to **repair** the painful area. Prolotherapy involves the proliferation of fibroblastic cells. This causes the regeneration of normal connective tissues, such as ligaments and tendons. The solution is injected into the fibro-osseous junction of the bone and connective tissue. The injections repair the painful area, by proliferating fibroblasts that regenerate normal ligament and tendon tissue at the fibro-osseous junction, by causing inflammation that simulates the natural healing process. Do not be fooled. Typical trigger point injections, epidural injections, cortisone shots, lidocaine shots, botulism injections, facet blocks, and nerve-root blocks are **not Prolotherapy.** They never were and never will be Prolotherapy. They have almost **nothing** in common with Prolotherapy except that they involve a syringe and a needle. *(See Figure 20-2.)*

You may be surprised to know that we do occasionally use cortisone, epidural injections, facet blocks, and a host of other injection techniques. There are select cases that may truly have a need for cortisone or a nerve block, but these are much fewer than most people realize. Our office has the tools needed to deal with all types of pain, which is unlike the average orthopedic or pain medicine office who is equipped with a prescription pad, cortisone, and nerve blocks. **Dr. Hauser loves giving injections!** During a typical day at Caring Medical he will give about 1,000+ injections. Dr. Hauser wrote to the *Guinness Book of World Records* to ask them to allow him to set the record for the most injections given in one hour. He felt with doing finger injections and other parts of the body where the bone is very close to the surface of the skin, that he could do one injection every three seconds which would amount to 1,200 injections in one hour. They wrote a nice letter back saying, "…don't call us, we'll call you." We wish Prolotherapy was just one large shot, but it isn't. *(See Figure 20-3.)*

GET IT OVER QUICKLY!

Nobody likes shots. Would you rather have a physician slowly inject the needle so that you feel every slow gradual progression of the needle? For shoulder injections, the needle first pierces the skin, then goes through the subcutaneous tissues, and passes through the fat to get to the deltoid muscle, then the fascia, and then down to the fibro-osseous junction of the supraspinatus tendon. The physician could perform this procedure so the patient feels the needle going through each layer, taking a break after every injection, with the patient still sweating after 10 minutes.

Medical Condition	Procedurist Thinking	Procedurist Treatment	Procedurist End Result
Knee osteoarthritis	Cause is wear and tear. Patient needs pain relief.	Give corticosteroid or hyaluronate injections. If fails, do knee replacement.	Knee replacement.
Hip labral tear	Labrum is sole problem. No treatment done to repair hip ligaments.	Labral debridement (remove part of labrum) or staple labrum to acetabulum (hip socket).	Current or future hip instability, leading to increased hip degeneration and possible hip replacement.
Lumbar radiculopathy	Space where nerve comes out (neural foramina) needs to be opened.	Steroid shot to nerve under fluoroscopy (x-ray guidance) or epidural steroid given. If fails, do surgery, which might include foraminotomy, laminectomy, or spinal fusion.	Foraminotomy, laminectomy, or spinal fusion.
Cervical degenerative disc disease (osteoarthritis)	Inflammation needs to be decreased or bone in disc needs to be removed for pain relief to occur.	Prescribe nonsteroid anti-inflammatory medication or perform cervical epidural. If no results, then do cervical spine fusion and/or disc replacement.	Cervical spine fusion or disc replacement causing adjacent segment disease.
Shoulder impingement syndrome	Overhead activities need to be eliminated and inflammation needs to be treated for pain relief to occur.	Steroid shot to the shoulder. If no help, then decompressive surgery (arthroscopy) or acromioplasty (bone removal) and/or debridement of rotator cuff tendons.	Arthroscopy or acromioplasty and/or rotator cuff debridement.
Medical Condition	**Prolotherapist Thinking**	**Prolotherapist Treatment**	**Prolotherapist End Result**
Knee osteoarthritis	Cause is joint instability from ligament laxity. A degenerated joint needs regeneration.	Comprehensive Prolotherapy to knee menisci, cartilage and ligaments.	Healed. Improved activity level.
Hip labral tear	Initial injury caused damage to ligaments, tendons and other structures around hip. The pain is from hip joint instability.	Comprehensive Prolotherapy to structures that provide stability in the front, side and back of hip, not just labrum.	Healed. Improved activity level.
Lumbar radiculopathy	Nerve irritation is from lumbar instability. Capsular ligaments that hold facet joints together need to be strengthened and tightened.	Comprehensive Prolotherapy to injured capsular ligaments.	Healed. Improved activity level.
Cervical degenerative disc disease (osteoarthritis)	Cervical discs and facet joints degenerate from cervical instability secondary to capsular ligament injury.	Stabilize cervical spine by performing Comprehensive Prolotherapy to the cervical facet joints and capsular ligaments.	Healed. Improved activity level.
Shoulder impingement syndrome	Impingement from shoulder instability from ligament laxity and/or labral tear.	Comprehensive Prolotherapy to structures causing the shoulder instability.	Healed. Improved activity level.

Figure 20-2: Thinking like a Prolotherapist versus a Procedurist for five common pain conditions. Prolotherapy treatments resolve joint instability and the root cause of joint pain. On the other hand, Procedurists utilize corticosteroid injections and surgeries that often lead to long-term problems, including increased joint instability and worsened arthritis.

INJURED LIGAMENTS: OVERLOOKED AS THE CAUSE OF TRIGGER POINTS, SUBLUXATIONS, SWELLING, AND CHRONIC MUSCLE SPASMS

Any physiotherapist or masseuse can massage away muscle spasms. A doctor can inject anesthetic into the muscles and immediately eliminate a muscle spasm. Doctors can also give muscle relaxants. The question is: Why do most of the people treated this way experience a recurrence of their pain? Most people with trigger points who get spray and stretch, ultrasound, physiotherapy, massage, traditional "trigger point" injections, or chiropractic/osteopathic manipulation experience continual recurrences of their pain and their trigger points.

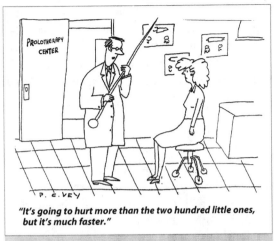

"It's going to hurt more than the two hundred little ones, but it's much faster."

Figure 20-3: Prolotherapy cartoon given to Dr. Hauser by a patient who had been successfully "Prolo'ed."

Bones only move out of alignment if the stabilizing structures themselves have been injured. **The main stabilizing structures in the joints of the body are the ligaments.** *(See Figure 20-4.)* This indicates that the cause of muscle spasm is not a problem in the muscle itself. It must be due to the fact that the sacroiliac joint will not stay in place.

The sacroiliac joint will not stay in place because the sacroiliac ligaments are weakened. When they are weakened, sacroiliac "slips or displacements" occur, which then lead to gluteus minimus muscle spasms.

If a patient has an underlying ligament injury causing chronic joint instability, traditional and nontraditional therapies would only address the secondary effects from this including muscle spasms (and resulting trigger points), joint swelling, and bone spurs. The frustrating fact for the physicians and other clinicians, and especially for the patient, is that no one identifies what is wrong. Most ligaments do not show up on radiographs or MRIs. Most physicians and other health care providers have little training in joint instability and ligament injury. In a comprehensive summary review on chronic pain, the overview noted "chronic pain remains intractable and minimally understood."[10] The mechanism is not understood and likely diagnostic tests are not helpful either. Plain radiographs show the cause of chronic pain in less than 1% of cases and MRIs are basically the same in people with chronic pain and those who are symptom free.[11-14] So what condition could account for the fact that clinicians can not document the cause objectively and definitively? It can't be the disc, or joint or cartilage because of all of

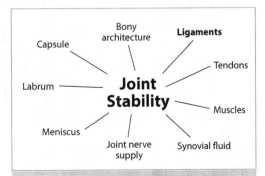

Figure 20-4: Structures involved in joint stability. The **major** structures involved in joint stability are the ligaments.

these structures show up clearly on the various tests. It is those which are injured most frequently: the ligaments. The ligaments also do not show up on diagnostic tests and as of yet there is no a universally accepted manner to diagnostically document ligament injury or the resultant joint instability. Thus, physical therapists, doctors, nurses, physician assistants and other people in the healing arts are not trained sufficiently to document ligament injuries and joint instability, thus these injuries in essence go *undetected and unobserved.*

From the chronic pain persisting, emotional factors start to enter such as depression, anxiety, hopelessness (of never getting better) and various fears. This is why cognitive behavior techniques, biofeedback, counseling, faith, anti-depressant and other central nervous system altering drugs are helpful to relieve symptoms but do little to cure the chronic pain. Structural, mechanical pain needs a structural solution. Both traditional and non-traditional therapies are temporarily helpful but not curative. The continued underlying initial ligament injury and resultant joint instability are the best explanation for this.

People in pain are injected with temporary pain relievers and muscle relaxers, manipulated, massaged, and physiotherapied to the tune of tens of thousands of dollars for only temporary effects. The treatments do provide temporary pain relief; but for permanent pain relief something else must be done. The something else is

Prolotherapy. Prolotherapy stimulates the growth of the ligaments, which provides the stimulus for the bony alignments to stay in place, resulting in no more slips or displacements; no more joint instability. *(See Figure 20-5.)*

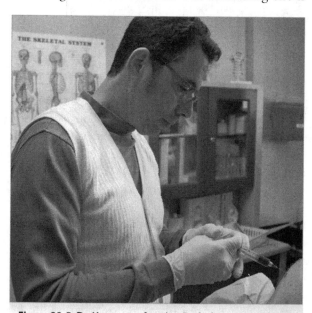

Figure 20-5: Dr. Hauser performing Prolotherapy on a knee.

MUSCLE PAIN IS DIFFERENT THAN LIGAMENT PAIN

Most people do not realize that the body's response to ligamentous injury is muscle spasm. The reason for this is two-fold: to provide joint protection/ stabilization and to notify the brain that the body is hurt. Unfortunately, the brains of many people register the pain signal as meaning, "I better take some anti-inflammatories or get a cortisone shot to stop the pain!" The muscle spasms are the body's secondary defense to stabilize the joints, if the ligaments are stretched.

When the ligaments become stretched, the muscles now have to act as joint stabilizers and movers. It is easy to see how they could become tense, knotty, and hyperirritable to electrical stimulation. **The muscles are now doing the job of both the ligaments and the muscles, and, therefore, may become increasingly fatigued.** By focusing on the muscles, the clinicians are missing the central factor in curing the problem. The cure lies in strengthening the ligaments and stopping the reason for the muscle spasms.

If you think about athletics and sports injuries, for example, how many times during rugby, soccer, hockey, basketball, or football matches are the players smashing each other's muscles? The thighs, back, chest, and calves are getting clobbered. After a few sessions in the hot tub and a couple of massages, the muscles feel great. Again, it goes back to the fact that muscle physiology and ligament physiology are **completely different.** Muscles have too big of an aerobic capacity and blood supply not to heal well after injury. Muscles are beefy red and the blood circulation in them can increase 20 times in a matter of minutes during a sprint, for instance. Ligaments, on the other hand, have a horribly slow metabolism, manifested by their white appearance and poor blood supply. You can exercise and receive physiotherapy day and night, and they will not have any substantial effect on ligament growth and regeneration. There is only one way to stimulate the proliferation of ligaments and that is by Prolotherapy.

LIGAMENT TRIGGER POINTS AND REFERRAL PATTERNS

Around the same time that Janet Travell, MD, was studying muscle trigger points and diagramming the referral pain patterns, George S. Hackett, MD, of Canton, Ohio, was doing the same thing for ligaments. *(See Figure 20-6.)* He published his work, as Dr. Travell did, in some of the best medical publications of the day, including the *Journal of the American Medical Association*, the *American Journal of Surgery*, and the AMA *Archives of Surgery*.[15-17] In 1956, he published the first edition of his book *Ligament and Tendon Relaxation Treated by Prolotherapy*.[18] So well-accepted was his work, that not only did the American Medical Association allow publication of his research in their journals, but Dr. Hackett himself sold his books and presented his research at AMA conventions in the late 1950s.

DR. GEORGE HACKETT: LIGAMENT REFERRAL PATTERNS

Dr. Hackett was the first one to coin the term Prolotherapy. After doing about 2,000 injections, he diagrammed the referral patterns of the neck and lower back ligaments. These drawings are very similar to the ones by Dr. Travell. The reason for this is that ligament laxity causes muscle trigger points to develop. The ligament laxity referral patterns and muscle trigger point patterns are very similar because they have the same etiology.

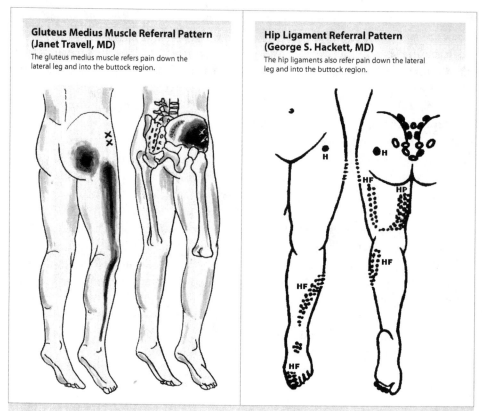

Figure 20-6: Components of Travell and Hackett referral patterns. Notice the similarities between the referral patterns.

Dr. Hackett is known for some famous lines such as these:

- "A joint is only as strong as its weakest ligament."
- "Most joint pain is ligament pain."
- "The evidence appears to be conclusive that relaxed supra- and interspinus ligaments are an etiological factor in the occurrence of ruptured disc."
- "The injection of a local anesthetic into the ligaments of an ankle for relief of pain following an injury...if given to enable an athlete to continue activity...is to be deplored."[17]

PROLOTHERAPY VERSUS TRIGGER POINT THERAPY

Understand that there is a significant difference between traditional trigger point injections and Prolotherapy. *(See Figure 20-7.)* Traditional trigger point injections are done directly into the muscles where the trigger points are located. Some physicians just stick the needle into the trigger point and do not inject any solution; a technique called dry needling. There are various trigger point solutions used, which can include procaine, lidocaine, longer-acting local anesthetics, isotonic

	Trigger Point Injections	**Prolotherapy**
Substance injected	Anesthetic/corticosteroid	Proliferant/anesthetic
Injection site	Muscle belly	Fibro-osseous junction
Mechanism of action	Relax muscles	Regenerate ligaments
Effect on joint stability	None	Enhanced
Immediate pain relief	Yes	Yes
Lasting pain relief	No	Yes
Recurrences	Frequent	Few

Figure 20-7: Trigger point injections versus Prolotherapy.

saline, corticosteroid, and botulin A toxin, depending on the experience of the physician. Some studies have shown that dry needling is as effective as injecting anesthetics in getting rid of trigger points.[19,20] The problem is that most people's trigger points return or are never permanently cured with dry needling or trigger point injections. Traditional trigger point injections do help decrease trigger point pain, and sometimes eliminate it, but rarely do they cure it, regardless of what is injected.

NEURAL THERAPY

Neural Therapy is a gentle healing technique developed in Germany that involves the injection of local anesthetics into autonomic ganglia, peripheral nerves, scars, glands, acupuncture points, trigger points, and other tissues.[21] What are autonomic ganglia? The body contains two nervous systems: the somatic and the autonomic. The somatic nervous system is under a person's voluntary control. The autonomic nervous system functions automatically. The autonomic ganglia is the place where the center of the autonomic nerves are located.

SOMATIC AND AUTONOMIC NERVOUS SYSTEMS

The nerves in the somatic nervous system control skin sensation and muscle movement. Picking up a cup of tea, for example, requires the somatic nervous system to sense the cup with the fingers and contract the muscles to lift the cup. These are the same nerves that are pinched in a herniated disc.

The autonomic nervous system is automatically activated. Life-sustaining functions like breathing, blood flow, pupil dilation, and perspiration are activated by the autonomic nervous system. People do not think about the blood vessels in their hands constricting when they are outside on a cold, winter day. This occurs automatically. The functioning of the autonomic nervous system is crucial, as it controls blood flow throughout the body. Illness often begins when the blood flow to an extremity or an organ is decreased.

Disturbed autonomic nervous system function has been implicated in the following diseases: headaches, migraines, dizziness, confusion, optic neuritis, chronic ear infections, tinnitus, vertigo, hay fever, sinusitis, tonsillitis, asthma, liver disease, gallbladder disease, menstrual pain, eczema, and a host of others. Neural Therapy, because it increases blood flow, may have profoundly positive effects on such conditions.[22]

INTERFERENCE FIELDS

The founder of Neural Therapy, Ferdinand Huneke, MD, felt one of its beneficial effects was the elimination of interference fields. An interference field is any pathologically damaged tissue which, on account of an excessively strong or long-standing stimulus or of a summation of stimuli that cannot be abated, is in a state of unphysiological permanent excitation.[23] In layman's terms, any time a tissue is injured it can continually excite the autonomic nervous system. These centers of irritation through the autonomic nervous system may cause disease in other parts of the body.

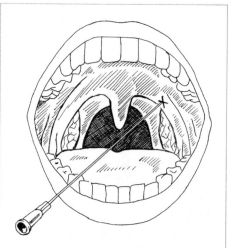

Figure 20-8: Neural therapy on the tonsils. Any previously traumatized, surgerized, or infected site or tissue can be an interference field for the autonomic nervous system.

Most interference fields are found in the head region. According to Dr. Huneke, teeth and tonsils are the two most common—probably because they are close to the brain and nerves. *(See Figure 20-8.)* An infected tooth can set up an interference field, causing a person to have chronic low back pain or a heart arrhythmia. A patient may have chronic low back pain that is unresponsive to surgical and conservative treatments because an interference field is present.

Scars are the next most common interference fields. Any scar, no matter how small or old, even if it dates back to early childhood, can be the interference field causing therapy-resistant rheumatoid arthritis, hearing loss, sciatica, or other serious disorders.[23]

NEURAL THERAPY AS PAIN MANAGEMENT

Neural Therapy involves the injection of anesthetic solutions, such as lidocaine or procaine, into these interference fields. The areas injected may include various areas of the teeth, tonsils, autonomic nervous system nerves, or ganglia, somatic or peripheral nerves, scars, or the area surrounding various organs. Immediate pain relief is often observed after the first injection because nerve irritation has been resolved.

Most traditional physicians are not aware of the role of the autonomic nervous system or do not diagnose problems involving it because an autonomic nervous system cannot be tested. The autonomic nervous system does not appear on x-rays; only somatic nervous system nerves can be seen.

To diagnose an autonomic nervous system problem, the clinician must understand interference fields as well as Neural Therapy. An autonomic nervous system disorder should be suspected if any of the following conditions are evident: burning pain, excessively cool or hot extremities, pale or red hands or feet, skin sensitivity to touch, scars, root canals, chronic problems occurring after an infection or accident, chronic pain not responsive to other forms of therapy, shooting burning nerve pain, pinched nerve, or a chronic medical condition that has not responded to other treatments.

While Neural Therapy is used more frequently as a healing modality in European countries than in the United States, nevertheless, Caring Medical offers this treatment, if appropriate, as an option after an initial consultation.

To learn more about Neural Therapy, consult the *Illustrated Atlas of the Techniques of Neural Therapy with Local Anesthetics*, a textbook from Germany.[24]

At our office, Neural Therapy has been a wonderful adjunctive therapy for the treatment of chronic pain and illness. A person with chronic pain often has evidence of both ligament laxity and autonomic nervous system dysfunction. In such a case, both Prolotherapy and Neural Therapy are warranted.

SUMMARY

When comparing other treatments to Prolotherapy for chronic pain, remember that most chronic pain is due to joint instability caused by ligament laxity. Most treatments focus on relieving muscle pain and swelling. However, these are really symptoms that lead back to the unresolved joint instability. Prolotherapy is the only regenerative treatment that addresses the cause of muscle spasms, joint swelling, cartilage deterioration, and more at the source. In some cases, it can be appropriate to use other injection therapies in combination with Prolotherapy, such as trigger point injections or Neural Therapy. ■

CHAPTER

THE EVOLUTION OF PROLOTHERAPY

It is difficult to believe that in this day and age we are still treating pain with NSAIDs, steroid shots, and narcotic medications, as well as using surgeries that often do not work to cure the pain problem. This is especially difficult to accept when one considers the work of just two men, George S. Hackett, MD, and Gustav A. Hemwall, MD, the Prolotherapy pioneers.

FROM SURGERY TO SUCCESS

George S. Hackett, MD, was a graduate of Cornell Medical School, class of 1916.[1] He was a busy consulting trauma surgeon at Mercy Hospital in Canton, Ohio. He describes it best. "During a period of over 20 years while engaged in a tremendous traumatic practice, I was also regularly called upon for special examinations by approximately 70 accident insurance companies to report accurate diagnoses and prognoses. I became aware of the indefinite and variable conclusions of our best diagnosticians in dealing with low back disability. Finally, in 1939, I arrived at the conclusion that relaxation of the articular ligaments was responsible for a considerable number of low back disabilities.

"I decided to attempt strengthening the ligaments by the injection of a proliferating solution within the fibrous bands to stimulate the production of fibrous tissue. The treatment proved to be satisfactory almost from the beginning, and it was cautiously extended until now, articular ligaments of the entire spine and pelvis and some other joints are treated with great satisfaction both to the patient and to me."[2]

THE SWITCH TO PROLOTHERAPY

Dr. Hackett, in his role as a trauma surgeon and consultant to insurance companies, was often asked his opinion of whether surgery would help people with their back pain and, if they had already had a back operation, could anything still be done for their pain that remained. Here are some of his observations that led to his belief that ligament laxity, especially around the sacroiliac joint, was where the answer lay. *(See Figure 21-1.)*

"Over two decades ago, three ideas appeared which definitely changed the course of events in low back treatment. One was the description of the ruptured nucleus pulposus in 1934 as described by Mixter and Barr. It is a definite scientific entity and will endure. However, **it has gotten out of control because of the confusion in diagnosis and has resulted in too many *unsatisfactory* operations.** Barr pointed out in 1951 that, 'Too many backs are being irretrievably damaged by ill-advised and ill-considered operations.' The mass production of unnecessary, unsatisfactory spinal operations that were turned out in the post-war decade by inexperienced surgeons, whose training was overemphasized on the mechanical side, helps to confuse the public and make them wary. I am frequently consulted by patients who have had disc

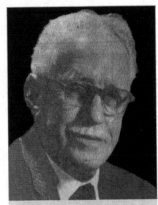

Figure 21-1: George S. Hackett, MD, coined the term Prolotherapy as well as pioneered the treatment.

and spinal fusion operations by surgeons who do not consider the sacroiliac joint and its ligaments as causing any trouble. These patients continue to have the same pain, referred pain and sciatica from relaxation of the ligaments that support the lumbosacral and sacroiliac articulations that they had previous to the operations."

"I have successfully treated them in cases that have not been too extensively **mutilated** by operations which sacrifice important ligaments and bone prominences that have been developed to give leverage for attached ligaments and tendons. The belief that the pain and disability of lumbosacral instability from ligament relaxation can be eliminated by lumbosacral fusion is **erroneous.** Even if the fifth lumbar vertebra was solidly fused by operation to the sacrum, there would remain the forward rotation of the upper sacrum at the sacroiliac joint. This would continue to place tension on the relaxed fibers of the iliolumbar and upper portion of the posterior sacroiliac ligaments, and frequently to a greater degree than before the fusion was performed."[2]

Dr. Hackett in the 1930s could see that spinal operations were not the answer to the chronic pain problem, and this was the impetus for him to look elsewhere for the answer. As he puts it, "No spinal fusion operation in the past has survived its originator, nor will probably any now in vogue, nor any in the future, for **most fusion operations impair function and usually result in limited activity and continued discomfort.** Eighteen years ago, I decided that much of the low back pain and disability was due to relaxation of the articular ligaments and considered methods of strengthening them. Having had some experience in operation on cases of hernia, which had previously been injected with a proliferating solution, I was impressed with the increased density and strength of the tissues which were encountered. I applied the proliferating injection treatment to the relaxed ligaments by injecting the solution within the fibrous bands, and within a short time I was impressed with the clinical results obtained and the patients were most enthusiastic."[2]

DEFINING THE TREATMENT

George S. Hackett, MD, coined the term Prolotherapy, fine-tuned the technique, and taught it to other physicians. *(See Figure 21-2.)* As he describes it,

"The treatment consists of the injection of a solution within the relaxed ligament and tendon which will stimulate the production of new fibrous tissue and bone cells that will strengthen the 'weld' of fibrous tissue and bone to stabilize the articulation and permanently eliminate the disability.

To the treatment of proliferating new cells, I have applied the name *Prolotherapy* from the word *proli* (Latin), meaning offspring; *proliferate*—to produce new cells in rapid succession (Webster's Dictionary). My definition of Prolotherapy as applied medically in the treatment of skeletal disability is 'the rehabilitation of an incompetent structure by the generation of new cellular tissue'...I have developed special techniques, particularly for lumbosacral and sacroiliac

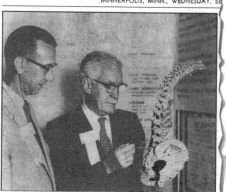

It Hurts Here
Dr. G.A. Hemwall, Chicago (left), got a lesson in back pain Tuesday from Dr. George S. Hackett, Canton , Ohio. The American Academy of Physical Medicine and Rehabilitation ended two days of meetings at the Leamington hotel, and the American Congress of Physical Medicine and Rehabilitation got ready for three days of meetings starting today. Hackett injects what he calls "an irritating solution" into weak backs to strengthen the ligaments—or, as he puts it, "stimulate production of new bone and fibrous tissue cells to strengthen the weld of ligament to bone." The method is not generally accepted, but Hackett claimed good results over 20 years.

Figure 21-2: Prolotherapy in history.
Doctors Hemwall and Hackett at the American Academy of Physical Medicine and Rehabilitation National meetings back in the 1950s.

joint stabilization, that make possible the injection of a small portion of the solution at from 10 to 15 places against bone from one insertion of the sharp needle through the skin... I am so confident of my diagnosis, the depth of the ligament, and my tactile sensation that I usually only use the proliferant combined with the anesthetic solution and no anesthetic solution alone before entering the ligament or tendon. Usually the needle is inserted at the trigger point of either ligament or tendon until the point of the needle contacts bone. The local pain is reproduced, confirming the diagnosis. The proliferating solution is injected while the point of the needle is held against the bone."[2]

THE HISTOLOGY

Histology might also be called microscopic anatomy. When put under a microscope, does Prolotherapy do everything that Dr. Hackett claims? He didn't wait to find out—he did most of the research on it himself! As he explains, "There was a need for this investigation because, although both the patients and I were satisfied that the clinical results of proliferation of ligaments in the stabilization of relaxed joints were entirely satisfactory, it became increasingly evident that **some physicians were skeptical of the method.** Also, no previous scientific work had been done which demonstrated the volume of strong fibrous tissue which could be generated by the introduction of a proliferant within the articular ligaments."[2]

Much of the research that Dr. Hackett performed was done in the 1950s on rabbit tendons. The first investigation was done using Sylnasol, a fatty acid proliferant, on the gastrocnemius and superficial flexor tendons, analogous to the Achilles tendon in man.[3] Microscopic slides were made through sections from the rabbit tendons following the Prolotherapy injection at various time intervals. The injections of proliferating solution were distributed throughout the tendon from its origin in the muscle to its insertion into the bone. The second injection was given six weeks after the first, and the third or last injection was given five months after the first, so that animals in all cases under two months' duration received only one injection, those under five months received two injections, and the longer cases received a total of three injections. The results of the experiments showed that there was **no** necrosis of any of the specimens and no destruction of any nerves, blood vessels or tendinous bands. It became evident from the histology that Prolotherapy stimulated the normal inflammatory reaction. *(See Figure 21-3.)*

Figure 21-4 shows the right and left tendons of two rabbits after nine and 12 months of proliferating treatment. In both cases, the left tendon was not injected

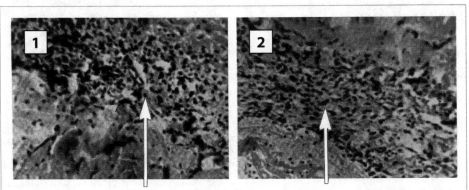

Arrow points to moderate infiltration of lymphocytes 48 hours after injection of proliferating solution. Note absence of cell-death in surrounding tissues.

Beginning fibroblastic organization present in adjacent tissues. Arrow points to capillary proliferation with moderate infiltration of lymphocytes. *Two weeks after injection, this microphotograph shows new tissue growth.*

Figure 21-3: Microphotographs of sections from rabbit Achilles tendons following the injection of the proliferant, Sylnasol. The same technique was done as that which is used clinically.

and was used as a control. The right tendon in each case received three injections. At the end of nine and 12 months, the injected right tendons in each case revealed an increase of 40% in diameter as compared with the controls, while the end of the bone with the attached tendon disclosed a 30% increase in diameter. *Figure 21-5* shows the proximal end of the tibial tarsal bone of the rabbit with the attached gastrocnemius and superficial flexor tendons. The films were made at one and three months after a single injection of proliferant solution had been distributed. It reveals that soft tissue increase at one month is pronounced due to the presence of inflammatory reaction, while at

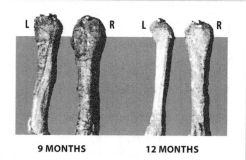

9 MONTHS   12 MONTHS

Left, controls; *right*, proliferated. The tendons on the right reveal an increase in diameter of 40%, which is estimated to double the strength of the tendon. The upper portion reveals the attachment of the ligament to the bone, which has increased 30% in diameter. The proliferating solution stimulates the production of new fibrous connective tissue cells, which become organized into permanent non-elastic fibrous tissue.

Figure 21-4: Photograph of rabbit tendons at 9 and 12 months after three injections of proliferating solution into the right tendons.

three months the increase is due to the production of permanent fibrous tissue. It also reveals a marked increase of bone at one month, as compared with the control, and a further increase of bone at three months. The increase of bone is significant because it results in a strong fibro–osseous union where sprains, tears, and relaxation

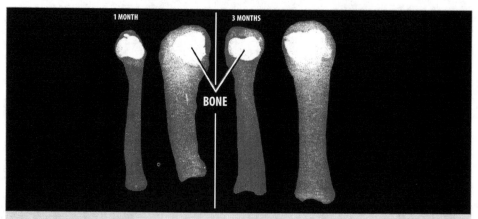

Figure 21-5: Roentgenograms of the proximal end of the tibial tarsal bone of the rabbit with the attached gastrocnemius and superficial flexor tendons. The films were made one and three months after a single injection of proliferant solution had been distributed throughout the tendon. They reveal a marked increase of bone at one month, as compared with the control, and a further increase of bone at three months. The increase in soft tissue at one month was pronounced, due to the presence of new fibrous tissue cells, while at three months the increase was due to the production of permanent fibrous tissue. The increase of bone was significant because it resulted in a strong fibro-osseous union ("weld") where sprains, tears, and relaxation of the ligament chiefly take place and where the sensory nerves are abundant.

of the ligament take place during proliferation.[3] Prolotherapy, besides inducing tendon growth and bone growth, was indeed causing fibro-osseous proliferation, just as Dr. Hackett said. **(See Figure 21-6.)**

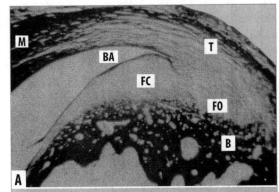

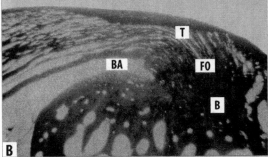

Figure 21-6: Microphotographs of induced fibro-osseous proliferation bone = B, Tendon = T, Muscle = M, Fibro-Osseous Junction = FO, Fibrocartilage = FC, Bursal Area = BA. Microphotographs of decalcified Achilles tendon attachments to the tibio-tarsal bones of a rabbit, two months after one injection of 0.5 cc of a proliferating solution (Sylnasol 25% in Pontocaine) was made into the right leg [B]. The injection was made against bone within the fibro-osseous attachment of the tendon. The control left leg [A] was not injected. **A. Control leg (above):** The tendon fibers (T) blend with the periosteum and continue into bone (B). They are firmly attached by calcification which extends outward into the fibro-osseous junction (FO). **B. Injected leg (below):** Proliferated new bone cells increase bone density (B), extend outward, and increase the area and density of the fibro-osseous junction (FO), and encroach on the fibrocartilage (FC) and bursal area (BA), without penetrating the tendon capsular sheath. The weld of tendon to bone is strengthened.

THE EARLY PROLOTHERAPY SOLUTIONS

After 21 years of clinical experience and eight years of doing animal experiments, Dr. Hackett published a study on the use of various solutions to induce fibro-osseous proliferation.[4] In regard to the technique of fibro-osseous proliferation he says, "The technic [technique] consists of injecting a combined proliferating and local anesthetic solution within the weak fibro-osseous attachment. A few drops are distributed in proximate positions while the point of the needle contacts bone. The new bone and fibrous tissue cells become strong in four to six weeks. The patient returns for re-evaluation in eight weeks and additional injections are given when indicated."[4] The study consisted of injections of proliferant within joints, at the site of fractures, at fibro-osseous junctions, and intrathecally (to monitor safety) in rabbits. Dr. Hackett noted that even when the Prolotherapy solution was injected into the spinal canal that no noticeable effect was seen. When purposely increasing the dose into the spinal canal, again no long-term consequences were found. In regard to healing fractures, he showed that Prolotherapy could hasten healing with the zinc sulfate and Sylnasol solutions. He found that cortisone had an inhibitory effect.

Dr. Hackett was mainly concerned with documenting fibro-osseous proliferation. He, therefore, used 192 rabbit Achilles tendons to determine the amount of new bone and fibrous tissue that was induced over variable periods from a few days to one year, following one or more injections of various solutions into the fibro-osseous junction of tendon to bone. *Figure 21-6* shows the comparative fibro-osseous proliferation that resulted over a period of eight weeks following a single injection of 0.5 cc of various solutions. Again, various solutions were found successful in inducing fibro-osseous proliferation. *(See Figure 21-7.)* In regards to the strength of the proliferation, he found Sylnasol, silica, and zinc sulfate to work the best. The proliferants Sotradegol®, Varisol, Q.U., and whole blood were modest in their proliferative effect. Calcium gluconate and daily exercise had minimal proliferating capabilities. Cortisone and estrogen had none. Cortisone, however, is not neutral but inhibitory. This can best be seen in the x-ray studies shown in *Figure 21-8*.

Solutions Used	Fibro-Osseous Proliferation
Controls	0
Sylnasol 33% in saline	5
Sylnasol 25% in pontocaine	4
Sylnasol 25% in pontocaine w/cortisone	1
Zinc sulfate (stock solution)	5
Calcium gluconate	1
Cortisone	0
Silica crystals	5
Silica oxidate	3
Whole blood	1
Effect of daily exercise	1

Rating Scale: 0 = control or no growth, 1 = slight growth, 2-4 = moderate growth, 5 = maximum growth or proliferation

Figure 21-7: Dr. George S. Hackett's animal research. Dr. George Hackett showed that Prolotherapy caused ligament and tendon growth, whereas cortisone did not.

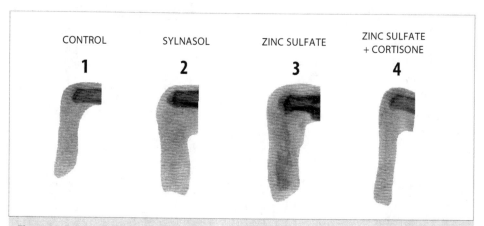

Figure 21-8: X-rays of induced fibro-osseous proliferation. X-rays of the Achilles tendon attachment to the tibio-tarsal bone of a rabbit, one month after one intraligamentous injection of 0.5 cc of fibro-osseous proliferants. **1.** Control. A faint shadow reveals bone extending into the tendons at the fibro-osseous junction where the tendon fibers enter the end of the bone and are firmly attached by ossification. **2.** and **3.** Injections of Sylnasol and zinc sulfate solutions have stimulated the proliferation of new bone as revealed by bone enlargement and increased density, which also extends further within the tendon where ossification of the fibers strengthens the weld of tendon to bone. **4.** Injection of zinc sulfate and cortisone solutions combined (3 to 1) reveal that cortisone inhibited the proliferative action of the zinc sulfate solution.

HACKETT REFERRAL PATTERNS

Besides doing the animal research which showed that fibro-osseous proliferation was possible, Dr. Hackett discovered a technique by which ligament and tendon relaxation could be documented. He describes it this way, "Ligament and tendon relaxation is diagnosed when trigger point tenderness is demonstrated by pressing the **thumb** over the attachment to bone. The diagnosis is invariably confirmed by intraligamentous injection of a local anesthetic solution. The anesthetic produces intense pain, which disappears within two minutes as the anesthetic takes effect. Knowledge of areas in which individual ligaments may produce referred pain is extremely valuable in diagnosis, as attention may be directed to the specific ligaments from which the pain originates. Dermatomes of referred pain have been determined from observations that were made while giving approximately 20,000 intraligamentous injections in diagnosis and treating ligament and tendon relaxation in 1,816 patients over a 20-year period."[5] **(See Figures 21-9, 21-10, 21-11.)**

Knowing the ligament referral patterns helps in determining the pain-producing structure for both the patient and the treating physician. By reproducing the pain during Prolotherapy and/or relieving the pain immediately after Prolotherapy (because of the anesthetic in the solution), the diagnosis is confirmed. This gives the patient and the doctor confidence that the correct structures were treated and a positive outcome will occur.

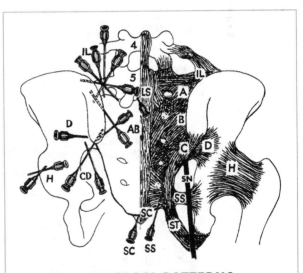

HACKETT REFERRAL PATTERNS
LOWER BACK AND HIP TRIGGER POINTS OF LIGAMENTS

IL:	Iliolumbar
LS:	Lumbosacral - Supra and Interspinus
A, B, C, D:	Posterior Sacroiliac
SS:	Sacrospinous
ST:	Sacrotuberus
SC:	Sacrococcygeal
H:	Hip - Articular
SN:	Sciatic Nerve

Figure 21-9: Ligamentous structures of the lower back and hip that refer pain down the lower leg. The illustration shows the trigger points of pain and the needles in position for confirmation of the diagnosis and for treatment of ligament relaxation of the lumbosacral and pelvic joints.

THE EARLY RESULTS

In regards to a medical therapeutic intervention, perhaps the most important factor is the benefit to side effect ratio. Is there

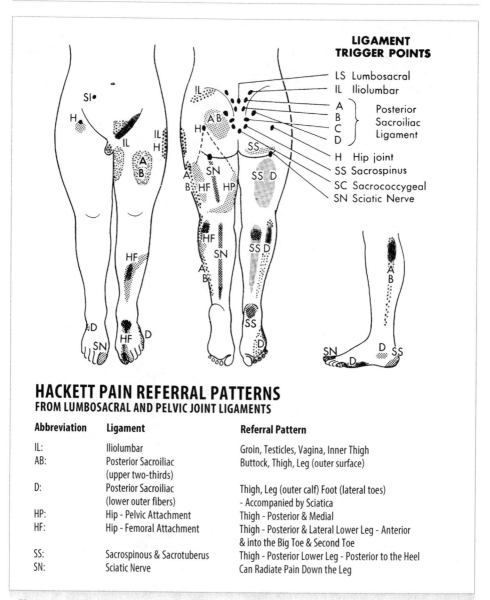

LIGAMENT TRIGGER POINTS

- LS Lumbosacral
- IL Iliolumbar
- A B C D } Posterior Sacroiliac Ligament
- H Hip joint
- SS Sacrospinus
- SC Sacrococcygeal
- SN Sciatic Nerve

HACKETT PAIN REFERRAL PATTERNS
FROM LUMBOSACRAL AND PELVIC JOINT LIGAMENTS

Abbreviation	Ligament	Referral Pattern
IL:	Iliolumbar	Groin, Testicles, Vagina, Inner Thigh
AB:	Posterior Sacroiliac (upper two-thirds)	Buttock, Thigh, Leg (outer surface)
D:	Posterior Sacroiliac (lower outer fibers)	Thigh, Leg (outer calf) Foot (lateral toes) - Accompanied by Sciatica
HP:	Hip - Pelvic Attachment	Thigh - Posterior & Medial
HF:	Hip - Femoral Attachment	Thigh - Posterior & Lateral Lower Leg - Anterior & into the Big Toe & Second Toe
SS:	Sacrospinous & Sacrotuberus	Thigh - Posterior Lower Leg - Posterior to the Heel
SN:	Sciatic Nerve	Can Radiate Pain Down the Leg

Figure 21-10: Ligament referral pain patterns from structures in Figure 22-9.

an excellent chance of benefit with very little risk of harm? It is clear from Dr. Hackett's research that the answer is a resounding yes. In his words, "In approximately 5,000 injections, no unfavourable incident has occurred."[6] "During a 21-year period, 1,857 patients with ligament/tendon disability were treated by Prolotherapy in our clinic and hospital. The technic of diagnosis and treatment was improved and extended from the low back to the occiput and into the extremities in collaboration with our colleagues to include several thousand patients in which a high degree of success continues. **Good to excellent results were reported**

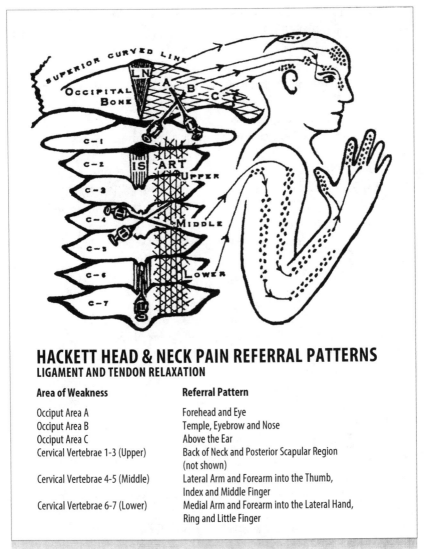

HACKETT HEAD & NECK PAIN REFERRAL PATTERNS
LIGAMENT AND TENDON RELAXATION

Area of Weakness	Referral Pattern
Occiput Area A	Forehead and Eye
Occiput Area B	Temple, Eyebrow and Nose
Occiput Area C	Above the Ear
Cervical Vertebrae 1-3 (Upper)	Back of Neck and Posterior Scapular Region (not shown)
Cervical Vertebrae 4-5 (Middle)	Lateral Arm and Forearm into the Thumb, Index and Middle Finger
Cervical Vertebrae 6-7 (Lower)	Medial Arm and Forearm into the Lateral Hand, Ring and Little Finger

Figure 21-11: Head and neck ligament referral pain patterns.

by 90%—82 consecutive patients with occipito-cervical disability treated by Prolotherapy during the past four years. There were no unfavorable sequelae."[7]

In a study of 206 traumatic headache patients done by Dr. Hackett and colleagues, 79% were completely relieved of their headaches and 89% of the participants in total had some decline in their headaches with the use of Prolotherapy.[8]

In regards to low back pain, Dr. Hackett found that about 90% of the patients had evidence of some type of ligament laxity, typically of the sacroiliac joint.[9,10] In one of his analyses, of the 1,857 patients treated for ligament laxity in the lower back, 1,583 experienced sacroiliac ligament relaxation.[11] In his experience, 82% of people with this condition are cured with Prolotherapy.[12] As he states it, "At the end of 14 years, a survey revealed that 82% of 1,178 patients treated with Prolotherapy considered themselves cured. I believe that I am now curing about 90% of the patients with instability of joints due to ligamentous relaxation to their satisfaction."[10] Guess where that last statement was published? Believe it or not, it was published in the *Journal of the American Medical Association* in 1957. A physician explained that in 82% of chronic low back cases the pain was cured by a simple, safe, office procedure, yet almost nobody in the medical profession paid attention. Nobody except a young Christian physician by the name of Gustav A. Hemwall, MD.

Fortunately for us, Dr. Hackett taught Dr. Hemwall the technique in the mid-1950s. *(See Figure 21-12.)* After Dr. Hackett died in 1969 at the age of 81, it was Dr. Hemwall who, until his death at the age of 90 in 1998, taught the majority of physicians the technique of Prolotherapy. This is why the technique of Prolotherapy utilized at Caring Medical is called the "Hackett-Hemwall Technique of Prolotherapy."

THE 1ST PROLOTHERAPY PIONEER

Those suffering from chronic pain owe George S. Hackett, MD, a great debt, as do all practitioners of Prolotherapy. His contribution to the field of pain management and Prolotherapy are monumental. Included in his achievements and discoveries are the following:

* Coined the term Prolotherapy.
* Showed through microscopic examination that Prolotherapy caused tendon growth.
* Documented histologically and via x-ray that Prolotherapy induced fibro-osseous proliferation.
* Quantified the amounts of tendon and fibro-osseous growth with various solutions.
* Proved cortisone inhibited fibro-osseous proliferation.
* Showed the safety through microscopic examination of the various proliferating solutions that he used.
* Discovered the referral pain patterns of the ligaments of the neck and lower back.
* Published his research in peer-reviewed journals.
* Presented his research at American Medical Association conventions.
* Documented the response of his patients over many years.
* Wrote a book on Prolotherapy and printed three editions.
* Taught the technique of Prolotherapy to other physicians.
* Presented Prolotherapy at various medical meetings across the country.
* Helped start The Prolotherapy Association.
* Over many decades, followed his patients to prove that Prolotherapy does indeed cure chronic pain.

TELEPHONE (708) 848-7773

G. A. HEMWALL, M.D.
715 LAKE STREET
OAK PARK, ILL. 60302

TO WHOM IT MAY CONCERN:

In 1955, I attended the annual AMA meeting in Atlantic City and in the Scientific Exhibits, Dr. George Hackett had an exhibit on Prolotherapy. I purchased his book and started to use the procedure with great success. In December, 1955 at the mid-year meeting of the AMA, I met Dr. Hackett again and he invited me to come and study with him in Canton, Ohio, which I did. We became friends, and I travelled with him to help in his exhibits. Later, with a few other doctors, we founded the Prolotherapy Association to further the teaching of the procedure.

Since that time, I have treated about 8000 patients in the U.S.A. and around the world with a 90% rate of cure or marked improvement of cases of head, neck, shoulder, low back, temporo-mandibular and joint pain of the extremities. Teaching seminars are held in various parts of the country each year.

G.A.Hemwall, M.D.
Associate Professor
Rush University
College of Medicine

Figure 21-12: Letter from Dr. Hemwall describing his training and long-term results.

The story of George S. Hackett, MD, has not been made into a Hollywood movie, because his technique of fibro-osseous proliferation is, in large part, ignored. One does wonder what the world would be like without headaches, back aches, or chronic pain. For that matter, what would your life be like without suffering from daily chronic pain? The powers that be may not shout out his name, but for the person who has seen Prolotherapy work or felt its benefits, to you, Dr. George S. Hackett, we say a most heart-felt "thank you."

GUSTAV A HEMWALL, MD:
PROLOTHERAPY PIONEER AND EVANGELIST

"Nothing was worse than a chronic low back pain patient walking into my office," said Gustav A. Hemwall, MD, the world's most experienced Prolotherapist. "I would try exercise, corsets, and surgery, but nothing really helped."

In 1955, when Dr. Hemwall visited a scientific exhibit at the national meeting of the American Medical Association, that all changed. Recalling the meeting, Dr. Hemwall said, "At one particular exhibit I noticed a crowd of doctors listening to a doctor say he had a cure for low back pain. This fellow had written a book on it as well." That fellow was George S. Hackett, MD, the father of Prolotherapy.

Once the crowd diminished, Dr. Hemwall asked Dr. Hackett how he could learn the treatment described in his book. Dr. Hackett responded by inviting Dr. Hemwall to observe him administering Prolotherapy. Dr. Hemwall became so proficient at administering the technique that Dr. Hackett would later refer patients to him.

Dr. Hemwall remembers, "When I returned from that meeting, I quickly read Dr. Hackett's book describing Prolotherapy and treated my first patient. After a few sessions of Prolotherapy, this patient, instead of coming into the office in a wheelchair, ran to catch four buses. From that point on, instead of dreading patients with low back pain, I began to look for them." That was 40 years before his death. Some 10,000 patients have received Prolotherapy from Dr. Hemwall since that first encounter with Dr. Hackett.

THE DECLINE OF PROLOTHERAPY DUE TO POOR TECHNIQUE

Chronic low back pain management took a drastic turn from when the American Medical Association presented Dr. Hackett's Prolotherapy work at their national meetings in 1955. Unfortunately, for the millions of Americans suffering from chronic back and body pain, several events led to the decline in the use of Prolotherapy in the late 1950s.

On August 8, 1959, the *Journal of the American Medical Association* reported a fatality after a Prolotherapy injection series. In the case report, Richard Schneider, MD, wrote, "...in the instance reported here, it must be emphasized that the sclerosing solution [Prolotherapy solution] was not the usual sodium salt of fatty acids and vegetable oil as described in the original monograph [by Dr. Hackett], but instead a solution of zinc sulfate in 2.5% phenol."[13]

This physician also apparently injected this solution into the spinal canal, not at the fibro-osseous junction where ligaments and tendons attach to bone. Dr. Schneider ended the case report with, "...this technique of precipitating fibro-osseous proliferation appears to be neither sound nor without extreme danger." It should be noted that the article was written by several physicians from the neurosurgery department at the University of Michigan Hospital.

This tragic case occurred because the physician used too strong a proliferant solution and did not follow a cardinal rule of Prolotherapy: Prolotherapy injections are given only when the needle is touching the bone at the fibro-osseous junction, with the only exception being joint injections. Unfortunately, early Prolotherapy physicians did not follow Dr. Hackett's technique. The flawed method these physicians utilized caused some harmful effects and discouraged other physicians from administering Prolotherapy. When properly administered, and the body possesses the ability to heal, Prolotherapy has few side effects and is effective in eliminating chronic pain. Since that time, pioneers such as Dr. Hemwall kept the Prolotherapy crusade going, successfully treating many patients, teaching the technique to other physicians, and continuing to promote Prolotherapy's effectiveness.

Today, Prolotherapy, although not as well known as we would hope, is definitely in the conversation as a treatment modality for pain and injury.

THE INSPIRATION FOR THIS BOOK

Dr. Hemwall had been the main proponent and teacher of Prolotherapy in the United States throughout the 1980s and 1990s. He was responsible for training more physicians and treating more people with Prolotherapy than anyone else. Without his perseverance, the Hackett technique of Prolotherapy may have vanished. We have been blessed to have worked under Dr. Hemwall as students, with him as partners, and beside him as colleagues. In this book, we hope to provide a glimpse of the man he was and the technique he so heartily supported. It has changed the way modern

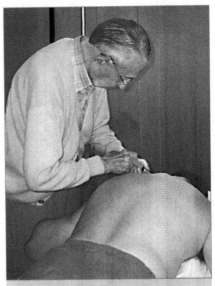

Figure 21-13: Dr. Hemwall doing what he did best—injecting and teaching Prolotherapy.
(Taken at Prolotherapy Course, Beulah Land Natural Medicine Clinic, 1998)

medicine treats pain patients. We have new and exciting techniques in the field of Prolotherapy or what others call regenerative injection therapy, much in part due to the work of Dr. Hemwall. *(See Figure 21-13.)*

DEVELOPMENT OF DIFFERENT PROLOTHERAPY SOLUTIONS

In his 19 years of using Sylnasol, a sodium salt of vegetable oil fatty acids, Dr. Hackett observed no side effects. Dr. Hemwall noted that a number of years after Dr. Hackett's original work was published, Sylnasol was taken off the market due to a lack of demand. After several years of using various solutions, Dr. Hemwall found that a simple dextrose and lidocaine solution was the ideal proliferant. It produced only a small amount of pain following the procedure, yet resulted in complete pain relief after only a few treatments. More dextrose solution could also be injected at one time than with the Sylnasol, allowing more areas of the body to be treated per visit.

Only recently has modern medicine figured out what Dr. Hemwall knew many years ago: that a simple dextrose solution is all that is needed to eliminate pain. Min-Young Kim, MD, and associates from Yonsei University Medical College in Seoul, South Korea, studied 64 patients with chronic pain. Dr. Kim compared using a 5% dextrose solution with the current standard trigger point injection solution of 0.5% lidocaine and placebo. The study found that not only did the dextrose solution prove to give statistically significant pain relief (P<.01) against placebo, it was that much better when compared to the lidocaine solution. The study also found that in follow-up, the pain relief with the dextrose solution remained.[14,15]

The basic Prolotherapy solution used for over 50 years includes hypertonic dextrose (10-25% concentration) along with an anesthetic. In our office, we often include other natural substances, such as Sarapin. The dextrose makes the solution more concentrated than blood (hypertonic), acting as a strong proliferant. Sarapin is used to treat nerve irritation and, in our experience, acts as a proliferant. Sarapin is an extract of the pitcher plant and is one of the few materials listed in the *Physicians' Desk Reference* that has no known side effects. Procaine is an anesthetic that helps reinforce the diagnosis because the patient will experience immediate pain relief after the Prolotherapy injections.

The current Prolotherapy technique described in this book, using these solutions, has been administered by Dr. Hemwall and our clinic to thousands of patients, administering millions of injections over the years. Not one case of permanent nerve injury, paralysis, or death has been documented. All medical treatments have potential benefits and potential risks. Prolotherapy risks may include

- Bleeding in the area
- Bruising in the area
- Increased pain
- Infection
- Joint effusion
- Nerve injury
- Puncture of a lung
- Spinal headache
- Stiffness
- Swelling
- Tendon/ligament injury

Since some of the risks with Prolotherapy relate to the actual technique performed, it is important to go to a clinic with a lot of experience. Surely a doctor can stick a needle into a nerve, ligament, or tendon and cause injury. A doctor can stick the needle into the lung when performing Prolotherapy to the thoracic vertebrae or ribs. A doctor could also stick the needle into the spinal canal when injecting any area of the spine and cause a cerebrospinal fluid leak. This is known as a spinal headache (which is a headache when you sit up). The risks of these side effects are rare, but do occur.

Even in the case of a punctured lung or a tickled nerve, it does not mean the technique of Prolotherapy was performed poorly. Everyone's anatomy is different. Technically, if a lung rides high (above first rib) or if a nerve is located in an unusual spot, these structures can be hit even though the Prolotherapy technique was good. Far and away, the benefits of relieving chronic pain and eliminating the need for medications and treatments that come with their own risks far outweigh the potential risks of Prolotherapy. The dextrose solution is safe, as it is the natural sugar d-glucose that is contained in, and nourishes, all cells of the body. It is the substance that is released when cells burst open after a trauma in order to attract the immune system to the area. Additional agents can be added to the basic solution, and include fatty acids, preservative-free zinc sulfate, manganese, pumice, or a dextrose-glycerine-phenol solution known as P2G. We are sometimes asked if dextrose Prolotherapy is still appropriate for special cases, such as if a patient also has diabetes or is pregnant. In diabetics, the blood sugar goes up about the same amount as after eating a normal lunch. So, Prolotherapy is safe even in diabetics. Pregnant and nursing mothers can also receive d-glucose. Of course, every patient's case must be individually reviewed and the proper solutions decided upon based on all aspects of his or her current health status.*

PROLOZONE™

Prolozone is a Prolotherapy technique developed by Frank Shallenberger, MD, that utilizes ozone gas, along with other therapeutic substances to stimulate healing and reduce pain in injured soft tissues and joints.[16] Dr. Shallenberger describes it as a regenerative and pain-relieving procedure that involves the proliferative principles of Prolotherapy, the cell membrane repolarizing principles of neural therapy, the stem cell stimulation of homeopathic therapy, and the metabolic principles of ozone therapy. The ozone gas is produced when oxygen is exposed to an electric spark via a corona discharge ozone generator. The concentration of ozone in the final gas mixture is between 1-3%.[17] Therapeutic injections of ozone into soft tissue structures, such as muscles, tendons and ligaments as well as arthritic joints for the relief of pain has been utilized for decades in medical clinics around the world.[18,19] Various case series have been published documenting the analgesic effect of ozone in osteoarthritis.[20-23] Double-blind randomized-controlled studies have also documented the therapeutic effects of Prolozone in the treatment of low back pain with and without sciatica.[24,25] As a powerful oxidizing agent, ozone has been found to have a pro-inflammatory as well as an anti-inflammatory effect, depending on the concentration utilized. Its proposed mechanisms for tissue repair and regeneration include the stimulating of growth factor production and release.[26-28]

LYFTOGT PERINEURAL INJECTION TECHNIQUE™

This Prolotherapy technique is also known as Subcutaneous Prolotherapy, Neurofascial, or Neural Prolotherapy. It involves the injection of 5% dextrose into the subcutaneous tissues to induce healing. Research into the healing effects of this type of Prolotherapy originated by a physician from New Zealand named John Lyftogt, MD.[29,30] The injections are given just underneath the skin at the location of sensitized peptidergic nerves. These nerves contain transient receptor potential vanilloid receptors (or capsaicin receptors) and are known as TRPV1 nerves. These nerves are sensitized because of trauma, injury or constriction and represent sites of neurogenic inflammation.[29,31-33] Neurogenic inflammation was first termed "inflammatory neuritis" by Dr. George Hackett in the 1950s.[7,34,35] Peptidergic sensory nerves are important because they maintain the health and renewal of joint structures, such as ligament and tendons. Injections of 5% dextrose at the sites of sensitized nerves can completely eliminate pain from neurogenic inflammation.[30,32] The injections are typically given weekly for 5-10 visits.

---

*Caring Medical Regenerative Medicine Clinics does not use or promote the use of each of these ingredients.

NERVE RELEASE INJECTION THERAPY

Pain can be attributed to the result of joint instability, excessive stretch of a primary ligament, neurogenic inflammation, nerve entrapment, or a combination of these. Most traditional dextrose and neurofascial Prolotherapy solve the problem of the first three. Nerve Release Injection Therapy (NRIT), also known as hydrodissection, addresses nerve entrapment. The treatment involves the injection of natural substances to mechanically release and nourish peripheral nerves. NRIT is done under ultrasound guidance to direct the solutions to the exact nerve entrapment location. Because the entrapment is resolved and the nourishment to the nerve is immediately restored, the symptom-relieving effects are often felt instantly after the procedure. This technique provides patients with the fastest, least invasive method to relieve nerve entrapment. Refer back to **Chapter 16** for more about nerve syndromes and entrapment.

CELLULAR SOLUTIONS - IS THE LATEST THE GREATEST?

As discussed in **Chapter 3**, one of the most significant advancements in the Prolotherapy world has been through the use of a person's own cells as the proliferant. These cells include blood, bone marrow, and fat. With these advanced solutions, we have to still remember the basic principles outlined by Drs. Hackett and Hemwall: the weakened ligaments and tendons are the cause of the pain. What is found on MRI or x-ray is generally the result of that weakness and joint instability. For example, to only inject the resultant meniscal tear with stem cells and not comprehensively treat the instability of the knee joint, is not thinking like a true Prolotherapist. Yes, there are positive outcome cases with some of these more simplistic forms of stem cell therapy. Some doctors focus on doing a single injection with "as many cells" or "the best cells" directed at the tear. However, the patient's joint instability goes unaddressed. This is why Caring Medical uses a combination of traditional Hackett-Hemwall Prolotherapy to address the supporting structures of the joint, as well as delivering cells directly to the tear, cartilage defect, and other areas that are deficient in healing cells.

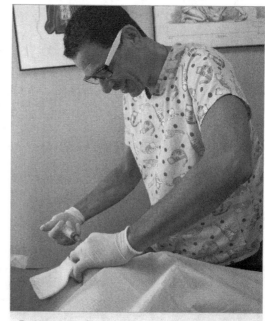

Dr. Hauser performing a lipoaspiration for Stem Cell Prolotherapy.

In most of the cases that we see at Caring Medical, a combination of regular Prolotherapy solutions and techniques can be used without the added cost of Cellular Prolotherapy kits and equipment, potentially saving the patient thousands. When cases call for cellular solutions, they are certainly recommended and used. However, we have treated many patients who spent a lot of money through orthopedic stem cell offices to get "the most cells" injected via a couple injections into the joint, but they did not get the relief they desired. When the Hackett-Hemwall technique is used, we were able to get most of those patients back to their desired activity level. It is great that many doctors are now seeing the power of Regenerative Medicine techniques and accelerating the possibilities of Prolotherapy for more advanced cases than ever before. With this we must remember to address the whole joint, not just inside the joint.

PROLOTHERAPY WITH GUIDANCE

The pioneers of Prolotherapy developed treatment techniques that were based on anatomical landmarks. Therefore, it is imperative that a good Prolotherapist be an expert in anatomy. Over the years, however, there have been advancements in devices like musculoskeletal ultrasound and x-ray that have allowed the average Prolotherapy office to have these technologies in-house. Their ability to visualize joint instability or help detail the extent of a tendon tear can prove helpful in diagnosing a patient. This may indicate to the practitioner what type of Prolotherapy solution would likely be most effective. It can also be used for needle placement, particularly when injecting Cellular Prolotherapy solutions at the exact site of a tear.

MUSCULOSKELETAL ULTRASOUND

Ultrasonography is an imaging modality that uses high frequency sound waves, to generate and record images of tissue boundaries. This allows visualization of structures including tendons, muscles, ligaments, cartilage, bone, and more. Patients love it because it is non-invasive, painless, convenient, and does not use radiation. For the practitioner, it can aid in diagnosing and identifying the extent of injured structures, such as tendon tears and degeneration, abnormal swelling,

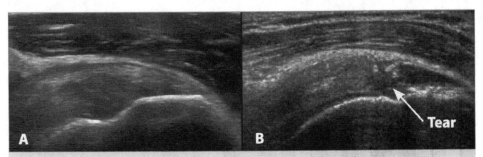

Figure 21-14: Ultrasound showing a normal (a) and a tear (b) in the supraspinatus tendon.

and cysts. Ultrasound is also used to document improvement in soft tissue healing. **(See Figure 21-14.)** When used during Prolotherapy, it can guide the practitioner to place cells and other proliferant solutions into a specific place, such as the exact site of a tear or cartilage defect. Ultrasound is also a key player in the Nerve Release Injection Therapy procedure, when trying to free up an entrapped nerve from the surrounding structures. Though it has many advantages, it is still used to enhance and verify, not replace, the findings from a thorough patient history and physical exam.

DIGITAL MOTION X-RAY (DMX)

In most cases of chronic pain, symptoms occur during movement or when the area is put under stress, and the symptoms remit upon rest. DMX is a motion picture of the bones while a person is moving and therefore, the ideal way to document

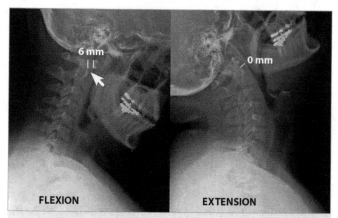

FLEXION   EXTENSION

Figure 21-15: Flexion-Extension views of a patient with C1-C2 (upper) cervical instability. During flexion (compared to extension) the distance between the odontoid (C2) and the posterior surface of C1 moves excessively. (arrow)

joint instability. **(See Figure 21-15.)** The scan is produced in real-time to show specifically what happens when the painful or injured area is put through a series of movements and full range of motion. The camera takes 30 individual x-ray frames per second, and the successive x-rays are digitized and sequenced to create a video representation. DMX produces a **fraction** of the radiation exposure of a regular x-ray, CT scan, or high-dose fluoroscopy, yet, for the average chronic pain patient, it shows a great deal more useful information than traditional still images.

SUMMARY

Regenerative Medicine would not be what it is today without the tireless work of the Prolotherapy pioneers. Throughout this book and every day in our clinic, we continue to honor their legacy. In the decades since Drs. Hackett and Hemwall were practicing medicine, Prolotherapy has seen some wonderful innovations, including the use of guidance and incorporating new ingredients to the tried and true dextrose proliferant. In our clinical experience and research, we find that the Hackett-Hemwall technique, which comprehensively treats the injured area using numerous injections, produces excellent patient results. We discuss these results in the next chapter. ■

CHAPTER

22

PROLOTHERAPY PROVIDES RESULTS

Not a day goes by that we are not asked "So, is there research on Prolotherapy?" This is a loaded question. Firstly, yes, there is a lot of research on Prolotherapy and all of the regenerative injection therapies, which include Platelet Rich Plasma, whole blood injections, bone marrow, etc... Much has been provided in the references throughout this book, and it is only a small sampling of what is available once one starts digging through the world-wide medical literature. Secondly, it often seems that the same people asking us to prove Prolotherapy are the same who never asked their surgeon the risks of cortisone, spinal fusion, and so forth. Treatments and surgeries are performed without discussion of why they where recommended when the long-term sequelae are well-known to cause further degeneration and arthritis. But we digress...

In this chapter, we present a summary of the research done by the Prolotherapy pioneers and our own research papers published since the initial edition of this book, as well as a sample of others who have helped advance the knowledge of Prolotherapy. For those interested in discovering more references on regenerative injection therapies, we invite you to check out the *Journal of Prolotherapy* online, as well as the studies available on PubMed.

PROLOTHERAPY PROVIDES RESULTS: THE RESEARCH

Prolotherapy repairs the painful area by proliferating fibroblasts, which regenerate normal ligament and tendon tissue at the fibro-osseous junction by causing inflammation that stimulates the natural healing process. In other words, **Prolotherapy stimulates your body to repair the painful areas.** There are two interesting studies to review here: one involving Prolotherapy to ligaments and the other on tendons. Both studies were done in the mid 1980s at the University of Iowa, in the department of orthopedics, and both studies show how Prolotherapy works.

RABBITS' KNEES

The first study, by Dr. Y. King Liu, was a double-blind study to assess the influence of a proliferant solution on rabbit medial collateral ligaments (MCL).[1] One rabbit knee was injected five separate times over a six-week period with the proliferant solution sodium morrhuate, an extract of cod liver oil. The other MCL of the knee was injected with saline. The animal was then sacrificed and the ligaments were measured, their strength determined, and the ligaments were examined under the microscope. The results are quite impressive. *(See Figure 22-1.)*

After six weeks, Prolotherapy caused an increase in ligament mass, ligament thickness, and fibro-osseous strength. The authors summarized their findings by stating, "We demonstrated that the strength of the bone-ligament junction (fibro-osseous junction) was **significantly increased** by repeated injections of sodium morrhuate. In addition, **significant increases** in the mass, thickness, and weigh-to-length ratio of injected ligaments were found. Morphological analysis of histological sections collectively showed a statistically significant increase in collagen fibril diameters of the experimental ligament."[1]

In a similar study using sodium morrhuate, J.A. Maynard and associates looked at the results of Prolotherapy in the patellar and Achilles tendons in rabbits. The primary purpose of this investigation was to see if more insight could be gained into the underlying mechanism related to the increased separation force (stronger connective tissue formed) in the Liu study, involving sodium morrhuate injected MCL. This study found that sodium morrhuate alters the morphometric features of tendons by **increasing** the gross circumference of the collagen fibrils. The researchers found that the increase in circumference appears to be due to an increase in cell population, water content, and ground substance. The researchers further clarified it by stating "the increased cell population is a common characteristic of other studies using sodium morrhuate and apparently is due to the formation of granulation tissue in the injected area. Consequently, not only is there an increase in the number of cells, but also a wider **variety** of cell types, fibroblasts, neutrophils, lymphocytes, plasma cells, and unidentifiable cells in the injected tissues. Interestingly, these findings are similar to dense connective tissues undergoing an injury-repair cycle in which the **proliferation** of cells from surrounding areolar tissue followed by granulation tissue

Effects of Five Prolotherapy Treatments

	Prolotherapy injected ligaments	Saline injected ligaments (control)	Percent improvement
Ligament mass (mg)	132.2	89.7	44
Ligament thickness (mm)	1.01	0.79	27
Ligament mass length (mg/mm)	6.45	4.39	47
Junction strength (N)	119.1	93.5	28

Figure 22-1: The effects of five Prolotherapy treatments to the medial collateral ligament. Prolotherapy causes a statistically significant increase in ligament mass and strength as well as bone-ligament junction strength.

has been well documented. This is followed by **fibroblast proliferation, increased vascular supply, and the deposition of new collagen.**"[2] In summary, Prolotherapy stimulates the normal repair process that occurs after a ligament, tendon, or other connective tissue is injured. Studying the tissue under the microscope revealed an increase in the blood circulation, which brings a myriad of immune cells including macrophages, neutrophils, lymphocytes, and fibroblasts. The end result being stronger and thicker connective tissues, such as ligaments and tendons, which are especially stronger at their fibro-osseous junctions.

GEORGE S. HACKETT, MD

Although chronic pain has many causes, the vast majority of chronic pain sufferers have loose joints caused by ligament weakness. This is evidenced by Dr. Hackett's research study described in the third edition of his book, *Ligament and Tendon Relaxation Treated by Prolotherapy*, published in 1958.[3] The study consisted of the following:

• sample size: 656 patients
• patient age range: 15 to 88 years-old
• duration of pain prior to treatment: three months to 65 years
• average duration of pain prior to treatment: four-and-a-half years
• duration of study: 19 years
• number of injections given: 18,000

Twelve years after the Prolotherapy treatment was completed, 82% of the patients considered themselves cured. Dr. Hackett believed that the cure rate with Prolotherapy was over 90% due to improvements in the technique over the years.

In 1955, Dr. Hackett analyzed 146 consecutive cases of undiagnosed low back disability during a two-month period. He found that 94% of the patients experienced joint ligament relaxation. In 1956, a similar survey of 124 consecutive cases of undiagnosed low back disability revealed that 97% of patients possessed joint instability from ligament weakness. The sacroiliac ligaments were involved in 75% of the low back ligament laxity cases. The lumbosacral ligaments were involved in 54%. He also noted that approximately 50% had already undergone back surgery for a previous diagnosis of a disc problem.[4]

At this time, Prolotherapy produced an 80% cure rate even though 50% of the people treated had undergone back surgery. Obviously, the surgical procedures did not relieve the patients' back pain. Rarely does a disc problem cause disabling back pain. Chronic pain in the lower back is most commonly due to ligament weakness—the reason Prolotherapy is so effective.

Dr. Hackett attributed ineffective response to Prolotherapy to the following:

- Inability to clearly confirm the diagnosis by the injection of a local anesthetic solution.
- Failure of the patient to return for completion of the treatment.
- Treatment in the presence of another disability.
- A less refined technique and less experience in the earlier studies.
- Lowered morale from years of suffering and disappointment from unsuccessful treatments and dependence on prescription pain medications.
- Non-responsiveness to the stimulation of proliferation.

Prolotherapy works because it causes ligament and tendon growth. Dr. Hackett used Sylnasol, a sodium salt fatty acid, as a proliferant in his original work. Animals were given between one and three injections of the proliferating solution into the tendon and the fibro-osseous junction. There was no necrosis (dead tissue) noted in any of the specimens. No destruction of nerves, blood vessels, or tendinous bands was noted. Compared to non-injected tendons, tendons treated with Prolotherapy showed a 40% increase in diameter. The fibro-osseous junction, where the tendon attaches to bone, increased by 30%, forming permanent tendon tissue. Dr. Hackett believed the 40% increase in diameter of the tendon represented a doubling of the tendon strength.[5]

GUSTAV A. HEMWALL, MD

Gustav A. Hemwall, MD, learned the technique of Prolotherapy from Dr. Hackett and then proceeded to treat more than 10,000 patients worldwide. He collected data on 8,000 of those patients. In 1974, Dr. Hemwall presented his largest survey of 2,007 Prolotherapy patients to The Prolotherapy Association. The survey related the following:

- 1,871 patients completed treatment
- 6,000 Prolotherapy treatments were administered
- 1,399 patients (75.5%) reported complete recovery and cure
- 413 patients (24.3%) reported general improvement
- 25 patients (0.2%) showed no improvement
- 170 patients were lost to follow-up

More than 99% of the patients who completed treatment with Prolotherapy found relief from their chronic pain. These results are similar to those published by Dr. Hackett, showing that Prolotherapy is completely curative in many cases and provides some pain relief in nearly all.[6]

ROBERT KLEIN, MD

In human studies, Robert Klein, MD, and associates, administered a series of six weekly injections in the lower back ligamentous supporting structures with a proliferant solution containing dextrose, glycerin, and phenol. Biopsies performed three months after completion of injections showed statistically significant increases in collagen fiber and ligament diameter of 60%. Statistically significant improvements in pain relief and back motion were also observed.[7]

THOMAS DORMAN, MD

In a 1989 study, Thomas Dorman, MD, noted, "I biopsied individuals before and after treatment with Prolotherapy and submitted the biopsy specimens to pathologists. Using modern analytic techniques, they showed that Prolotherapy caused regrowth of tissue, an increased number of fibroblast nuclei (the major cell type in ligaments and other connective tissue), an increased amount of collagen, and an absence of inflammatory changes or other types of tissue damage."[8]

Dr. Dorman performed a retrospective survey of 80 patients treated with Prolotherapy for cervical, thoracic, and lumbar spine pain, or a combination of these. Of these patients, 31% were involved in litigation or workers' compensation cases. The patients were evaluated up to five years after their Prolotherapy treatment. Analysis of the 80 patients showed a statistical significance of $P<.001$ for improvements in severity of pain, daily living activities, and influence of sleep pattern. Prolotherapy was shown to eliminate pain, improve activity level, and help the patients get a good night's sleep.[9]

MILNE ONGLEY, MD

Using the same solution as Dr. Klein, Milne Ongley, MD, and associates, demonstrated a stabilization of the collateral and cruciate ligaments of the knee joint with Prolotherapy. All subjects treated showed an increase in activity and reduction in pain.[10] Two double-blind studies where patients received either an injected proliferant solution or a solution without proliferant concluded that Prolotherapy was effective in eliminating pain.[11,12]

A problem with controlled studies using Prolotherapy injections is that the control group still receives an injection, though without any proliferant. An injection into a tender area is a treatment utilized in pain management. The result is that the control group actually receives a therapeutic intervention. Despite these concerns, Prolotherapy in the above two studies was shown to be an effective treatment for chronic low back pain.

K. DEAN REEVES, MD

For many years, K. Dean Reeves, MD, has been at the forefront of Prolotherapy research. Dr. Reeves has helped Prolotherapy penetrate allopathic medicine by writing whole chapters on Prolotherapy that were published in mainstream medical journals and books including *Physical Medicine and Rehabilitation Clinics of North America*, *Physiatric Procedures*, and *Pain Procedures in Clinical Practice*.[13-15]

He was the primary researcher performing two randomized, prospective, placebo-controlled, double-blind clinical trials of dextrose Prolotherapy injections on osteoarthritic joints.[16,17] The first was on 77 patients (111 knees) who had radiographically confirmed evidence of symptomatic knee osteoarthritis.[16] These patients had an average weight of 193 pounds and pain for more than 10 years in the qualifying knees. This study included 38 knees with **no cartilage** remaining in at least one compartment.

Dr. Reeves was also the primary researcher performing randomized, prospective, placebo-controlled, double-blind clinical trials of dextrose Prolotherapy injections on osteoarthritic fingers and knee joints.[18,19] Other notable studies headed up by Dr. Reeves including the use of dextrose Prolotherapy for ACL and fibromyalgia.[20,21] Dr. Reeves has also teamed up with Prolotherapy physician, researcher, and educator from Argentina, Gaston A. Topol, MD, to produce some excellent studies on Prolotherapy for conditions including Osgood-Schlatter disease, knee osteoarthritis, and groin pain.[22-25] Anyone interested in delving further into the Prolotherapy research should review Dr. Reeves' wonderful contributions in the field.

DAVID RABAGO, MD

One of the most respected Prolotherapy research contributors currently is Dr. Rabago, Board-Certified family physician and Assistant Professor at the University of Wisconsin-Madison. He has contributed numerous articles on Prolotherapy for chronic pain, many of which can be found on PubMed. One of his most notable studies is a randomized control trial on utilizing dextrose Prolotherapy for knee osteoarthritis. Ninety patients were studied who had at least three months of knee pain due to osteoarthritis. The participants were randomized to blinded injections of either dextrose Prolotherapy or saline, or at-home exercise instruction. Injections were done at 1, 5, and 9 weeks with as-needed additional treatments at 13 and 17 weeks. All groups reported improvement composite WOMAC scores (Western Ontario McMaster University Osteoarthritis Index) compared to baseline status at 52 weeks. Adjusted for sex, age, and body mass index, WOMAC scores for patients receiving dextrose Prolotherapy improved more ($P < .05$) at 52 weeks than did scores for patients receiving saline and exercise (score change: 15.3 ± 3.5 vs 7.6 ± 3.4, and 8.2 ± 3.3 points, respectively), and exceeded the WOMAC-based minimal clinically important difference. Patient satisfaction with Prolotherapy was high. The study resulted in clinically meaningful sustained improvement of pain, function, and stiffness scores for knee osteoarthritis compared with blinded saline injections and at-home exercises.[26]

ROSS HAUSER, MD

Our team has been dedicated to furthering the research on Prolotherapy for a variety of painful conditions and body areas. The following is a short sampling of our research, study results, and notable published articles. We invite you to read the articles in full, as well as see new research as it gets released, by visiting CaringMedical.com/prolotherapy-research/.

USE OF PROLOTHERAPY FOR INDIVIDUAL JOINTS

For 10 years, we ran a quarterly charity clinic in southern Illinois, which concentrated on providing Prolotherapy services for the underserved population. To our team, this represented the worst case scenario for Prolotherapy efficacy results for a number of reasons:

1. Patients were seen an average of three months apart instead of at the normal 4-6 week interval.
2. There were no additional solution ingredients available other than the basic dextrose solution, such as what would be available in a private practice armamentarium.
3. There was no use of Cellular Prolotherapy which would have been a preferred treatment for the more advanced cases.
4. Patients were not advised on diet, exercise habits, or other lifestyle factors, as would happen in our private practice.
5. The majority of patients who attended the clinic sessions had very few resources or options for treating their pain, or had exhausted other avenues.

Thus, the patients who were contacted after the clinic ended acted as their own control, so to speak, because they had degenerative conditions which were either non-responsive to previous treatments, or they could not obtain additional care for various reasons.

Our team performed retrospective analysis on a total of 709 cases covering 11 body areas: ankle[27], back[28], elbow[29], foot and toe[30], hand and finger[31], hip[32], knee[33], neck[34], shoulder[35], temporomandibular joint[36], and wrist.[37] Of the 11 studies, the average pain level prior to Prolotherapy was 6.3 with an average pain level after Prolotherapy of 2.2, on a scale of 1-10. Eighty-nine percent of patients reported greater than 50% pain relief. *(See Figure 22-2.)*

GLENOID LABRUM AND ACETABULAR LABRUM LESION STUDIES

The first scientific papers detailing the use of Prolotherapy for lesions of both the glenoid labrum and the acetabular labrum, were published in the *Open*

Pain Levels Before and After Prolotherapy

Area treated	Average pain level prior to Prolotherapy	Average pain level after Prolotherapy	Percent of patients who reported > 50% pain relief
Ankle	7.9	1.6	90%
Back	5.6	2.7	89%
Elbow	5.1	1.6	94%
Foot	7.1	2.3	84%
Hand	5.9	2.6	82%
Hip	7.0	2.4	89%
Knee	6.5	2.5	88%
Neck	5.6	2.3	89%
Shoulder	7.1	2.3	87%
TMJ	5.9	2.5	93%
Wrist	5.5	1.4	90%
Overall average	6.3	2.2	89%

Figure 22-2: Use of Prolotherapy for pain in individual joints.
Prolotherapy caused a statistically significant decline in pain.

Rehabilitation Journal.[38,39] In the glenoid labrum study, 33 patients with labral tears were treated in our clinic with intra-articular injections of hypertonic dextrose. Patient-reported assessments were collected by questionnaire at a mean follow-up time of 16 months. Treated patients reported highly significant improvements with respect to pain, stiffness, range of motion, crunching, exercise and need for medication. All 31 patients who reported pain at baseline experienced pain relief, and all 31 who reported exercise impairment at baseline reported improved exercise capability. Patients reported complete relief of 69% of recorded symptoms. One patient reported worsening of some symptoms.

In the acetabular labrum study, 19 patients with labral tears were treated in our clinic with intra-articular injections of hypertonic dextrose. Patient-reported assessments were collected by questionnaire between 1 and 60 months post-treatment (mean = 12 months). All patients reported improvements in pain relief and functionality. Patients reported complete relief of 54% of recorded symptoms. Improvements did not show dependence on the time between treatment and follow-up. No adverse events were reported.

KNEE STUDIES: CHONDROMALACIA PATELLA AND MENISCAL PATHOLOGY

Two of our highlighted knee studies focused on chondromalacia patella, and the other on meniscal pathology.[40,41] We retrospectively evaluated the effectiveness of Prolotherapy in resolving pain, stiffness, and crepitus, and improving physical activity in 69 knees in 61 patients' chondromalacia. At least 6 weeks after their last Prolotherapy session (average length of time from last Prolotherapy session was 14.7 months), patients provided self-evaluation of knee pain upon rest, activities of daily living (ADL) and exercise. Symptom severity, sustained improvement of symptoms, number of pain pills needed, and patient satisfaction before treatment and improvement after treatment were recorded. Following Prolotherapy, patients experienced statistically significant decreases in pain at rest, during ADL, and exercise. For daily pain level, ROM, daily stiffness, crepitus, and walking and exercise ability, sustained improvement of over 75% was reported by 85% of patients. Fewer patients required pain medication. Only 3 of 16 knees were still recommended for surgery after Prolotherapy.

Another retrospective study was done involving 24 patients, representing 28 knees, whose primary knee complaints were due to meniscal pathology documented by MRI. The average number of Prolotherapy treatments received was six and the patients were interviewed on average 18 months after their last Prolotherapy visit. Prolotherapy caused a statistically significant decline in the patients' knee pain and stiffness. Starting and ending knee pain declined from 7.2 to 1.6, while stiffness went from 6.0 to 1.8. Prolotherapy caused large improvements in other clinically relevant areas such as range of motion, crepitation, exercise, and walking ability. Patients stated that the response to Prolotherapy met their expectations in 27 out of the 28 knees (96%). Only 1 out of the 28 patients ended up getting surgery after Prolotherapy.

REGENERATION OF ARTICULAR CARTILAGE WITH PROLOTHERAPY

Most patients who come to our office worried about their x-ray or MRI before Prolotherapy eventually realize that it does not always matter what is found on imaging, so long as the joint has good motion, is able to function, and does not hurt. Then after experiencing Prolotherapy, and starting to feel better, who has the time for repeat imaging? But because we are asked frequently about this, we published two interesting articles that address the regeneration of articular cartilage with Prolotherapy—a scientific editorial on the cellular science as well as patient case studies with before and after x-rays.[42,43]

JOINT INSTABILITY

An ongoing part of our research and clinical experience reveals that most patients with chronic pain have underlying joint instability. It is a missing, but critical, diagnosis that leads to all of the problems covered in this book and in our other research articles. These articles examine ligaments as the primary stabilizers of joints, and what happens to them upon injury. Additionally, what happens during the subsequent healing phases and how Prolotherapy is an effective modality for correcting joint instability.[44-46]

CERVICAL INSTABILITY

As discussed in the earlier chapters, an especially debilitating condition is cervical spine instability, and particularly upper-cervical spine instability. Prolotherapy has proven to have excellent results in eliminating the clusters of symptoms, including headaches, vertigo, facial pain, and a host of other symptoms caused by cervical spine instability, also known as Barré-Lieou or cervicocranial syndrome. To date, we have published four scientific articles on Prolotherapy for cervical instability.[47-50]

ADDITIONAL STUDIES BY HAUSER ET AL. ON PROLOTHERAPY
AND REGENERATIVE INJECTION TREATMENTS:

- Arcuate ligament of the knee[51]
- Avascular necrosis of the talus[52]
- Barré-Lieou syndrome/cervicocranial syndrome[49]
- Basal thumb osteoarthritis[53]
- Bone Marrow Prolotherapy research and case studies[54-56]
- Bunion/first metatarsophalengeal pain[57]
- Chronic pain and degeneration in an incomplete C4-C5 spinal cord injury[58]
- Chronic regional pain syndrome/reflex sympathetic dystrophy[59]
- Headache and migraine[60]
- Joint hypermobility syndrome/Ehlers-Danlos syndrome[61]
- Ligament injury and healing[44-46]
- Morton's neuroma[62]
- Non-operative treatment of cervical radiculopathy[63]
- Osteoarthritis[64]
- Osteochondritis dissecans[65]
- Over-manipulation syndrome[66]
- Platelet Rich Plasma Prolotherapy for meniscal pathology[67]
- Prolotherapy as an alternative to surgery[68]
- Scientific literature review and systematic review of dextrose Prolotherapy[69,70]

THE CASE FOR PROLOTHERAPY

Over the years, a number of prominent Prolotherapy practitioners have dedicated tremendous time and resources proving via published research that Prolotherapy is a superior treatment for musculoskeletal pain.

In the December 2011 issue of the *Journal of Prolotherapy*, our team, along with others in the field, made *The Case for Prolotherapy*. One of the key articles was titled, "Journal of Prolotherapy International Medical Editorial Board Consensus Statement on the Use of Prolotherapy for Musculoskeletal Pain."[71] The goal was to prove, once and for all, that Prolotherapy is a successful and safe treatment for a wide variety of chronic pain conditions. Though individual study designs and treatment techniques vary, the data is overwhelmingly positive. Following are the studies amassed for that article.

CONDITIONS SUCCESSFULLY TREATED BY PROLOTHERAPY:

Degenerative Arthritis

Prolotherapy is indicated for the following degenerative arthritis (osteoarthritis or osteoarthrosis) conditions:

- Degenerative joint disease involving all peripheral joints including the knees, hips and fingers[21,27-37,41,72,73,177]
- Degenerative spinal disease including spondylosis, spondylolisthesis and degenerative disc disease[74-79,178]
- Osteochondral defects[80-85]

Joint Instability

Prolotherapy is indicated for these ligamentous injuries and other conditions that can cause joint instability and pain:

- Ligament tears and injury[73,86-89]
- Labral tears and degeneration[39]
- Meniscus tears and degeneration[41,67]
- Congenital conditions such as joint hypermobility syndrome and Ehlers-Danlos syndrome[61]

Tendinopathy

Prolotherapy is indicated for the following conditions involving tendons, and the entheses:

- Tendinopathy[90-96]
- Tendinosis[97-100]
- Tendinitis[101-105]
- Grade one and two tears (partial tears)[106,107]
- Enthesopathies including osteitis pubis and medial tibial stress syndrome[108-110]
- Muscle origin pain and tears[23,93,107]

Prolotherapy in rare situations can be used for complete tendon tears such as when a patient is not a surgical candidate or has strong desires/reasons not to get surgery. Two case reports show repair of a complete tear/rupture, an Achilles tendon and anterior cruciate ligament tear.[111,112]

OTHER MUSCULOSKELETAL CONDITIONS

Prolotherapy can be successfully used, along with other therapies for the following musculoskeletal conditions:
- Post-surgical pain syndrome[113,114]
- Myofascial pain syndrome[115-118]

- Fibromyalgia[20]
- Complex regional pain syndrome[59]
- Chronic headaches[36,60,119,120]
- Radiculopathy[121,122]
- Autonomic symptoms, including Barré-Lieou syndrome[120,123-125]
- Apophyseal growth plate injuries, including Osgood- Schlatter disease[25,126]
- Other[74,95,127-134]

PROLOTHERAPY AS AN ALTERNATIVE TREATMENT

Prolotherapy is a viable alternative to pain medications including NSAIDs, physiotherapy, and/or cortisone (steroid) injection for the following conditions:

- Tendinitis or bursitis[92,96,118]
- Epicondylitis (epicondylosis)[99,102,135]
- Plantar fasciitis (fasciosis)[90,96,981,136]
- Tendinopathy (tendinosis or other enthesopathy)[137-142]
- Ligament injury (tear or laxity)[21,73,87,116,143,144]
- Degenerative arthritis (degenerative joint and spinal disease)[15,75,76,79,133,145]
- Neuritis[91,123,146,147]
- Temporomandibular joint syndrome[36,148-150]
- Myofascial pain syndrome[95,96,117,139,146,151,152]
- Fracture pain[131,134]

Prolotherapy can be used as alternative to surgery for the following conditions:

- Degenerative arthritis (degenerative joint disease)[32,33,39,41,72,81,82,145]
- Degenerative spinal arthritis (spondylosis and degenerative disc disease)[133,153-157]
- Tendon or ligament tear[106,107,158,159]

PROLOTHERAPY TO ENHANCE SURGICAL OUTCOMES

Prolotherapy can be used to potentially enhance outcomes in the following surgical procedures:

- Tendon repairs[106,158,160-162]

- Fusion[163,164]
- Ligament repairs[155,165,166]
- Bone fractures and other lesions[65,167-170]
- Osteochondral defects[168,171-176]

SUMMARY

We love to see the resulting positive strides in the evolution of pain management. Through the research, as well as our own clinical experience doing Prolotherapy since 1993, we believe that regenerative injection therapy, including Prolotherapy and orthobiologics treatments, should become the first-line treatment in the vast array of conditions discussed in this book. With every new research paper published, it is our hope that it reaches those people suffering with sports injuries, arthritis, and other chronic pain and they will find renewed hope that there is a regenerative treatment that can help them. That treatment is, of course, Prolotherapy! ∎

CHAPTER

23

ANSWERS TO COMMON QUESTIONS ABOUT PROLOTHERAPY

We hope that you have found the information presented on Prolotherapy as a viable first-line treatment helpful thus far. No matter what medical procedure, Prolotherapy or otherwise, you should have all of your questions answered. In this chapter, we summarize some of the top questions about Prolotherapy that we are asked every day. If you have more questions that are not covered in this book, remember that we would love to hear from you. Email us at DrHauser@caringmedical.com.

1. DO PROLOTHERAPY INJECTIONS HURT?

As the saying goes with bodybuilders, it also goes with Prolotherapy, "No pain, no gain." Shots are shots. "Do they hurt?" every new patient asks. All doctors were taught the appropriate answer to this question in medical school: "It hurts a little." Some people have many Prolotherapy injections and do not flinch, while others receive a few shots and have a rough time.

Being hesitant about receiving injections should not be a reason to shy away from Prolotherapy because there are a lot of options for assisting with the pain of the procedure. At Caring Medical, we apply a lidocaine cream on the skin prior to treatment, which is all that most people need. You may be surprised at how well most people handle the procedure with just the lidocaine cream, some deep breathing, or essential oils. When more assistance is needed to help a person through the treatment, we can inject extra anesthetic around the area prior to the actual Prolotherapy injections, as well as prescribe oral medication for pain or anxiety, or use nitrous oxide, similar to what is used in dental practices.

For those requiring injections in many areas at one time or in delicate areas, intravenous conscious sedation may be used. The sedation does make a person "woozy" but some people prefer it because it eliminates the pain of the procedure. Nearly all of our patients receive Prolotherapy without any sedation and do quite well.

2. HOW SAFE IS PROLOTHERAPY?

Prolotherapy is a very safe procedure when performed by a practitioner who has been properly trained in the anatomical targets, and who uses ingredients with a high safety record, and who emphasizes safe practices for medical injections, and makes the solutions fresh each day.

In his study published in 1961, Abraham Myers, MD, states that in treating 267 patients with low back pain, with and without sciatica, from May 1956 to October 1960, "Over 4,500 [Prolotherapy] injections have been given without the occurrence of any complication."[1]

It would be nice to believe that Prolotherapy is 100% safe like Dr. Myers' report indicated, but like all invasive procedures in the body, Prolotherapy has risks. The major risk with Prolotherapy is infection. Prolotherapy involves a lot of injections. Just like in surgery, no matter how much you clean the skin, infection can result. This includes skin, blood and joint infections. This risk is rare but real. Other risks include increased pain, bleeding, bruising, swelling, nerve/tendon/ligament injury, puncture of the lung (for thoracic/rib injections), and spinal headache (spine injections).

While on the subject of safety, one must also consider the safety of living with chronic pain. This may be a new concept to some, but living with pain is not wise. Pain not only decreases one's enjoyment of life, it creates stress in the body. Stress is the worst detriment to good health. A body under stress triggers the "fight or flight" response, which means the adrenal gland begins excreting hormones such as cortisol and adrenaline. The same thing occurs when a gun is pointed at you during a robbery, but for a shorter period of time.

The adrenal gland, also known as the stress gland, secretes cortisol to increase the amount of white blood cells that are activated, as in cases of allergic or infectious stress. It puts the body "on alert." The adrenal gland is one of the reasons a person wakes up in the morning. Chronic pain causes the adrenal gland to be in a continual "alert mode," secreting cortisol as would occur with an infection or when a person is being robbed. As the chronic pain lingers, cortisol is continually produced. Cortisol levels are supposed to be low at nighttime, putting the body in the sleep mode. With chronic pain, high cortisol levels put the body in the alert mode and insomnia results. The increased cortisol production eventually wears the body down, resulting in increased fatigue. This explains why many chronic pain patients have difficulty sleeping and complain of non-restful sleep.

The adrenal gland also secretes adrenaline, more properly named epinephrine, which is the hormone that stimulates the sympathetic nervous system. When adrenaline is secreted it causes the body to produce free radicals, causing oxidative damage to the body. Long-term stress from chronic pain results in long-term oxidative damage. This is one reason that people who suffer from chronic pain are ill more frequently and age prematurely. This can also explain why they seem "stressed-out." Physiologically, they are! It becomes a vicious cycle. Many of you reading this are probably nodding your head because you or your loved one are stuck in this cycle. Chronic pain changes a person on so many levels. It has been shown to decrease the gray matter in the brain.

Pain causes enormous stress on the body which further enhances the need to rid the body of the pain. Prolotherapy is recommended for nearly every patient with structural chronic pain. Structural pain from a loose joint, cartilage, muscle, tendon, or ligament weakness can be eliminated with Prolotherapy.

Prolotherapy, in our opinion, is much safer than taking an anti-inflammatory medication. But like all medical procedures there are risks. This is why it is important to seek a Prolotherapist who has helped cases like yours. It is not recommended to have just any doctor inject you, especially if they have only trained by watching videos or on cadavers. We find that the best Prolotherapists have been trained on real patients and are able to treat all areas of the body comprehensively. During a consultation, they can more clearly define any particular risks that would potentially apply to you or any counter-indication based on your other health conditions. The safest Prolotherapy specialists do what we've termed as "think like a Prolotherapist." You don't want someone who just "thinks like an injectionist." This is a traditional doctor posing as a Prolotherapist. They tell you they can try a couple Prolotherapy injections, not even comprehensively treating the joint, and then tell you about how their other specialties are cortisone and joint replacement surgery.

3. HOW MANY TREATMENTS ARE NECESSARY AND HOW OFTEN?

The anesthetic in the solution used during Prolotherapy sessions often provides immediate pain relief. The pain relief may continue after the effect of the anesthetic subsides, due to the stabilizing of the treated joints because of the inflammation caused by the Prolotherapy injections. This pain relief normally continues for a few weeks after the first treatment.

Between the second and fourth weeks, the initial stabilization induced by the Prolotherapy subsides and, because the initial growth of ligament tissue is not complete, some of the original pain may return during this "window period" of healing. Follow-up is typically recommended at four to six weeks after each treatment to ensure an accurate assessment of results, avoiding an evaluation of a patient during the "window period." Prolotherapy is performed every four to six weeks because most ligaments heal over a four to six-week period.[2] *(See Figure 23-1.)*

As healing progresses, the quantity of injections required per treatment usually decreases. The pain generally continues to diminish with each treatment until it is completely eliminated. Three to six treatments are normally required to eliminate pain. Because everyone is unique, some people may only require one treatment while others will require six to eight treatments. Rarely are more needed.

In some cases, patients will experience no pain relief after their first or second Prolotherapy treatment. This does not mean the therapy is not working, rather it is an indication that the ligaments and tendons are not yet strong enough to stabilize the joints. The amount of collagen growth required for stabilization of the joint is

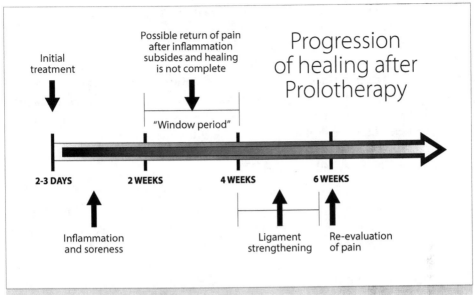

Figure 23-1: Progression of healing after Prolotherapy.

different for each person. A patient who experiences pain relief at rest but not during activity, requires further treatment to strengthen the area. If Prolotherapy treatments are continued, there is an excellent chance of achieving total pain relief with the resumption of all previous activities.

4. WHEN CAN I RETURN TO WORK?

Most patients return to work the next day, and some even go to work after treatment. Marion is a perfect example of this when she gets a sports injury. She can get a treatment and go back to her desk and work. What a champ! She has obviously been around Prolotherapy for a very long time. She barely flinches! For most of us, however, heading home after treatment and taking it easy after all those shots may sound more appealing. Of course, taking any additional time off depends on your job and how physically demanding it is on the area you are having treated. The area is a little stiff and swollen for the first couple days after treatment, and can be tender for a few days after treatment. We typically recommend that our patients not aggressively exercise for approximately 4 days post-treatment.

All prospective patients who receive disability insurance or workers' compensation, who are involved in a legal matter, or are on a leave of absence from work, are told that the ultimate goal of Prolotherapy treatments is to help them return to normal function, including returning to work. For individuals who do not have a real desire to return to work or discontinue receiving disability insurance, Prolotherapy is not indicated. In such cases, the individuals do not possess a "real" desire to heal and Prolotherapy will not ease the pain, as pain relief would be an admission that disability checks are no longer needed.

Though cases of patients who find it more appealing to continue life "in the system" exist, the overwhelming majority of people we treat who are suffering from chronic pain desire to find a solution in order to return to work. A few patients have a phobia of needles. For those individuals, other Natural Medicine treatments are prescribed, but the results are significantly less dramatic than what is expected with Prolotherapy. Herbs and vitamins will not stabilize a chronically loose joint. Exercise will not stabilize a chronically loose joint. Prolotherapy is the one treatment that will. There is no substitute for Prolotherapy with regard to curing pain.

5. WHAT IF I'M SCARED OF SHOTS?

No one really loves getting injections, but this should not be a reason to not get Prolotherapy. Most people feel the results are completely worth overcoming a fear of needles. Plus, there are so many ways that a patient can be helped through the treatment, such as pre-procedure anti-anxiety medication, numbing the area prior to the treatment, nitrous oxide gas, or in some cases, conscious sedation.

Patients who do not attain pain relief because of a phobia of needles, or give up on Prolotherapy after one or two sessions because of slower than expected pain relief are needlessly living with chronic pain, especially when a conservative, curative treatment is available. The number one reason for partial pain relief with Prolotherapy is not completing the full course of Prolotherapy sessions. It is important that the patient does not become disappointed if the pain is not relieved after one or two sessions, especially a patient who has been in pain for decades. We have seen severe pain cases that require only one treatment and relatively simple cases that require six sessions.

Overcoming phobias and fears is difficult but worthwhile, and it often produces the most happiness. Dr. Hauser's phobia was girls. In high school, he was often too scared to ask a girl for a date. There was one particular girl's picture he fell in love with when he was 12 years of age while looking through his yearbook at Jack Benny Junior High School in Waukegan, Illinois. It wasn't until after high school graduation that he was brave enough to call her. We talked and laughed for hours at Bevier Park in Waukegan, Illinois, on July 19, 1980. Many years later, we are still talking and laughing. We're sure glad that he had the courage to call Marion that day. Our lives would be pretty empty without each other! We must often overcome our fears to enjoy the true happiness that life offers.

6. WHAT ENHANCES OR LIMITS LIGAMENT AND TENDON TISSUE HEALING?

There are many factors that are involved in a person's ability to heal after Prolotherapy. Age, obesity, hormones, nutrition, sleep, physical activity, medications, concurrent treatment regimens used, and infections are some of these factors. All of these have an effect on a person's immune function. Good immune function is needed for a person to adequately heal soft tissue injuries and respond well to Prolotherapy.

Immune function declines with age and endocrine or nutritional inadequacies. Immobility, RICE, NSAIDs, infections, allergies, acid blood, and poor tissue oxygenation all cause a decline in the immune response. This poor immune response causes poor ligament and tissue healing, resulting in chronic pain. Chronic pain may lead to immobility and subsequent use of NSAIDs, which leads to insomnia and depression, which causes some people to eat poorly, which can lead to acid blood and poor tissue oxygenation, producing further tissue and tendon weakness.

Prolotherapy initiates the growth of ligament and tendon tissue, but the body actually grows the tissue. If the body is deprived of the necessary building blocks to grow strong new tissue, the response to Prolotherapy will be reduced. Therefore all factors that decrease tendon and ligament growth should be increased before and during Prolotherapy to ensure complete healing. Prolotherapy's effectiveness and the body's ability to complete the healing process is different for each individual.[3-7]

7. WHAT IS THE EFFECT OF AGE ON HEALING?

Prolotherapy patients in our office range from 4-94 years of age. Children and adolescents usually require only one Prolotherapy treatment to resolve a ligament or tendon injury. The young body is already primed to grow new tissue, making Prolotherapy treatments extremely effective.

Adults and the elderly may require more treatments because they are not in the growth mode of life. An adult being treated for chronic pain will receive an average of four to six sessions of Prolotherapy per area. Those with excellent immune systems will grow more ligament and tendon tissue per session and will, therefore, require fewer sessions. Those with poor immune systems, especially smokers, require more than the average four sessions. The Prolotherapy treatments are generally given every six weeks to allow the treated area ample time to grow strong ligaments and tendons.

We so often wish that more elderly folks who are suffering in pain would seek Prolotherapy. Most of these people worked so hard earlier in life, only to retire but be in too much physical pain to take full advantage of retirement. It appears that the feeling among the older generation is that pain is just a normal part of the aging process. There is no honor in suffering needlessly from pain.

Losing the ability to be mobile and active is possibly the worst thing that can happen to people as they age. Activity truly keeps the blood flowing. Joints, like the hips and knees, depend on walking and weight-bearing activities to provide nourishment to the joint cartilage. No walking, no nourishment. No nourishment, no cartilage. No cartilage, no movement. Walking keeps people alive and keeps the body functioning. If stiffness sets in, the grave may follow.

Because most bodily functions decline with age, the ability to heal an injury and the immune system response are slower. With age, the ligament and tendon tissue contains less water, noncollagenous protein, and proteoglycans. Proteoglycans are a proteinaceous material containing a large quantity of water. The proteoglycans and subcomponents, such as glucosamine and chondroitin sulfate, allow structures like ligaments, intervertebral discs, and articular cartilage to withstand intense pressure.[8-10] *(See Figure 23-2.)* The collagen matrix becomes disorganized and prone to injury. Chronic ligament and tendon laxity is a reason for chronic pain in the aging population. For these reasons, older people may respond slower and, because of this slower healing, more Prolotherapy sessions may be needed. Teenagers, because they are in the growing phase of life, rarely need more than one or two Prolotherapy treatments to eliminate chronic pain. People in their 90s will heal slower because of their age and often require more than the typical four Prolotherapy sessions to cure their chronic pain.

Pain is not a normal part of the aging process. Chronic pain always has a cause and that cause is not "old age syndrome." Chronic pain is almost always due to ligament weakness. Prolotherapy can help strengthen ligaments at any age and is the treatment of choice for chronic pain, regardless of age.

8. WHAT IS THE EFFECT OF OBESITY ON HEALING?

Ligaments, which provide stability to the joints, resist stretching (good tensile strength). Tensile strength of ligaments is much less than the tensile strength of bone. Thus, when a joint is stressed, the ligament will be injured prior to the bone because it is the weak link of the bone-ligament complex.[11] The ligament will stretch and sprain before the bone will fracture. The area where the ligament is injured is the fibro-osseous junction.

The strength of the ligament required to maintain the stability of the joint depends directly on the pressure applied. The heavier the force applied to the joint, the stronger the ligament must be to hold the joint in place. Getting tackled by a Chicago Bears football player would require ligaments to withstand more pressure

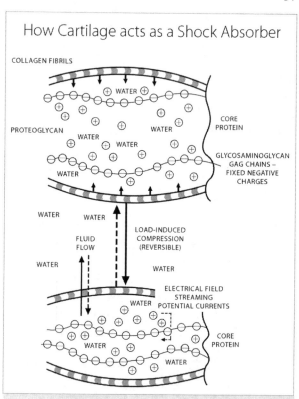

Figure 23-2: The proteoglycan structure of articular cartilage. The high content of water in proteoglycans help the cartilage act as a shock absorber.

than getting tackled by the average 12 year-old. This explains why overweight people, exhibiting a positive "basketball-belly sign," are prone to chronic pain and impaired healing. The excess weight places increased pressure on the ligaments, especially in the lower back, hip, and knee areas.

Weight loss is effective for decreasing the pain of osteoarthritis and chronic ligament and tendon weakness because it diminishes the stress on the joints. Stabilization and movement of the joint requires less work by the ligaments and tendons, resulting in reduced pain. However, in our experience, obese patients still benefit from Prolotherapy greatly. We do our best to help them with a combined approach of Prolotherapy for restoring the ligament strength, and a healthy diet plan to maintain a healthier and more active lifestyle as they are able to exercise longer due to less pain.

9. DO HORMONES PLAY A ROLE IN HEALING?

The endocrine system produces and secretes hormones for the body, including adrenal hormones such as cortisol, thyroid hormones, Growth Hormone, melatonin, prostaglandins, and insulin. Hormones such as testosterone, cortisol, and thyroxine regulate the growth of tissue. An inadequate endocrine system will propagate ligament and tendon weakness. Soft tissue healing of ligaments and tendons will be compromised if any of these hormones are deficient.[7,12,13] Hormone levels also naturally decrease with age. Therefore, these hormones may need to be supplemented in order to ensure complete healing.

To be evaluated for hormone deficiencies and the use of natural hormones, an evaluation by a Natural Medicine physician should be considered.

10. WHAT IS THE ROLE OF NUTRITION IN HEALING?

Nutritional deficiencies are epidemic in modern society affecting both overall health and the healing of ligaments and tendons. Ligaments and tendons consist of water, proteoglycans, and collagen. Collagen represents 70-90% of the weight of connective tissues and is the most abundant protein in the human body, approximately 30% of total proteins and 6% of human body weight.

Collagen synthesis requires specific nutrients including iron, copper, manganese, calcium, zinc, vitamin C, and various amino acids.[14] Proteoglycan synthesis requires the coordination of protein, carbohydrate polymer, and collagen synthesis, along with trace minerals such as manganese, copper, and zinc. Proper nutrition is an essential factor in soft tissue healing. A diet lacking in adequate nutrients such as vitamin A, vitamin C, zinc, and protein will hinder the healing process and the formation of collagen tissue. For these reasons, everyone should take a good multivitamin and mineral supplement.

Water is the most necessary nutrient in the body. The human body is composed of 25% solid matter and 75% water. Many of the supporting structures of the body, including the articular cartilage surfaces of joints and the intervertebral discs, contain a significant amount of water. Seventy-five percent of the weight of the upper part of the body is supported by the water volume stored in the disc core.[15] Inadequate intake of water may lead to inadequate fluid support to these areas, resulting in weakened structures that may produce chronic pain. We recommend purified water as the primary beverage for optimal health.

One aspect of your life you should really take control over is the food you put in your body. This is the fuel you are giving yourself to heal. We cannot emphasize this enough. Everyone needs to eat fresh foods, not only while undergoing a Prolotherapy treatment series, but for better overall health. The majority of your food should not come from

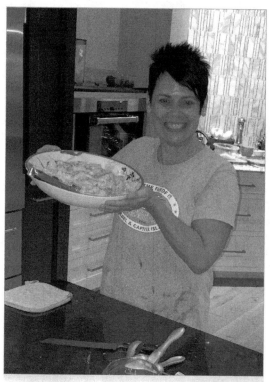

Marion serving up a delicious homemade dinner.

boxes, freezer, a restaurant, or a microwave if you want to maximize your healing with Prolotherapy. If fresh protein and vegetables are the basis of each of your meals, you are on a pretty great start! This should be the basis for most people. Two other considerations for healing are to cut out sugar, as it dampens your immune function and to increase your vegetables, since they help boost your immune function.

We developed The Hauser Diet® which is comprised of five unique Diet Types, spanning from high protein and fat with very low carbohydrates, to balanced, all the way to vegan vegetarian. What we realized early in our individual practices was that traditional low fat diet recommendations were not for everyone. There are certain tendencies and metabolic markers that indicate what type of diet is best for each individual. This is a concept we use for helping our patients determine the best healing foods for them. For those of you who are interested in learning more about the Hauser Diet, you can read Marion's book: *The Hauser Diet: A Fresh Look at Healthy Living*, as well as HauserDiet.com.

11. WHAT IS THE ROLE OF SLEEP IN HEALING?

Chronic pain patients are often prescribed antidepressant medications, like Elavil, to aid sleep. These medicines provide some temporary pain relief and aid sleep. However, chronic pain is not due to an Elavil or other pharmaceutical drug deficiency. Chronic pain has a cause. Until the etiology is determined and treated, all therapeutic modalities will provide only temporary relief. Prolotherapy injections to strengthen the ligament and tendon attachments to bone cause permanent healing.

Chronic pain and chronic insomnia go hand in hand. The adrenal gland secretion of the hormone cortisol normally decreases at night, and the pineal gland secretion of melatonin increases, thereby enabling sleep. Unfortunately, the chronic pain patient's secretion of cortisol does not decline because chronic pain is seen by the body as stress, thereby stimulating the adrenal gland, which reacts to stress, to produce cortisol. This results in chronic insomnia. The secretion of cortisol will stop only when the chronic pain is relieved. Chronic insomnia increases chronic pain. Prolotherapy breaks this cycle. Pain relief leads to a good night's sleep.

Sleep is vital to health maintenance. Sleep stimulates the anterior pituitary to produce Growth Hormone. Growth Hormone is one of the main anabolic, meaning to grow or repair, hormones in the body whose job is to repair the damage done to the body during the day. Every day, soft tissues including ligaments and tendons are damaged. It is vital to obtain deep stages of sleep, as during this time Growth Hormone is secreted.

Without deep stages of sleep, inadequate Growth Hormone is secreted and soft tissue healing is inadequate. *(See Figure 23-3.)* Growth Hormone levels also appear to

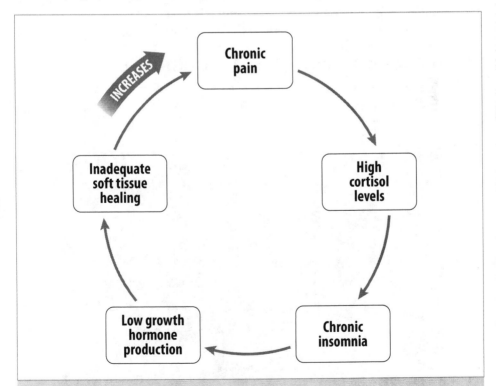

Figure 23-3: The effect of chronic insomnia on soft tissue healing. Chronic insomnia causes low Growth Hormone production which leads to inadequate soft tissue production.

be increased with exercise and amino acid supplementation with ornithine, arginine, or glutamine.[16,17]

A natural way to increase sleep and improve deep sleep is aerobic exercise, like cycling, walking, or running. Melatonin, L-tryptophan (an amino acid), valerian root, and gamma hydroxybutyrate are also beneficial natural sleep aids.

12. WHAT IS THE ROLE OF PHYSICAL ACTIVITY IN HEALING?

Exercise is currently the traditional treatment of choice for chronic pain. Chronic pain patients often experience an exacerbation of their pain when exercising. This is an indication that ligament laxity is the cause of the pain. Ligament laxity generally causes pain when the joint is stressed, which occurs with activity. The proper treatment is not to "work through the pain," but to correct the source of the pain. The main function of exercise is to strengthen muscle, not to grow ligament tissue.

Aggressive exercise may worsen ligament injury and is not recommended until Prolotherapy has strengthened the joint sufficiently to provide pain relief. A good rule-of-thumb is if doing something hurts, don't do it. Once healing begins and the pain has decreased, dynamic range-of-motion exercises, like walking, cycling, and swimming, are more helpful than static-resistive exercises like weight lifting.[18] A more formal exercise program is necessary after the ligaments strengthen and the joint stabilizes. This exercise program will strengthen the muscles around the joint and increase the flexibility of the muscles which protect the joint from reinjury.

13. IS PROLOTHERAPY USEFUL FOR ACUTE INJURIES?

If inflammation is so beneficial, why not use Prolotherapy for the treatment of an acute injury? Prolotherapy is beneficial and will speed the recovery process of an acute injury. However, the first treatment course should always be the most conservative

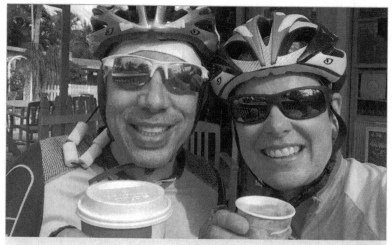

Enjoying a cup of coffee during a long bike ride. Cycling has helped us both stay fit and recover from injuries.

one. A more conservative approach to treating acute injuries to ligaments and tendons is Movement, Exercise, Analgesics, and Treatment, also known as MEAT. While immobility is detrimental to soft tissue healing, movement is beneficial.[19] Movement and gentle range-of-motion exercises improve blood flow to the area, removing debris. Heat also increases blood flow so this is recommended after an acute injury. If movement of the joint is painful, then isometric exercises should be performed. Isometric exercising involves contracting a muscle without movement of the affected joint. An example of this is a handshake. Both parties squeeze, creating a muscle contraction without joint movement.

Natural analgesics or pain relievers that are not synthetic anti-inflammatories may be used. Natural substances, such as the enzymes bromelain, trypsin, and papain, aid soft tissue healing by reducing the viscosity of extracellular fluid. This increases nutrient and waste transport from the injured site, reducing swelling or edema.[20] A narcotic, such as codeine, may be prescribed short-term for an extremely painful acute injury. Narcotics are wonderful pain relievers and do not interfere with the natural healing mechanisms of the body, if used in the short-term. Your body produces its own narcotics, called endorphins, which work to reduce pain from an acute injury. Other options for pain control include acetaminophen or tramadol. As previously mentioned, these can be used, as they relieve pain but do not decrease inflammation.

The "T" in MEAT stands for specific Treatments that increase blood flow and immune cell migration to the damaged area, which will aid in ligament and tendon healing. Treatments such as physical therapy, massage, chiropractic care, ultrasound, myofascial release, and electrical stimulation all improve blood flow and assist soft tissue healing. *(See Figure 23-4.)*

If circumstances are such that time is a factor, we often use Prolotherapy as an initial treatment for acute pain or injury, particularly related to sports injuries. An individual who would normally wait two to three months for an acute injury to heal, may heal in only two to three weeks if given Prolotherapy. We have seen this increased speed of recovery in a multitude of injuries, including ACL (anterior cruciate ligament) sprains of the knee, shin splints, back injuries such as herniated discs, and many more. We have even used Prolotherapy to help pregnant women get through the back pain of pregnancy. So Prolotherapy is a great choice for acute, as well as chronic injuries and pain.

Grade of ligament injury	Specific injury	Return to play using RICE	Return to play using MEAT
One	Ligament sprain	7-14 days	2-4 days
Two	Ligament partial tear	3-7 weeks	1-3 weeks
Three	Complete tear	12-16 weeks after surgery	4-8 weeks after surgery

Figure 23-4: Average healing rate and grade of ligament injury relative to RICE and MEAT treatments. Athletes can typically return to sports much faster using MEAT than RICE.

14. DON'T I NEED AN MRI IF I HAVE PAIN?

Nope. If an MRI is ordered for you, find out the reason why! There is almost no other reason to get one except to prepare you for surgery. MRIs cannot tell you what is causing the pain, just confirm what is known by history and physical exam.

Most MRI findings have nothing to do with the person's pain, and is thus the reason for most "failed surgery syndromes." Once you receive surgery, that region will never be the same. For example, during arthroscopy, shaving cartilage and meniscal tissue in the knee accelerates arthritis. Surgery for pain, in the best scenario, should be done only after all conservative treatments have been tried and failed, including Prolotherapy.

Remember, MRIs see the result of wear and tear, a trauma, etc. The findings are typically the result of joint instability. The treatment for joint instability is Prolotherapy. In most cases we see, the patient could have had a head start on healing if they would have skipped the MRI. Any good Regenerative Medicine practitioner will recommend an MRI if the case warrants it. But with the high cost to get an MRI and the high rate of inaccuracy,

MRI Versus the Thumb			
		MRI	**THUMB**
False-positive rate of static MRI positive in asymptomatic middle-aged persons (conservative estimate)	Lower back	64%	0
	Neck	50%	0
	Shoulder	54%	0
	Knee	62%	0
Cost		$3,200	Free (Included in office visit)
Time involved		45 minutes	45 seconds
Ability to reproduce pain		None	100%
Enjoyment by clinician		None	Lots
Likelihood of progression to surgery		Very high	Very low

Figure 23-5: MRI versus the thumb. Which do you want diagnosing your injury?

the practitioner may recommend other, more specific tests that can see the joint in motion or give a better picture than a static MRI, such as a Digital Motion X-ray or musculoskeletal ultrasound. Still, even with some of the other imaging options available, "My Reproducibility Instrument" will always come out on top. **(See Figure 23-5.)**

15. WHY SHOULDN'T I JUST CONTINUE TAKING PAIN MEDICATION?

Most people understand the addictive quality of narcotics. This is a good reason not to use narcotics for more than a few days. Another reason to avoid narcotics is that narcotic medications suppress the immune system.

Chronic use of narcotics has been shown to decrease both B-cell and T-cell function, reduce the effectiveness of phagocytes to kill organisms like Candida and cause atrophy of such important immune organs as the spleen and thymus.[21,22] The spleen and thymus glands are two structures in the body that are vital to helping the immune system fight off infections. Another study on the use of narcotics concluded that people with the potential for bacterial or viral infections should be cautioned against the use of narcotic medication.[3]

Narcotic medications, because of their potential immune-suppressing effect as well as their addictive properties, should be used as little as possible. Narcotic medications, as indicated above, can cause the shrinking of such important glands as the thymus and spleen.

If pain medicine is needed, Tylenol® or Ultram® can be used because they do not suppress inflammation. Anti-inflammatory medications, such as Motrin®, Advil®, or Aleve®, cannot be used because they suppress inflammation and block the beneficial effects of the Prolotherapy. Most people with chronic pain admit that they want to stop using pain medications. Often they say, "I just don't feel right being on those." Of course not. Would you feel "right" if your spleen and thymus were shrinking?

As previously stated, nonsteroidal anti-inflammatory drugs (NSAIDs) have been shown to produce short-term pain benefit but leave long-term loss of function.[23] NSAIDs also inhibit proteoglycan synthesis, a component of ligament and cartilage tissue. Proteoglycans are essential for the elasticity and compressive stiffness of articular cartilage. Suppression of their synthesis has significant adverse effects on the joint.[24-26] NSAIDs are the mainstay treatment for acute ligament and tendon injuries, yet efficacy in their usefulness is lacking.[27] Worse yet is the long-term use by people with chronic pain. Studies in the use of NSAIDs for chronic hip pain revealed an acceleration of arthritis in the people taking NSAIDs.[28-30]

In one study, NSAID use was associated with progressive formation of multiple small acetabular and femoral subcortical cysts and subchondral bone-thinning. In this study, 84% of the people who had progressive arthritis were long-term NSAID users. The conclusion of the study was, "This highly significant association between NSAID use and acetabular destruction gives cause for concern."[28] As it should, acetabular destruction, femoral subcortical cysts, and subchondral bone-thinning are all signs that the NSAIDs were causing arthritis to form more quickly. This is one explanation why people taking Motrin®, Advil®, Aleve®, or any other NSAID will likely require more medicine to decrease their pain. Eventually the medicine does not stop the pain because the arthritis process is actually accelerating while taking the medicine. *(See Figure 23-6.)*

The end result of taking NSAIDs for pain relief is an arthritic joint. How many times has an NSAID cured a person of his or her pain? Even long-term aspirin use has been associated with accelerating hip damage from arthritis.[31] When comparing the long-term use of indomethacin in the treatment of osteoarthritis of the hip, it was clearly shown that the disease progressed more frequently and the destruction within the hip joint was more severe with drug use than without.[32]

NSAIDs are truly anti-inflammatory in their mechanism of action. Since all tissues heal by inflammation, one can see why long-term use of these medications will have harmful effects. Osteoarthritis and other chronic pain disorders are not an indomethacin or other NSAID deficiency. This is why the use of these drugs will

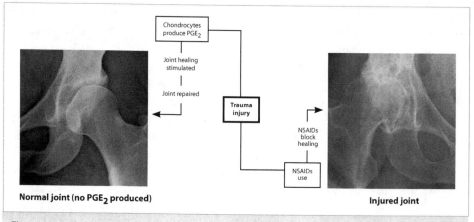

Figure 23-6. Chondrocytes produce Prostaglandin E2 (PGE$_2$) in response to injury. NSAIDs, especially those that block COX-2 inhibit PGE$_2$ synthesis in chondrocytes thereby stalling the body's main inflammatory repair mechanism. Long-term, this will accelerate degenerative osteoarthritis of the joint.

never cure any disease. Their chronic long-term use will not cure; it will hamper soft tissue healing and accelerate the arthritic process.

NSAIDs should not be taken while undergoing Prolotherapy because they inhibit the inflammation caused by the treatment. For that matter, anyone with chronic pain should seriously consider stopping NSAIDs and starting Prolotherapy.

SUMMARY

We are excited for you! Throughout this book, you have learned a lot about Prolotherapy and the wide array of conditions it helps, as well as how it compares to other popular pain management techniques. Prolotherapy offers a pain cure! It is the regenerative treatment that makes the most sense for patients of any age who want to return to work and sports quickly, whether suffering from acute or chronic injuries. It is safe, quick, and effective! Even if you have struggled with poor nutrition, weight issues, insomnia, or other stumbling blocks that aggravate your pain; there are Natural Medicine techniques that can help you obtain better health to assist in the healing process. We would love to help you accomplish your goals of a healthier, pain-free life! Now that you understand the principles of how Prolotherapy works, it is time to take action! We would love to hear from you with questions about your own case. You can contact us directly through our website CaringMedical.com or email DrHauser@caringmedical.com. Our team of professionals is ready to answer your questions and help you Prolo your pain away! ■

CHAPTER

MAXIMIZE YOUR PROLOTHERAPY POTENTIAL

If you have been reading this book thinking "This all sounds great, but I'm not sure that I'm a good candidate," we will review some of the factors that help determine the likelihood of success with Comprehensive Prolotherapy based on our clinical findings.

The "ideal" Prolotherapy candidate has the following:
• Pain originating from a ligament or tendon.
• Good range of motion.
• Strong immune system.
• Ability to receive the recommended number of treatment sessions.
• Healthy diet.
• Positive mental outlook and willingness to improve.

We can tell you that most of the new patients who come to our office do not necessarily represent the "ideal" Prolotherapy candidate. There are factors beyond Prolotherapy that should be addressed or corrected, if needed, in order to optimize results, as we have discussed throughout this book. The primary indication for Prolotherapy is #1: pain originating from joint instability due to a ligament or tendon weakness. This is what Prolotherapy treats. Common painful signs indicate that a problem resides with ligament laxity, including tenderness, clicking and grinding of the joint, muscle spasms and more. *(See Figure 24-1.)*

POWER OF REGENERATIVE MEDICINE

We have been blessed to take on some of the world's toughest pain cases. Think about the power of Prolotherapy if it can take patients who have been told "you've got no cartilage left," "you're one of the worst cases I've seen," or even "there's nothing more we can do for you" and get most of those people back to walking without pain, able to work, and participating in sports and hobbies again. This is the reality of what we see all day long at Caring Medical. Prolotherapy can be a life-changing

Common Signs & Symptoms as Possible Indications for Prolotherapy

- Aching, burning or tingling pain or sensation that is referred into an upper or lower extremity
- Chronic muscle spasms
- Distinct tender points at the entheses where tendons or ligaments attach to the bones
- Laxity of a tested joint, especially compared to the non-painful side
- Popping, clicking, grinding, or catching sensations in joints
- Recurrent joint subluxations or dislocations
- Recurrent swelling or fullness in a joint
- Temporary benefit from chiropractic, osteopathic, or self-manipulation that fails to resolve

Figure 24-1: Common signs and symptoms as possible indications for Prolotherapy.

treatment! Many of the new patients we treat have seen at least 5 other practitioners and been run through the mill of traditional care: they have been put on a number of immunosuppressant medications, they have been given one joint-destroying cortisone injection after another, their joint has lost a considerable amount of motion, they waited until they were nearly disabled to seek treatment, they are feeling hopeless or depressed about their situation, or they eat poorly for one reason or another. It is often like trying to reverse a freight train, but Prolotherapy has proven to be the most effective tool for helping these chronic pain cases.

WHAT IF I'M NOT A GOOD PROLOTHERAPY CANDIDATE? YOU MIGHT ACTUALLY BE ONE!

In our experience, seeking Prolotherapy from a clinic that addresses the reasons why a patient may not heal can help their chances of success with the treatment. This is what we strive for at Caring Medical. We also know when a patient may not be a good candidate for Prolotherapy and other options need to be sought. In those cases, most patients would say that it was still worth consulting with a Prolotherapy practitioner before doing anything drastic and irreversible such as joint replacement surgery, nerve ablation, fusion or laminectomy. If there is a reason why you would not be a good candidate for regenerative treatments, we will make the best suggestions we can for a comprehensive approach, as if you were our own family member. As with any treatment, there are limitations as to what would make someone a good candidate for the treatment. In addition, there are some conditions that may initially sound like they would not be appropriate for Prolotherapy, but may actually respond well to it.

TENDONITIS OR TENDINOSIS

True tendonitis is a short-lived inflammatory condition. However, most people diagnosed with tendonitis actually have developed tendinosis. When the tendon problem has become chronic, and the person continues to use ice and anti-inflammatory medications, this is now a case of tendinosis—which, of course, responds well to Prolotherapy.

BONE SPURS

We've already discussed that bone spurs are a direct result of joint instability. The body overgrows bone in an attempt to stabilize the joint. Most of these cases, if caught early, are still good candidates for Prolotherapy. There are, however, some cases where the bone spur is restricting almost all joint motion and the joint damage is too severe for Prolotherapy. For instance, the bone that used to be round becomes flattened through continued pressure on the unstable joint. Again, this is why turning off the pain signal with cortisone and pain medication is so dangerous in the long-term. It can leave you with irreversible bone and joint damage. *(See Figure 24-2.)*

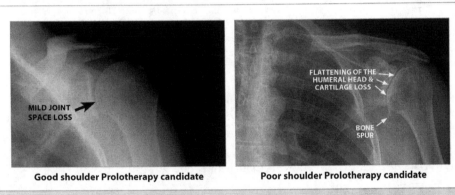

Good shoulder Prolotherapy candidate   Poor shoulder Prolotherapy candidate

Figure 24-2. A good vs. poor shoulder Prolotherapy candidate. Joint architecture and range of motion are important considerations to determine if a patient is a good Prolotherapy candidate. The patient on the left was a good candidate who presented with full range of motion and only mild loss of joint space. The patient on the right presented with very limited range of motion, loss of cartilage, and a large bone spur. In addition, there is a flattening of the humeral head in the patient on the right, compared to the patient on the left. Prolotherapy cannot make a flattened bone round again. Therefore, the patient on the right was a poor candidate for Prolotherapy. Avoiding bone destruction is one of the many reasons to seek Prolotherapy sooner than later.

AVASCULAR NECROSIS OR OSTEONECROSIS

Avascular necrosis, or bone death, is an example of a condition that may be due to joint instability or may be due to lifestyle or medication. There are two reasons why someone develops avascular necrosis: a systemic problem or joint instability. The bone can die due to large doses of medications needed to treat certain systemic conditions, such as chemotherapy or prednisone. Or, avascular necrosis can occur in cases of excessive alcohol use. These cases are not due to joint instability and would not be appropriate Prolotherapy candidates. However, very often people develop avascular necrosis due to joint instability, since avascular necrosis occurs at the end of the bone which is the same place where the ligaments attach. If there is ligament damage, this can interrupt the blood supply. After continued pressure, bone can die. Therefore, avascular necrosis can be yet another MRI finding that really indicates that the person's pain is coming from joint instability. Prolotherapy, and specifically Cellular Prolotherapy, is a good option for these cases. *(See Figure 24-3.)*

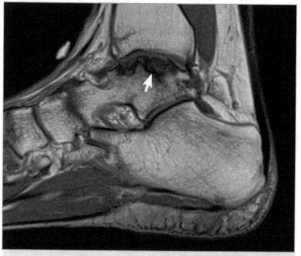

Figure 24-3: A young mom with a long-term history of oral steroid use which led to AVN (arrow) in her ankle. After four Bone Marrow Prolotherapy treatments the patient is now able to do all activities and exercise without pain.

GOUT AND PSEUDOGOUT

Gout is another good example of a case that may or may not be a good Prolotherapy candidate. People with gout can generally control the condition with proper nutrition and Natural Medicine intervention, including a purine-restricted diet with plenty of fresh foods and nutritional supplements to ward off a painful gout attack. But we have seen a lot of cases of pseudo-gout where, upon exam, they have tenderness and weakness at the ligament attachments. These people may have an appropriate case for Prolotherapy, if their pain is due to ligament laxity.

ARACHNOIDITIS

Arachnoiditis is typically diagnosed in someone who has undergone back surgery and still suffers severe back pain that radiates down the legs and often to the feet. The pain has a persistent burning, stinging, or aching quality.[1] The diagnosis is occasionally made when similar symptoms are felt in the neck, arms, or the mid back with radiation into the chest. This pain is typically unresponsive to pain medications and muscle relaxants.

The term arachnoiditis signifies an inflammation of the arachnoid membrane which covers the spinal cord. The diagnosis of arachnoiditis is generally inaccurate because no signs of inflammation, such as redness, fever, or an elevated sed rate (blood test that identifies inflammation), are seen in these patients. All that is seen is scar tissue on the MRI. What percentage of people will develop a scar as evidenced on x-ray after back surgery? If you said 100%, you are correct. Each time a person undergoes surgery, a scar will develop. It is that simple.

The scar tissue was not present before the surgery, but the back and leg pains were. The surgery did not address the cause of the back and leg pain. Furthermore, the scar tissue seen on the scan most likely has nothing to do with the current pain complaints of the patient.

In one study consisting of 36 patients with arachnoiditis, each patient averaged three previous myelograms and three back surgeries. Don't you think your x-ray would show scar tissue after all of that?! In this study, 88% of the patients were diagnosed with arachnoiditis by x-ray and the other 12% by surgery. The most startling result observed from the study was that the average life span was shortened by 12 years.[2] Anyone who has had back surgery with recurrent pain should be evaluated for another cause of the pain besides arachnoiditis. Epidural steroid injections, more surgeries, spinal cord stimulator implantation, or other invasive treatments for arachnoiditis are only marginally helpful.[2,3]

The primary cause of radiating pain is joint instability due to ligament laxity. Therefore, a patient diagnosed with arachnoiditis should see a Prolotherapist to relieve the pain, not a surgeon.

NERVE PAIN

Most cases that involve a nerve being pinched, inflamed, or entrapped do not necessarily need surgery to open up space. A skilled Prolotherapist knows that most nerves become irritated due to joint instability. This is common with radiculopathy where the capsular ligaments of the spine have allowed the vertebra to pinch the nerve when the person moves, sending wildfire-like pain down the arm or leg. With the various Prolotherapy solutions and techniques available, including Nerve Release Injection Therapy, there are non-surgical ways to free up nerves that are getting compressed. *(See Figure 24-4.)*

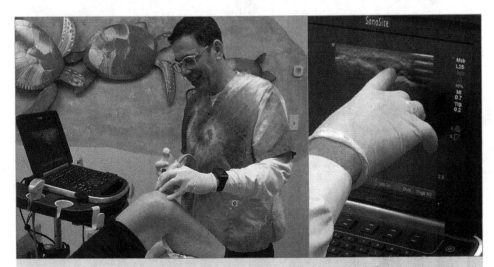

Figure 24-4: Swollen peroneal nerve resolved with Nerve Release Injection Therapy. Once the nerve is identified with ultrasound, nourishing solutions are injected around it to release the entrapment.

MAXIMIZING YOUR PROLOTHERAPY POTENTIAL

As we tell our patients, success with Prolotherapy is a two-way street. Our part is to properly identify all the pain-causing structures and to comprehensively treat them. The patient's responsibility is to do everything within reason to promote physical and emotional wellbeing. You are an active participant in your recovery. Beyond making the trip to receive Prolotherapy, you are actively making choices in your life that support your own physical, emotional, mental, and spiritual health. This may mean making some "uncomfortable" or even downright "difficult" changes to create new healthy habits and relationships. Know who your support team is, including family and friends, who want to see you succeed and will do their best to support your efforts. If you are dedicated to getting rid of your pain once and for all, this is a necessary part of the journey.

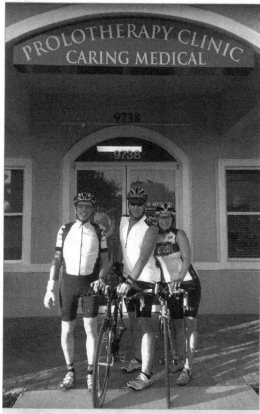

Oasis of hope! Dr. Hauser and Marion riding in to the Florida office with a great friend, Dr. Bill Sawyer, who has used Prolotherapy for numerous sports injuries. Caring Medical strives to be an oasis of hope for cases that would have otherwise needed multiple surgeries, extended time off work and sports, or ever increasing amounts of pain medication.

DIET

If we had to summarize the basic Hauser Diet rules for everyone to follow, it would include adequate protein, fresh vegetables, and purified water, in addition to avoiding processed foods, sugar, and excessive alcohol intake. If you are struggling with your overall health and ability to heal, the first place to look is what fuel you are putting in your body. This could mean finding out which Diet Type is best for you. Many of our patients are surprised to find out that their real metabolic needs are a high protein and high fat diet with very few carbohydrates, and they had been previously trying to eat a very low fat diet with a lot of fruit. Or there are people who have been following a higher protein diet, carbohydrate-restricted only to find out that they function better on a more vegetarian diet. The main point here is that most people need to clean up their diets. It is our wish that people will decide to make these improved eating habits part of their lives forever, and not just during a

Prolotherapy treatment series. Never underestimate the power of food!

To learn more about The Hauser Diet principles, check out the book *The Hauser Diet: A Fresh Look at Healthy Living*, or visit HauserDiet.com.

EXERCISE

In order to nourish a joint, it needs motion. In our office, we guide patients on what types of exercises are best for their condition, and typically allow patients to restart exercising in approximately 4 days after treatment. There are a variety of ways to keep up your fitness level without necessarily hurting the joint further. Gradually increasing back up to high impact sports is typically recommended. Some preferred exercises include swimming, aqua jogging, cycling, balance and core work. The general rule of thumb is to not aggravate the pain. Some dull pain is normal after exercise. But if the pain is lingering more than a couple hours, it likely means you did too much.

Exercise is supposed to strain muscles not joints. Joints are not supposed to be hot or swollen after exercise or activity. Exercise that causes sharp joint pain or results in joint pain lasting longer than two hours after the exercise has stopped, has put too much pressure on the joint and is part of the chronic pain problem, not solution. Sometimes improvement in exercise technique is needed to reduce the joint stress. This is where an athlete can benefit from working with a trainer or therapist who can re-train the body to do proper form and movements that do not cause sheer force on the joints. Sheer forces put strain on ligaments, menisci and labrum as well as the joint capsule. Sheer forces occur when one bone is rotating while the adjacent bone is stationary. This puts strain on joint structures and increases joint instability and may even cause Prolotherapy to be less effective. Make sure exercise is done with stress on the muscles not on the joints and no sheer or torque forces are applied on the joint with exercise.

Balance work can be beneficial for everyone, and especially during rehabilitation of a joint. Ligaments affect the proprioception or balance sensation of the joint. The muscles don't work right and the joint does not function quite right. Balance work can be very gentle on the ligaments and often can be started right away after the first Prolotherapy session. Balance work can be as simple as standing on one leg, doing one legged mini-squats, or balancing on discs or other gym equipment. The lower limb will not feel normal until the ligaments and joint are strong and stable, respectively, but also the muscle strength in the injured extremity must be back to normal. What is often forgotten is balance work, as this works the nervous system receptors in and around the joint. Balance deficits must also be resolved especially for the athlete to be able to say the injury is 100% cured.

Exercise ability is an excellent gauge for determining the true status of the joint. When people cover up the pain for years with NSAIDs and cortisone shots, they do not truly know how the joint is doing because they keep exercising on an injured joint, and therefore continue the wear and tear process. With Prolotherapy, those items are taken out of the equation, and the person knows the joint is getting stronger because activities are gradually increased without the aid of pain pills. In essence, the person acts as his or her own control for the success of the treatment.

APPROPRIATE BRACING

There are times where a joint needs to be braced. Someone who walks all day on the job, may need a knee brace after Prolotherapy. As the ligament tightens, the brace is used less and less. One area of the body where bracing is especially important is when the upper neck is unstable. Often with C1-C2 instability, some bracing is required. A person can be braced in one of three positions: neutral, head slightly flexed or slightly extended. The position that feels the best for a prolonged period of time would be the one that is chosen, unless bracing in a position based on optimal joint positioning found under x-ray. Since eating in cervical brace causing extension or movement of C1-C2 area, the brace is taken off while eating.

STOP MANIPULATING THE JOINT

Whether this is self-manipulation or through a practitioner, the joint should not be continuously manipulated. This works against what Prolotherapy is trying to achieve. The ligaments are encouraged to strengthen and tighten the joint in to proper alignment, eliminating constant subluxations and instability, and thereby halting the vicious cycle of feeling the need to crack or pop the joints and spine.

ANCILLARY THERAPIES

Prolotherapy is an excellent stand alone treatment, though some people who are really passionate about Natural Medicine also like to use certain ancillary therapies to aid in their rehabilitation. Acupuncture, massage, reflexology, hyperbaric oxygen, cold laser, infrared heat, and IV nutrients are among some of the most common ancillary treatments. There are also some conditions, such as a frozen shoulder, where physical therapy exercises must accompany Prolotherapy to restore proper motion to the shoulder. In general, therapies that encourage circulation to the injured or painful area are helpful at encouraging healing while undergoing Prolotherapy. However, it is important that the other therapists know you are receiving Prolotherapy and they understand how it works in order to not interrupt or stop the progress made with Prolotherapy. It is also wise to make the Prolotherapist aware of exactly what type of therapies are being done between Prolotherapy visits, and even to have some communication with the other therapist, in a letter, phone call, or email. The Prolotherapist will need to give some overall guidance, particularly in regard to chiropractic and physical therapy, so the ancillary therapies are controlled and do not adversely affect the Prolotherapy. This is the ideal way to build a team that works for your benefit and can get you past the pain and on with your life.

SURROUND YOURSELF WITH POSITIVITY AND SUPPORT

Having unresolved chronic pain can cause you to take an overall inventory of how you live your life. It is astounding how many of our patients who improve with Prolotherapy, after years of negativity surrounding their lives with chronic pain, look back and see the ordeal as a wake-up call. During their fight to come back from an injury, to get off narcotic pain medication, or to restore mobility that was lost, they find that the need to confront other areas of their life that were holding them back. This could be mending broken relationships, forgiving past offenses, and having the courage to make new friendships and focus on being positive and grateful for all the things in life. We see that patients who don't sweat the small stuff tend to have the better outcomes. They are not focused on whether the 2mm tear they had has completely repaired as much as they are happy that now they can go down a flight of stairs without the knee giving out. A Chiari malformation found on MRI isn't the focus, rather, rejoicing that their migraines have ceased. The person who cut you off in traffic can be forgiven because you are driving to work, a job that you were unable to perform only a few months ago. A little positivity goes a long way.

THE END...

Let us just say "thank you" for your interest in learning the concepts provided here. It has been a remarkable journey since the original printing of this book, seeing so many lives transformed through Prolotherapy and Regenerative Medicine. We have been blessed to use these principles to help alleviate chronic pain and injuries in our patients, friends, family, and in our own sports injuries. We hope that you will apply the principles discussed in this book to your life. If you do, you should soon agree that no matter how bad the pain, you can always *"Prolo Your Pain Away!"* ∎

Sincerely, with warm regards...until our next book...

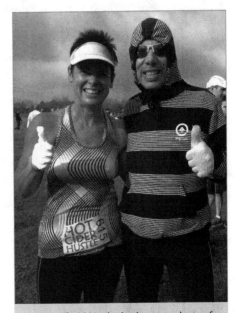

You can do it! No doubt there are plenty of obstacles to navigate when you have chronic pain or sports injuries. But every obstacle that you overcome, large or small, can make you feel incredible. Enjoy the journey! We thank you for being a part of ours!

Ross and Marion Hauser
The Doctor and the Dietitian®

REFERENCES

CHAPTER 1
WHY SHOULD YOU CONSIDER PROLOTHERAPY?

1. Hackett G, et al. *Ligament and Tendon Relaxation Treated by Prolotherapy.* Third Edition. Springfield, IL: Charles C. Thomas, 1958, pp. 5.

2. Babcock P, et al. *Webster's Third New International Dictionary.* Springfield, MA: G. & C. Merriam Co., 1971. pp. 1815.

3. Benajmin M, et al. The "enthesis organ" concept. Why enthesopathies may not present as focal insertional disorders. *Arthritis Rheum.* 2004;50:3306-13.

4. Slobodin G, et al. Varied presentations of enthesopathy. *Seminars in Arthritis and Rheum.* 2007;37:119-126.

5. Shaibani A et al. The significance of enthesopathy as a skeletal phenomenon. *Clin Exp Rheum.* 1993; 11:399-403.

6. Corrao G, et al. Evidence of tendinitis provoked by fluoroquinolone treatment: a case-control study. *Drug Safety.* 2006;29:889-96.

7. Blanco I, et al. Corticosteroid-associated tendinopathies: an analysis of the published literature and spontaneous pharmacovigilance data. *Drug Safety.* 2005;28:633-43.

8. Haradsson BT, et al. Corticosteroids reduce the tensile strength of isolated collagen fascicles. *American Journal of Sports Medicine.* 2006;34:1992-7.

9. Browner B. *Skeletal Trauma.* Volume 1. Philadelphia, PA: W.B. Saunders, 1992, pp. 87-88.

10. Deese J. Compressive neuropathies of the lower extremity. *Journal of Musculoskeletal Medicine.* 1988; November: 68-91.

11. Wheaton MT, et al. The ligament injury-osteoarthritis connection: the role of prolotherapy in ligament repair and the prevention of osteoarthritis. *J Prolotherapy.* 2011;3(4):790-812.

12. The diagnosis and management of soft tissue knee injuries: internal derangements. Best practice evidence-based guideline. New Zealand Guidelines Group Incorporated. 2002. Available at: http://www.acc.co.nz/PRD_EXT_CSMP/groups/external_communications/documents/guide/wcmz002488.pdf

13. Hauser RA, et al. Structural basis of joint instability as cause for chronic musculoskeletal pain and its successful treatment with regenerative injection therapy (Prolotherapy). *The Open Pain Journal.* 2014;7:9-22.

14. Rhalmi S, et al. Immunohistochemical study of nerves in lumbar spine ligaments. *Spine.* 1993;18:264-267.

15. Ahmed M, et al. Neuropeptide Y, tyrosine hydroxylase and vasoactive intestinal polypeptide-immunoreactive nerve fibers in the vertebral bodies, discs, dura matter, and spinal ligaments of the rat lumbar spine. *Spine.* 1993;18(2):268-273.

16. Hackett G, et al. *Ligament and Tendon Relaxation Treated by Prolotherapy.* Fifth Edition. Oak Park, IL: Gustav A Hemwall, Publisher, 1993, pp. 20.

17. Robbins S. *Pathologic Basis of Disease.* Third Edition. Philadelphia, PA: W.B. Saunders, 1984, p. 40.

CHAPTER 2
PROLOTHERAPY, INFLAMMATION, AND HEALING: WHAT'S THE CONNECTION?

1. Bruckner P. *Clinical Sports Medicine.* NY, NY. McGraw-Hill Book Company. 1995, pp 105-109.

2. Mirkin G. Why ice delays recovery. Available at: http://www.drmirkin.com/fitness/why-ice-delays-recovery.html. Accessed on April 28, 2016.

3. Greene J. Cost-conscious prescribing of nonsteroidal anti-inflammatory drugs for adults with arthritis. *Archives of Internal Medicine.* 1992;152:1995-2002.

4. Robbins S. *Pathologic Basis of Disease.* Third Edition. Philadelphia, PA: W.B. Saunders, 1984, p. 40.

5. Greenfield B. *Rehabilitation of the Knee: A Problem-Solving Approach.* Philadelphia, PA: F.A. Davis, 1993.

6. Woo S. Injury and repair of the musculoskeletal soft tissues. *American Academy of Orthopaedic Surgeons.* 1987.

7. Mankin H. Localization of tritiated thymidine in articular cartilage of rabbits inhibits growth in immature cartilage. *Journal of Bone and Joint Surgery.* 1962;44A:682.

8. Robbins S. *Pathologic Basis of Disease.* Third Edition. Philadelphia, PA: W.B. Saunders, 1984, p. 40.

9. Benedetti R. Clinical results of simultaneous adjacent interdigital neurectomy in the foot. *Foot and Ankle International.* 1996;17:264-268.

10. Salter R. The effects of continuous compression on living articular cartilage. An experimental investigation. *Journal of Bone and Joint Surgery.* 1960;42A:31.

11. Salter R. The pathological changes in articular cartilage associated with persistent joint deformity: an experimental investigation. In Gordon, D. (ed.), *Studies of Rheumatoid Disease: Proceedings of the Third Canadian Conference on Research in the Rheumatic Diseases.* Toronto: University of Toronto Press, 1965, p. 33.

12. Kuettner K. *Articular Cartilage and Osteoarthritis.* New York, NY: Raven Press, 1992.

13. Salter R. The biological concept of continuous passive motion of synovial joints. *Clinical Orthopaedics and Related Research.* 1989;242:12-25

14. Salter R. Continuous passive motion and the repair of full-thickness defects—a one-year follow-up (Abstract). *Orthop. Trans.* 1982;6:266.

15. Salter R. The healing of intra-articular fractures with continuous passive motion. In Copper R. (ed.) *American Academy of Orthopaedic Surgeons Instructional Course Lectures.* St. Louis, MO: C.V. Mosby, 1979.

16. Palmoski M. Effects of some nonsteroidal anti-inflammatory drugs on proteoglycan metabolism and organization in canine articular cartilage. *Arthritis and Rheumatism.* 1980;23:1010-1020.

17. Bleakley C, et al. The use of ice in the treatment of acute soft-tissue injury: a systematic review of randomized controlled trials. *Am J Sport Med.* 2004;32:251–261.

18. Newton P. The effect of lifelong exercise on canine articular cartilage. *American Journal of Sports Medicine.* 1997;25:282-287.

19. Tornkvist H. Effect of ibuprofen and indomethacin on bone metabolism reflected in bone strength. *Clinical Orthopedics.* 1984;187:225.

20. Lindholm T. Ibuprofen: effect on bone formation and calcification exerted by the anti-inflammatory drug ibuprofen. *Scandinavian Journal of Rheumatology.* 1981;10:38.

21. Williams R. Ibuprofen: an inhibitor of alveolar bone resorption in beagles. *J. Periodont. Res.* 1988;23:225.

22. Tornkvist H. Effect of ibuprofen and indomethacin on bone metabolism reflected in bone strength. *Clinical Orthopedics.* 1984;187:225.

23. Obeid G. Effect of ibuprofen on the healing and remodeling of bone and articular cartilage in the rabbit temporomandibular joint. *Journal of Maxillofacial Surgery.* 1992, pp. 843-849.

24. Brandt K. The effects of salicylates and other nonsteroidal anti-inflammatory drugs on articular cartilage. *American Journal of Medicine.* 1984;77:65-69.

25. Palmoski M. Effect of salicylate on proteoglycan metabolism in normal canine articular cartilage in vitro. *Arthritis and Rheumatism.* 1979;22:746-754.

26. Palmoski M. Marked suppression by salicylate of the augmented proteoglycan synthesis in osteoarthritic cartilage. *Arthritis and Rheumatism.* 1980;23:83-91.

27. Hugenberg S. Suppression by nonsteroidal anti-inflammatory drugs on proteoglycan synthesis in articular cartilage. *Arthritis and Rheumatism.* 1992;35:R29.

28. Brandt K. Should osteoarthritis be treated with nonsteroidal anti-inflammatory drugs? *Rheumatic Disease Clinics of North America.* 1993;19:697-712.

29. Palmoski M. In vitro effect of aspirin on canine osteoarthritic cartilage. *Arthritis and Rheumatism.* 1983;26:994-1001.

30. Coke H. Long-term indomethacin therapy of coxarthrosis. *Annals of Rheumatic Diseases.* 1967; 26:346-347.

31. Solomon L. Drug-induced arthropathy and neurosis of the femoral head. *Journal of Bone and Joint Surgery (Britian).* 1973;55:246-261.

32. Newman N. Acetabular bone destruction related to nonsteroidal anti-inflammatory drugs. *Lancet.* 1985;2:11-14.

33. Rashad S. Effects of nonsteroidal anti-inflammatory drugs on the course of osteoarthritis. *Lancet.* 1989;2:519-522.

34. Huskisson HC, et al. Effects of anti-inflammatory drugs on the progression of osteoarthritis of the knee. *Journal of Rheumatology.* 1995;22:1941-1946.

35. Williams K. Evidence on NSAID use in soft tissue injuries. *Nursing Times.* 2012;108:12-14.

36. Connizzo B, et al. The detrimental effects of systemic Ibuprofen delivery on tendon healing are time-dependent. *J Bone Joint Surg Am.* 2003;85:1914-20.

37. van Esch R. NSAIDs can have adverse effects on bone healing. *Med Hypotheses.* 2013;81:343-6.

38. Hauser R. The acceleration of articular cartilage degeneration in osteoarthritis by non steroidal anti-inflammatory drugs. *Journal of Prolotherapy.* 2010;(2)1:305-322.

39. Gossec L, et al. Predictive factors of total hip replacement due to primary osteoarthritis: a prospective 2 year study of 505 patients. *Annals of Rheumatic Diseases.* 2005;64:1028-1032.

40. Hauser R. Degeneration of articular cartilage in osteoarthritis by corticosteroid injections. *Journal of Prolotherapy.* 2009;2:107-123.

41. Wrenn R. An experimental study on the effect of cortisone on the healing process and tensile strength of tendons. *Journal of Bone and Joint Surgery.* 1954;36A:588-601.

42. Truhan A. Corticosteroids: a review with emphasis on complication of prolonged systemic therapy. *Annals of Allergy.* 1989;62:375-390.

43. Roenigk R. *Dermatologic Surgery.* Marcel Dekker, Inc., p. 155.

44. Davis G. Adverse effects of corticosteroids. *Systemic Clinical Dermatology.* 1986;4:161-169.

45. Gogia P. Hydrocortisone and exercise effects on articular cartilage in rats. *Archives of Physical Medicine and Rehabilitation.* 1993;74:463-467.

46. Chandler G. Deleterious effect of intra-articular hydrocortisone. *Lancet.* 1958;2:661-663.

47. Chunekamrai S. Changes in articular cartilage after intra-articular injections of methylprednisolone acetate in horses. *American Journal of Veterinary Research.* 1989;50:1733-1741.

48. Pool R. Corticosteroid therapy in common joint and tendon injuries of the horse: effect on joints. *Proceedings of the American Association of Equine Practice.* 1980;26:397-406.

49. From personal correspondence between the authors and Michael Herron, DVM.

50. Scutt N, et al. Glucocorticoids inhibit tenocyte proliferation and tendon progenitor cell recruitment. *J Orthop Res.* 2006 Feb;24(2):173-82.

51. Zhang J, et al. The effects of dexamethasone on human patellar tendon stem cells: implications for dexamethasone treatment of tendon injury. *J Orthop Res.* 2013;31(1):105-10.

52. Coombes BK. Efficacy and safety of corticosteroid injections and other injections for management of tendinopathy: a systematic review of randomised controlled trials. *Lancet.* 2010; 376:1751-67.

53. Borowsky CD. Sources of sacroiliac region pain: insights gained from a study comparing standard intra-articular injection with a technique combining intra- and peri-articular injection. *Arch Phys Med Rehabil.* 2008;89:2048-56.

54. Wong MW. Dexamethasone significantly decreased cell viability, suppressed cell proliferation, and reduced collage synthesis in cultured human tenoccytes. *J Rheumatol.* 2005;32(2):307-19.

55. Behrens F. Alteration of rabbit articular cartilage of intra-articular injections of glucocorticoids. *Journal of Bone and Joint Surgery.* 1975;57A:70-76.

56. Eklhom R. On the relationship between articular changes and function. *Acta Ortho. Scand.* 1951; 21:81-98.

57. Lanier R. Effects of exercise on the knee joints of inbred mice. *Anat. Rec.* 1946;94:311-319.

58. Saaf J. Effects of exercise on articular cartilage. *Acta Ortho. Scand.* 1950;20:1-83.

59. Gogia P. Hydrocortisone and exercise effects on articular cartilage in rats. *Archives of Physical Medicine and Rehabilitation.* 1993;74:463-467.

CHAPTER 3

CELLULAR PROLOTHERAPY

1. Murphy J, et al. Reduced chondrogenic and adipogenic activity of mesenchymal stem cells from patients with advance osteoarthritis. *Arthritis Rheumatology.* 2002;46:704-13.

2. Luyten F. Mesenchymal stem cells in osteoarthritis. *Current Opinion in Rheumatology.* 2004;16:559-603.

3. Pittenger MF, et al. Multilineage potential of adult human mesenchymal stem cells. *Science.* 1999;284:143-147.

4. Yoo JU, et al. The chondrogenic potential of human bone-marrow-derived mesenchymal progenitor cells. *American Journal of Bone and Joint Surgery.* 1998;80:1745-1757.

5. Rios C, et al. Biologics in shoulder surgery: the role of adult mesenchymal stem cells in tendon repair. *Techniques in Orthopaedics.* 2007;22(1)2-9.

6. Uysal AC, et al. Tendon regeneration and repair with adipose derived stem cells. *Current Stem Cell Research and Therapy.* 2010;5(2):161-167.

7. Little D, et al. Ligament derived matrix stimulates a ligamentous phenotype in human adipose-derived stem cells. *Tissue Engineering Part A.* 2010;15(7):2307-2319.

8. Pereira RF, et al. Marrow stromal cells as a source of progenitor cells for nonhematopoietic tissues in transgenic mice with a phenotype of osteogenesis imperfecta. *Proceedings of the National Academy of Sciences.* 1998;95:1142-1147.

9. Hoffstetter CP, et al. Marrow stromal cells from guiding strands in the injured spinal cord and promote recovery. *Proceedings of the National Academy of Sciences.* 2002;99:2199-2204.

10. Ma T. Mesenchymal stem cells: from bench to bedside. *World Journal of Stem Cells.* 2010;2(2):13-17.

11. Mishra, et al. Buffered platelet-rich plasma enhances mesenchymal stem cell proliferation and chondrogenic differentiation. *Tissue Engineering, Part C.* 2009;15(3).

12. Kakudo N, et al. Proliferation-promoting effect of platelet-rich plasma on human adipose-derived stem cells and human dermal fibroblasts. *Plastic & Reconstructive Surgery.* 2008;122(5):1352-1360.

13. Tatebe M. Differentiation of transplanted mesenchymal stem cells in large osteochondral defect in rabbit. *Cytotherapy.* 2005;7:520-530.

14. Edwards SG, et al. Autologous blood injections for refractory lateral epicondylitis. *Journal of Hand Surg (Am).* 2003;28:272-8.

15. Raeissadat SA, et al. Effect of platelet-rich plasma versus autologous whole blood on pain and function improvement in tennis elbow: a randomized clinical trial. *Pain Res Treat.* 2014;2014:191525. Doi: 10.1155/2014/191525. Epub 2014 Jan 2.

16. Kazemi M, et al. Autologous blood versus corticosteroid local injection in the short-term treatment of elbow tendinopathy: a randomized clinical trial of efficacy. *American Journal of Physical Medicine and Rehabilitation.* 2010;89:660-667.

17. Candrili C, et al. Autologous blood injection to the temporomandibular joint: magnetic resonance imagining findings. *Imaging Sci Dent.* 2012;42:13-8.

18. Candrili C, et al. The effect of chronic temporomandibular joint dislocation: frequence on the success of autologous blood injection. *Maxillofac Oral Surg.* 2013;12:414-7.

19. Foster T, et al. Platelet-rich plasma: from basic science to clinical applications. *The American Journal of Sports Medicine.* 2009;37(11):2259-2272.

20. Haynesworth SE, et al. Mitogenic stimulation of human mesenchymal stem cells by platlet release suggest a mechanism for enhancement of bone repair by platelet concentrates. Presented at the 48th meeting of the Orthopedic Research Society, Boston, MA 2002.

21. Marx R, et al. Platelet rich plasma (PRP): a primer. *Practical Pain Management.* March 2008;8(2):46-47.

22. Hall M, et al. Platelet-rich plasma: current concepts and application in sports medicine. *Journal of the American Academy of Orthopedic Surgeons.* 2009;27:602-608.

23. Marx R. Platelet-rich plasma: evidence to support its use. *J Oral Maxillofac Surg.* 2004;62:489-96.

24. Caplan A, et al. Mesenchymal stem cells and tissue repair. In: *The Anterior Cruciate Ligament: Current and Future Concepts.* Ed. By DW Jackson. New York, Raven press, 1993, p. 405-417.

25. Rigotti G, et al. Adipose-derived mesenchymal stem cells: past, present and future. *Aesth Plast Surg.* 2009;33:271-273.

26. Fraser J, et al. Fat tissue: an underappreciated source of stem cells for biotechnology. *Trends Biotechol.* 2006;24:150-154.

27. Santiago L, et al. Delivery of adipose-derived precursor cells for peripheral nerve repair. *Cell Transplant.* 2009;18(2):145-58.

28. Wakitani S, et al. Mesenchymal cell-based repair of large, full-thickness defects of articular cartilage. *J. Bone Joint Surg.* (Am) 1994;76:579-592.

29. Wakitani S, et al. Human autologous culture expanded bone marrow mesenchymal cell transplantation for repair of cartilage defects in osteoarthritic knees. *Osteoarthritis Cartilage.* 2002;10:199-206.

30. Murphy J, et al. Stem cell therapy in a caprine model of osteoarthritis. *Arthritis Rheum.* 2003;48:3464-3474.

31. Centeno C, et al. Increased knee cartilage volume in degenerative joint disease using percutaneously implanted, autologous mesenchymal stem cells. *Pain Physician.* 2008;11:3:343-353.

32. Albano J, et al. Autologous fat grafting as mesenchymal stem cell source and living bioscaffold in a patellar tendon tear: a case report. *Clinical J Sports Medicine.* 2011 Jul;21(4):359-61.

33. Alderman D, et al. Stem cell Prolotherapy in regenerative medicine: background, theory and protocols. *Journal of Prolotherapy.* 2011;3(3):689-708.

34. Alderman D, et al. Advances in regenerative medicine: high-density platelet rich plasma and stem cell Prolotherapy for musculoskeletal pain. *Practical Pain Management.* Oct 2011;11(8).

35. Izadpanah R, et al. Biologic properties of mesenchymal stem cells derived from bone marrow and adipose tissue. *J Cell Biochem.* 2006;99:1285-1297.

36. Kern S, et al. Comparative analysis of mesenchymal stem cells from bone marrow, umbelicial cord blood or adipose tissue. *Stem Cells.* 2006;24:1294-1301.

37. Strem B, et al. Multipotential differentiation of adipose tissue-derived stem cells. *Keio J Med.* 2005;54:132-139.

38. Prockop D, et al. *Mesenchymal Stem Cells, Methods and Protocols.* Humana Press, a part of Springer Science, NJ. 2008.

39. Chen X, et al. Tendon tissue engineering with mesenchymal stem cells and biografts: an option for large tendon defects? *Front Biosci (School Ed).* 2009 Jun;1:1:23-32.

40. Uysal A, et al. Differentiation of adipose-derived stem cells for tendon repair. *Methods Mol Biol.* 2011;702:443-51.

41. Jung M, et al. Enhanced early tissue regeneration after matrix-assisted autologous mesenchymal stem cell transplantation in full thickness chondral defects in a minipig model. *Cell Transplantation.* 2009;18(8):923-932.

42. Lee K, et al. Injectable mesenchymal stem cell therapy for large cartilage defects-a porcine model. *Stem Cells.* 2007;25:2965-2971.

43. Dragoo J, et al. Tissue-engineered cartilage and bone using stem cells from human infrapatellar fat pads. *J. Bone Joint Surg. Br.* 2003;85:740-747.

44. Hsu W, et al. Stem cells from human fat as cellular delivery vehicles in an athymic rat posterolateral spine fusion model. *J. Bone Joint Surg. Am.* 2008;90:1043-1052.

45. Bacou F, et al. Transplantation of adipose tissue-derived stromal cells increases mass and functional capacity of damaged skeletal muscle. *Cell Transplant.* 2004;13:103-111.

46. Rodriguez L, et al. Clonogenic multipotent stem cells in human adipose tissue differentiate into functional smooth muscle cells. *Proc Natl Acad Sci USA.* 2006;108:12167–12172.

47. Goudenege S, et al. Enhancement of myogenic and muscle repair capacities of human adipose-derived stem cells with forced expression of MyoD. *Mol Ther.* 2009;17:1064–1072.

48. Di Summa P, et al. Adipose-derived stem cells enhance peripheral nerve regeneration. *J. Plast Reconstr Aesthet Surg.* 2010 Sept;63(9):1544-52.

49. Nakada A, et al. Regeneration of central nervous tissue using a collagen scaffold and adipose-derived stromal cells. *Cells Tissues Organs.* 2009;190:326–335.

50. Cowan C, et al. Adipose-derived adult stromal cells heal critical-size mouse calvarial defects. *Nat. Biotechnol.* 2004;22:560–567.

51. Dudas J, et al. The osteogenic potential of adipose-derived stem cells for the repair of rabbit calvarial defects. *Ann. Plast. Surg.* 2006;56:543–548.

Yoon E, et al. In vivo osteogenic potential of human adipose-derived stem cells/poly lactide-co-glycolic acid constructs for bone regeneration in a rat critical-sized calvarial defect model. *Tissue Eng.* 2007;13:619–627.

52. Rosenbaum A, et al. The use of mesenchymal stem cells in tissue engineering: a global assessment. *Organogenesis.* 2008 Jan-Mar;4(1):23-37.

53. Cousin B, et al. Reconstitution of lethally irradiated mice by cells isolated from adipose tissue. *Biochem Biophys Res Commun.* 2003;21:1016–1022.

54. Puissant B, et al. Immunomodulatory effect of human adipose tissue-derived adult stem cells: comparison with bone marrow mesenchymal stem cells. *Br. J. Haematol.* 2005;129:118–129.

55. Kim W, et al. Wound healing effect of adipose-derived stem cells: a critical role of secretory factors on human dermal fibroblasts. *J Dermatol Sci.* 2007 Oct;48(1):15-24.

56. Ebrahimian T, et al. Cell therapy based on adipose tissue-derived stromal cells promotes physiological and pathological wound healing. *Arterioscler Thromb Vasc Biol.* 2009;29(4):503-510.

57. Trottier V, et al. IFATS collection: using human adipose-derived stem/stromal cells for the production of new skin substitutes. *Stem Cell.* 2008;26:2713–2723.

58. Connoly J, et al. Development of an osteogenic bone-marrow preparation. *Journal of Bone and Joint Surgery America.* 1989;71:684-691.

59. Gangji V, et al. Treatment of osteonecrosis of the femoral head with implantation of autologous bone-marrow cells. *A pilot study. Journal of Bone and Joint Surgery America.* 2004;86A:1153-1160.

60. Hernigou P, et al. Treatment of osteonecrosis with autologous bone marrow grafting. *Clinical Orthopaedic and Related Research.* 2002;14-23.

61. Hernigou P, et al. Percutaneous atulogous bone-marrow grafting for nonunions. Influence of the number and concentration of progenitor cells. *Journal of Bone and Joint Surgery America.* 2005;87:1430-1437.

62. Hernigou P, et al. The use of percutaneous autologous bone marrow transplantation in nonunion and avascular necrosis of bone. *Journal of Bone and Joint Surgery British.* 2005;87:896-902.

63. McLain R, et al. Aspiration of osteoprogenitor cells for augmenting spinal fusion: comparison of progenitor cell concentrations from the vertebral body and iliac crest. *Journal of Bone and Joint Surgery America.* 2005;87:2655-2661.

64. Muschler G, et al. Spine fusion using cell matrix composites enriched in bone marrow-derived cells. *Clinical Orthopedics and Related Research.* 2003;102-118.

65. Kevy S, et al. Point of care concentration of bone marrow. In: *Orthopedic Research Society.* Chicago Illinois: 2006.

66. Muschler G, et al. Aspiration to obtain osteoblast progenitor cells from human bone marrow: the influence of aspiration volume. *Journal of Bone and Joint Surgery.* 1997;70A:1699-1709.

67. Connoly J. Injectable bone marrow preparations to stimulate osteogenic repair. *Clinical Orthopaedics and Related Research.* 1995;313:8-18.

68. Shenaq D, et al. Mesenchymal progenitor cells and their orthopedic applications: forging a path towards clinical trials. *Stem Cell International.* 2010;519028. doi:10.4061/2010/519028.

69. Chanda D, et al. Therapeutic potential of adult bone marrow-derived mesenchymal stem cells in diseases of the skeleton. *Journal of Cellular Biology.* 2010;111:249-257.

70. Vats A, et al. The stem cell in orthopaedic surgery. *The Journal of Bone and Joint Surgery British.* 2004;86B:159-164.

71. Muschler G, et al. Selective retention of bone marrow-derived cells to enhance spinal fusion. *Clinical Orthopedics and Related Research.* 2005;432:242-251.

72. Pittenger M, et al. Multilineage potential of adult human mesenchymal stem cells. *Science.* 1999;284(5411):143-147.

Caplan A, et al. Mesenchymal stem cells and tissue repair. In: *The Anterior Cruciate Ligament: Current and Future Concepts.* Jackson DW (ed). Raven Press. New York. 1993. pp 405-417.

73. Young R, et al. Use of mesenchymal stem cells in a collagen matrix for Achilles tendon repair. *J. Orthop Res.* 1998;16:406-413.

74. Fortier L, et al. Concentrated bone marrow aspirate improves full-thickness cartilage repair compared with microfracture in the equine model. *Journal of Bone and Joint Surgery America.* 2010;92:1927-1937.

75. Im G, et al. Do adipose tissue-derived mesenchymal stem cells have the same osteogenic and chondrogenic potential as bone marrow-derived cells? Osteoarthritis Cartilage/OARS. *Osteoarthritis Research Society.* 2005;13:845-853.

76. Afizah H, et al. A comparison between the chondrogenic potential of human bone marrow stem cells and adipose-derived stem cells taken from the same donors. *Tissue Engineering.* 2007;13:659-666.

77. Huang J, et al. Chondrogenic potential of progenitor cells derived from human bone marrow and a patient-matched comparison. *Journal of Orthopedic Research.* 2005;23:1383-1389.

78. Winter A, et al. Cartilage-like gene expression in differentiated human stem cell spheroids: a comparison of bone marrow-derived and adipose tissue-derived stromal cells. *Arthritis and Rheumatism.* 2003;48:418-429.

79. Diekman B, et al. Chondrogenesis of adult stem cells from adipose tissue and bone marrow: induction by growth factors and cartilage-derived matrix. *Tissue Engineering: Part A.* 2010;16:523-533.

80. Bernardo M, et al. Human mesenchymal stem cells derived from bone marrow display a better chondrogenic differentiation compared with other sources. *Connective Tissue Research.* 2007;48:132-140.

81. Khan S, et al. Bone growth factors. *Orthopedic Clinics of North America.* 2000;31:375-388.

82. Muschler G, et al. Practical modeling concepts for connective tissue stem cell and progenitor compartment kinetics. *Journal of Biomedical Biotechnology*. 2003;170-193.

83. Bruder S, et al. Mesenchymal stem cells in osteobiology and applied bone regeneration. *Clinical Orthopaedics and Related Research*. 1998;355S:S247-S256.

84. Granero-Molto F, et al. Role of mesenchymal stem cells in regenerative medicine: application to bone and cartilage repair. *Cell & Tissue-based Therapy*. 2008;255-268.

85. Clark B, et al. Biology of bone marrow stroma. *Annals of New York Academy of Sciences*. 1995;770:70-78.

86. Hauser RA. et al. Treating osteoarthritic joints using dextrose Prolotherapy and direct bone marrow aspirate injection therapy. *The Open Arthritis Journal*. 2014;7:1-9.

87. Hauser RA. et al. Regenerative injection therapy with whole bone marrow aspirate for degenerative joint disease: A case series. *Clinical Medicine Insights: Arthritis and Musculoskeletal Disorders*. 2013;6:65–72.

CHAPTER 4

PROLO YOUR BACK PAIN AWAY!

1. Katz J. A randomized, placebo controlled trial of bupropion sustained release in chronic low back pain. *J Pain*. 2005;6:656-661.

2. Assendelft W. Spinal manipulative therapy for low back pain. A meta-analysis of effectiveness relative to other therapies. *Ann Intern Med*. 2003;138:871-881.

3. Cherkin DC. A review of the evidence for the effectiveness, safety, and cost of acupuncture, massage therapy, and spinal manipulation for back pain. *Ann Intern Med*. 2003;138:898-906.

4. Freeman B. Intradiscal electrothermal therapy versus placebo for the treatment of chronic discogenic low back pain. *Spine*. 2005;30:2369-2377.

5. Turner J, et al. Patient outcomes after lumbar spinal fusions. *JAMA*. 1992;286(7):907-910.

6. Schwarzer AC, et al. The sacroiliac joint in chronic low back pain. *Spine*. 1995;20(1):31-37.

7. Jensen MC, et al. Magnetic resonance imaging of the lumbar spine in people without back pain. *New Engl J Med*. 1994;331(2);69-73.

8. Weiner BK, et al. The accuracy of MRI in the detection of Lumbar disc containment. *Journal of Orthopaedic Surgery and Research*. 20083:46. DOI: 10.1186/1749-799X-3-46.

9. Jensen M. Magnetic resonance imaging of the lumbar spine in people without back pain. *New England Journal of Medicine*. 1994;331:69-73.

10. Hackett,G. Shearing injury to the sacroiliac joint. *Journal of the International College of Surgeons*. 1954;22:631-639.

11. Bellamy N. What do we know about the sacroiliac joint? *Seminars in Arthritis and Rheumatism*. 1983;12:282-313.

12. Paris S. Physical signs of instability. *Spine*. 1985;10:277-279.

13. Schwartz R. Prolotherapy: a literature review and retrospective study. *Journal of Orthopaedic Medicine and Surgery*. 1991;12:220-223.

14. Hauser RA, et al. Evidence-based use of dextrose Prolotherapy for musculoskeletal pain: a scientific literature review. *Journal of Prolotherapy*. 2011;3(4):765-789.

15. Hauser RA, et al. Dextrose Prolotherapy for unresolved low back pain: a retrospective case series study. *Journal of Prolotherapy*. 2009;1(3):145-155.

16. Steuer J, et al. Quantitative radiologic criteria for the diagnosis of lumbar spinal stenosis: a systematic literature review. *BMC Musculoskeletal Disorders*. 2011;12:175. Doi:10.1186/1471-2474-12-175.

17. Mueller R. *Anesthesia in Current Surgical Diagnosis and Treatment*. Seventh Edition. Los Altos, CA: 1983, pp. 162-169.

18. Modic MT, et al. Lumbar degenerative disk disease. *Radiology*. 2007;245(1):43-61.

19. Burton, C. Conservative management of low back pain. *Postgraduate Medicine*. 5:168-183.

20. Blackley HR, et al. Determining the sagittal dimensions of the canal of the cervical spine. The reliability of ratios of anatomical measurements. *J Bone Joint Surg British.* 1999 Jan;81(1):110-112.

21. Moskovich R, et al. Does the cervical canal to body ratio predict spinal stenosis? *Bull Hosp Jt Dis.* 1996;55(2):61-71.

22. Merriman J. Prolotherapy versus operative fusion in the treatment of joint instability of the spine and pelvis. *Journal of the International College of Surgeons.* 1964;42:150-159.

23. U.S. Preventive Services Task Force. Screening for adolescent idiopathic scoliosis. *Journal of the American Medical Association.* 1993;269:2667-2672.

24. Gunnoe BA. Adolescent idiopathic scoliosis. *Orthopaedic Review.* 1990;19:35-43.

25. Scoliosis Research Society. Conditions and Treatment. Available at: http://www.srs.org/patients-and-families/conditions-and-treatments/parents/scoliosis/adolescent-idiopathic-scoliosis. Accessed October 20, 2016.

26. Winter R. Pain patterns in adult scoliosis. *Orthopedic Clinics of North America.* 1988;19:339-345.

27. Mengert W. Referred pelvic pain. *Southern Medical Journal.* 1943;36:256-263.

28. Pitikin H. Sacrathrogenetic telagia, part two: a study of referred pain. *Journal of Bone and Joint Surgery.* 1936;18:365-374.

29. Traycoff R. Sacrococcygeal pain syndromes: diagnosis and treatment. *Orthopedics.* 1989;12:1373-1377.

CHAPTER 5

PROLO YOUR HEAD AND NECK PAIN AWAY!

1. Hauser RA, et al. Chronic neck pain: making the connection between capsular ligament laxity and cervical instability. *The Open Orthopaedics Journal.* 2014;8:326-345.

2. Frank CB. Ligament structure, physiology, and function. *J Musculoskelet Neuronal Interact.* 2004;4(2):199-201.

3. Winkelstein BA, et al. An intact facet capsular ligament modulates behavioral sensitivity and spinal glial activation produced by cervical facet joint tension. *Spine* (Phila Pa 1976). 2008;33(8):856-62.

4. Stemper BD, et al. Effects of abnormal posture on capsular ligament elongations in a computational model subjected to whiplash loading. *J Biomech Eng.* 2005; 38(6): 1313-23.

5. Ivancic PC, et al. Whiplash causes increased laxity of cervical capsular ligament. *Clin Biomech.* 2008;23(2):159-65.

6. Bellamy N. What do we know about the sacroiliac joint? *Seminars in Arthritis and Rheumatism.* 1983;12:282-313.

7. Hauser RA, et al. Dextrose Prolotherapy for recurring headache and migraine pain. *Practical Pain Management.* 2009 Jun;58-65.

8. Dextrose Prolotherapy for unresolved neck pain. *Practical Pain Management.* 2007 Oct;56-69.

9. Hauser RA. The biology of Prolotherapy and its application in clinical cervical spine instability and chronic neck pain: a retrospective study. *European Journal of Preventive Medicine.* 2015:3(4):85-102. doi: 10.11648/j.ejpm.20150304.1.

10. Barré J. Le syndrome sympathique cervical postérieur et sa cause frequent l'arthrite cervicale. *Rev. Neurol.* 33:1246–1254.

11. Tamura T. Cranial symptoms after cervical injury—aetiology and treatment of the Barré-Lieou Syndrome. *Journal of Bone and Joint Surgery.* 1989;71B:283-287.

12. Bland J. *Disorders of the Cervical Spine.* Philadelphia, PA: W.B. Saunders, 1987.

13. Qian J, et al. Dynamic radiographic analysis of sympathetic cervical spondulosis instability. *Chinese Medical Sciences Journal.* 2008;24(1):46-49.

14. Kayfetz D. Occipito-cervical (whiplash) injuries treated by Prolotherapy. *Meidcal Trial Technique Quarterly.* 1963 June;9-29.

15. Claussen,CF, et al. Neurootological contributions to the diagnostic follow-up after whiplash injuries. *Acta Otolaryngology (Stockh).* 1995; Suppl. 520:53-56.

16. Hauser RA, et al. Cervical instability as a cause of Barré-Lieou syndrome and definitive treatment with Prolotherapy: a case series. *European Journal of Preventive Medicine.* 2015;3(5):155-166. doi: 10.11648/j.ejpm.20150305.1.

17. Hackett G. Prolotherapy for headache. *Headache.* 1962;1:3-11.

18. Hackett G. Prolotherapy in whiplash and low back pain. *Postgraduate Medicine.* 1960, pp. 214-219.

19. Kayfetz D. Whiplash injury and other ligamentous headache—its management with Prolotherapy. *Headache.* 1963;3:1-8.

20. Merriman J. Presentation at the Hackett Foundation Prolotherapy meeting, Indianapolis, IN, October 1995.

21. Cook C, et al. Identifiers Suggestive of Clinical Cervical Spine Instability: A Delphi Study of Physical Therapists. *Journal of the American Physical Therapy Association.* 2005;85:895-906.

22. Meadows J, et al. *Cervical Spine. Orthopedic Physical Assessment.* 5 ed. Saunders Elsevier; 2008. pp. 17-44.

23. Hino H, et al. Dynamic motion analysis of normal and unstable cervical spines using cineradiography. An in vivo study. *Spine.* 1999;15(24):163-168.

24. Dvorak J, et al. Functional diagnostics of the cervical spine used computer tomography. *Neuroradiology.* 1988;30:132-137.

25. Radcliff K, et al. CT and MRI-based diagnosis of craniocervical dislocations: the role of the occipitoatlantal ligament. *Clinical Orthopedics and Related Reserach.* 2012;470(6):1602-1613.

26. Antinnes J, et al. The value of functional computed tomography in the evaluation of soft-tissue injury in the upper cervical spine. *European Spine Journal.* 1994;3:98-101.

27. Bogduk N, et al. The cervical zygapophysial joints as a source of neck pain. *Spine.* 1988;13(6):610-617.

28. Manchikanti L, et al. Prevalence of facet joint pain in chronic spinal pain of cervical, thoracic, and lumbar regions. *BMC Musculoskeletal Disorders.* 2004;5(15).

29. Peh W. Image-guided facet joint injection. *Biomedical Imaging and Intervention Journal.* 2011;7(1).

30. Hauser RA, et al. Upper cervical instability of traumatic origin treated with dextrose Prolotherapy: a case report. *Journal of Prolotherapy.* 2015;7:e932-e935.

31. Leddy J, et al. Rehabilitation of concussion and post-concussion syndrome. *Sports Health: A Multidisciplinary Approach.* 2012;4(2):147-154.

32. Winkelstein B, et al. The cervical facet capsule and its role in whiplash injury: a biomechanical investigation. *Spine.* 2000;25(10):1238-1246.

33. Siegmund GP, et al. Head-turned postures increase the risk of cervical facet capsule injury during whiplash. *Spine* (Phila PA 1976). 2008;33(15):1643-9.

34. Storvik SG, et al. Axial head rotation increases facet joint capsular ligament strains in automotive rear impact. *Med Bio Eng Comput.* 2011;49(2):153-61.

35. Kubala M, et al. Diagnosis, pathogenesis, and treatment of "drop attacks." *JAMA Neurology.* 1964;11(2):107-113.

36. Hauser RA, et al. Non-operative treatment of cervical radiculopathy: a three part article from the approach of a physiatrist, chiropractor, and physical therapist. *JOP.* 2009;1(4):217-231.

37. Darnell M. A proposed chronology of events for forward-head posture. *Journal of Craniomandibular Practice.* 1983;1:49-54.

38. Rocabado M. Biomechanical relationship of the cranial, cervical and hyoid regions. *Physical Therapy.* 1983;1:62-66.

39. Schultz L. A treatment for subluxation of the temporomandibular joint. *Journal of the American Medical Association.* September 25, 1937, pp. 1032-1035.

40. Schultz L. Twenty years' experience in treating hypermobility of the temporomandibular joints. *American Journal of Surgery.* 1956;92:925-928.

41. Hauser RA, et al. Evidence-based use of dextrose Prolotherapy for musculoskeletal pain. *JOP.* 2011;3(4):765-789.

42. Hakala R. Prolotherapy in the treatment of TMD. *The Journal of Craniomandibular Practice.* 2005;23:1-6.

43. Hakala R, et al. The use of Prolotherapy for temporomandibular joint dysfunction. *Journal of Prolotherapy.* 2010;(2)3:439-446.

44. Refai H, et al. The efficacy of dextrose Prolotherapy for temporomandibular joint hypermobility: a preliminary perspective, randomized, double-blind, placebo-controlled clinical trial. *Journal of Oral and Maxillofacial Surgery.* 2011. Doi:10.1016j. joms.2011.02.128.

45. Hauser RA, et al. Dextrose Prolotherapy and pain of chronic TMJ dysfunction. *Practical Pain Management.* 2007;October:56-69.

46. Cheshire W. Botulin toxin in the treatment of myofascial pain syndrome. *Pain.* 1994; 59:65-69.

47. Headache Relief Newsletter, Edition 13, Philadelphia, PA: The Pain Center, 1995.

48. Thigpen C. The styloid process. *Trans American Laryngological Rhinology Otology Association.* 1932;28:408-412.

49. Eagle W. Elongated styloid process. *Archives of Otolaryngology.* 1937;25:584-587.

50. Shankland W. Differential diagnosis of headaches. *Journal of Craniomandibular Practice.* 1986;4:47-53.

51. Ernest E. Three disorders that frequently cause temporomandibular joint pain: internal derangement, temporal tendonitis, and Ernest syndrome. *Journal of Neurological Orthopedic Surgery.* 1986; 7:189-191.

52. Shankland,W. Ernest syndrome as a consequence of stylomandibular -ligament injury: a report of 68 patients. *Journal of Prosthetic Dentistry.* 1987;57:501-506.

53. Wong E. Temporal headaches and associated symptoms relating to the styloid process and its attachments. *Annals of Academic Medicine (Singapore).* 1995;24:124-128.

54. DeLisa J. *Rehabilitation Medicine.* Philadelphia, PA: J.B. Lippincott, 1988.

CHAPTER 6
PROLO YOUR SHOULDER PAIN AWAY!

1. Bot SD, et al. Incidence and prevalence of complaints of the neck and upper extremity in general practice. *Annals of Rheumatic Diseases.* 005;64:118-123.

2. Hakala P, et al. Back, neck, and shoulder pain in Finnish adolescents: national cross section surveys. *British Medical Journal.* 2002;325:390-398.

3. Van der Windt DA, et al. Shoulder disorders in general practice: incidence, patient characteristics and management. *Annals of Rheumatic Diseases.* 1995;54:959-964.

4. Matsen, F. Anterior glenohumeral instability. *Clinics in Sports Medicine.* 1983;2:319-336.

5. Hauser RA, et al. Prolotherapy: a non-invasive approach to lesions of the glenoid labrum; a non-contArolled questionnaire based study. *The Open Rehabilitation Journal.* 2013;6:69-76.

6. Andersen L. Shoulder pain in hemiplegia. *American Journal of Occupational Therapy.* 1985;39:11-18.

7. Scott J. Injuries to the acromioclavicular joint. Injury. *The British Journal of Accident Surgery.* 1967;5:13-18.

8. Butters K. Office evaluation and management of the shoulder impingement syndrome. *Orthopedic Clinics of North America.* 1988;19:755-765.

9. Hauser RA, et al. A retrospective study on Hackett-Hemwall dextrose Prolotherapy for chronic shoulder pain at an outpatient charity clinic in rural Illinois. *Journal of Prolotherapy.* 2009;1(4):205-216.

10. Sefidbakht S, et al. MRI-arthroscopic correlation in rotator cuff tendon pathologies; a comparison between various centers. *Archives of Bone and Joint Surgery.* 2016;4(2):141-144.

11. Farley TE, et al.The coracoacromial arch: MR evaluation and correlation with rotator cuff pathology. *Skeletal Radiol.* 1994 Nov;23(8):641-5.

12. Bencardino JT, et al. Pain related to rotator cuff abnormalities: MRI findings without clinical significance. *J Magn Reson Imaging.* 2010 Jun;31(6):1286-99.

13. Chandnani V. MRI findings in asymptomatic shoulders: a blind analysis using symptomatic shoulders as controls. *Clinical Imaging.* 1992;16:25-30.

14. Neumann C. MR imaging of the shoulder: appearance of the supraspinatus tendon in asymptomatic volunteers. *American Journal of Radiology.* 1992;158:1281-1287.

15. Sher J. Abnormal findings on magnetic resonance images of asymptomatic shoulders. *Journal of Bone and Joint Surgery.* 1995;77A:10-15.

CHAPTER 7

PROLO YOUR KNEE PAIN AWAY!

1. Ongley M. Ligament instability of knees: a new approach to treatment. *Manual Medicine.* 1988; 3:152-154.

2. Hashemi M, et al. The effects of Prolotherapy with hypertonic dextrose versus Prolozone (intraarticular ozone) in patients with knee osteoarthritis. *Anesth Pain Med.* 015;17;5(5):e27585.

3. Topol GA, et al. Chondrogenic effect of intra-articular hypertonic-dextrose (Prolotherapy) in severe knee osteoarthritis. *PM R.* 2016 Apr 4. pii: S1934-1482(16)30054-5.

4. Eslamian F, et al. Therapeutic effects of prolotherapy with intra-articular dextrose injection in patients with moderate knee osteoarthritis: a single-arm study with 6 months follow up. *Ther Adv Musculoskelet Dis.* 2015 Apr;7(2):35-44.

5. Rabago D, et al. Dextrose prolotherapy for knee osteoarthritis: a randomized controlled trial. *Ann Fam Med.* 2013 May-Jun; 11(3):229-237.

6. Rabago D, et al. Hypertonic dextrose injections (prolotherapy) for knee osteoarthritis: results of a single-arm uncontrolled study with 1-year follow-up. *J Altern Complement Med.* 2012 Apr;18(4):408-14. doi: 10.1089/acm.2011.0030.

7. Rabago D, et al. Hypertonic dextrose injection (prolotherapy) for knee osteoarthritis: Long term outcomes. *Complement Ther Med.* 2015 Jun;23(3):388-95. doi: 10.1016/j.ctim.2015.04.003. Epub 2015 Apr 8.

8. Ada AM. Treatment of a medial collateral ligament sprain using prolotherapy: a case study. *Altern Ther Health Med.* 2015 Jul-Aug;21(4):68-71.

9. Reeves K, et al. Long term effects of dextrose Prolotherapy for anterior cruciate laxity. *Alternative Therapies.* 2003;9:58-62.

10. Kim J. The effect of Prolotherapy for osteoarthritis of the knee. *Journal of the Korean Academy of Rehabilitation Medicine.* 2002;26:445-448.

11. Grote W, et al. Repair of a complete anterior cruciate tear using Prolotherapy: a case report. *International Musculoskeletal Medicine.* 2009;1:31(4):159-165.

12. Kim J. Effects of Prolotherapy on knee joint pain due to ligament laxity. *The Journal of the Korean Pain Society.* 2004;17:47-50.

13. Reeves K, et al. Randomized prospective double-blind placebo-controlled study of dextrose Prolotherapy for knee osteoarthritis with or without ACL laxity. *Alternative Therapy Health Medicine.* 2000;6:77-80.

14. Hauser RA, et al. A retrospective study on dextrose Prolotherapy for unresolved knee pain at an outpatient charity clinic in rural Illinois. *Journal of Prolotherapy.* 2009;1(1):11-21.

15. Graham, G. Early osteoarthritis in young sportsmen with severe anterolateral instability of the knee. *Inury: British Journal of Accident Surgery.* 1988; 19:247-248.

16. Kidd, R. Recent developments in the understanding of Osgood-Schlatter disease: a literature review. *Journal of Orthopaedic Medicine.* 1993; 15:59-63.

17. Hauser RA, et al. Outcomes of Prolotherapy in chondromalacia patella patients: improvements in pain level and function. *Clinical Medicine Insights: Arthritis and Musculoskeletal Disorders.* 2014;7:13-20.

18. Brindle T, et al. The meniscus: review of basic principles with application to surgery and rehabilitation. *Journal of Athletic Training.* 2001;36(2):160-169.

19. Trias A. Effect of persistent pressure on articular cartilage: an experimental study. *J Bone Joint Surg.* 1961;43-B(2):376-386.

20. Shrive, N. Load-bearing in the knee joint. *Clinical Orthopaedics.* 1978; 131:279-287.

21. Radin, E. Role of menisci in the distribution of stress in the knee. *Clinical Orthopaedics.* 1984; 185:290-294.

22. Greis PE, et al. Meniscal injury I: basic science and evaluation. *J Am Acad Orthop Surg.* 2002;10(3):168-176.

23. Shakespeare DT, et al. The bucket-handle tear of the meniscus: a clinical and arthrographic study. *J Bone Joint Surg Br.* 1983;65-B(4):383-387.

24. Andrish H. Meniscal injuries in children and adolescents: diagnosis and management. *J Am Acad Orthop Surg.* 1996;4(5):231-237.

25. Englund M, et al. Incidental meniscal findings on knee MRI in middle-aged and elderly persons. *N Engl J Med.* 2008;359(11):1108-1115.

26. Ahmed, A. In vitro measurements of the static pressure distribution in synovial joints. Part one: tibial surface of the knee. *Journal of Biomechanical Engineering.* 1983; 105:216-225.

27. Baratz M. Meniscal tears: the effect of meniscectomy and of repair on intra-articular contact areas and stress in the human knee. *American Journal of Sports Medicine.* 1986; 14:270-275.

28. Bessette G. The meniscus. *Orthopaedics.* 1992; 15:35-42.

29. Radin E. Role of the menisci in the distribution of stress in the knee. *Clinical Orthopaedics.* 1984; 185:290-294.

30. Seedhom B. Transmission of the load in the knee joint with special reference to the role of the menisci. *Eng. Med.* 1979: 8:220-228.

31. Dandy D. The diagnosis of problems after meniscectomy. *Journal of Bone and Joint Surgery.* 1975; 57B:349-352.

32. Maletius, W. The effect of partial meniscectomy on the long-term prognosis of knees with localized, severe chondral damage. *American Journal of Sports Medicine.* 1996; 24:258-262.

33. Bolano L. Isolated arthroscopic partial meniscectomy. *American Journal of Sports Medicine.* 1993; 21:432-437.

34. Hauser RA, et al. The case for utilizing Prolotherapy as first-line treatment of meniscal pathology: a retrospective study shows Prolotherapy is effective in treatment of MRI-documented meniscal tears and degeneration. *Journal of Prolotherapy.* 2010;2(3):416-437.

CHAPTER 8
PROLO YOUR HIP PAIN AWAY

1. Friberg O. Clinical symptoms and biomechanics of lumbar spine and hip joint in leg-length inequality. *Spine.* 1983;18:643-651.

2. Cummings G. The effect of imposed leg-length difference on pelvic bone symmetry. *Spine.* 1993;18:368-373.

3. Ober F. The role of the iliotibial band and fascia lata as a factor in the causation of low-back disabilities and sciatica. *Journal of Bone and Joint Surgery.* 1936; p. 18.

4. Swezey R. Pseudo-radiculopathy in subacute trochanteric bursitis of the subgluteus maximus bursa. *Archives of Physical Medicine and Rehabilitation.* 1976;57:387-390.

5. National Instititues of Health Total hip replacement. Consensus Development Conference Statement. 1994.

6. Smith TO, et al. The clinical and radiological outcomes of hip resurfacing versus total hip arthroplasty: a meta-analysis and systematic review. *Acta Orthopedica.* 2010 Dec;81(6):684-695.

7. Health Quality Ontario. Metal on metal total hip resurfacing arthroplasty. An evidence-based analysis. *Ont Health Technol Assess Ser.* 2006; 6(4):1–57.

8. Kurtz SM et al. Do ceramic femoral heads reduce taper fretting corrosion in hip arthroplasty? A retrieval study. *Clinical Orthopaedics and Related Research.* 2013 Oct; 471(10): 3270–3282.

9. Reito A, et al. High prevalence of adverse reactions to metal debris in small-headed ASR hips. *Clinical Orthopaedics and Related Research.* 2013 Sep;471(9):2954-2961.

10. Kramer WC, et al. Pathogenetic mechanisms of prosttraumatic osteoarthritis: opportunities for every intervention. *Inter J Clinical and Experimental Med.* 2011;4(4):285-298.

11. Henak CR. Subject-specific analysis of joint contact mechanics: application to the study of osteoarthritis and surgical planning. *J Biomech En.* 2013;135(2):0210031-02100326.

12. Ochoa LM et al. Radiographic prevalence of femoroacetabular impingement in a young population with hip complaints is high. *Clin Orthop Rel Res.* 2010;468(10):2710-2714.

13. McCarthy JC, et al. The role of labral lesions to development of early degenerative hip disease. *Clinical Orthopaedics and Related Research.* 2001;393:25-37.

14. Reid GD, et al. Femoroacetabular impingement syndrome: an underrecognized cause of hip pain and premature osteoarthritis? *Topics in Integrative Health.* 2012:3 ID: 3.2004.

15. Hauser RA, et al. A retrospective study on Hackett-Hemwall dextrose Prolotherapy for chronic hip pain at an outpatient charity clinic in rural Illinois. *Journal of Prolotherapy.* 2009;1(2):76-88.

16. Hauser RA, et al. Regenerative injection therapy (Prolotherapy) for hip labrum lesions: rationale and retrospective study. *The Open Rehabilitation Journal.* 2013;6:59-68.

17. Groh MM. A comprehensive review of hip labral tears. *Curr Rev Musculoskeletal Med.* 2009;2:105-117.

CHAPTER 9
PROLO YOUR PELVIC AND GROIN PAIN AWAY!

1. Topol GA, et al. Regenerative injection of elite athletes with career-altering chronic groin pain who fail conservative treatment: a consecutive case series. *Am J Phys Med Rehabil.* 2008;87(11):890-902.

2. Topol GA, et al. Efficacy of dextrose Prolotherapy in elite male kicking-sport athletes with chronic groin pain. *Archives Phys Med Rehabil.* 2005;86:697-702.

3. Schwarzer, A. The sacroiliac joint in chronic low back pain. *Spine.* 1995;20:31-37.

4. Harrison DD, et al. Sitting biomechanics, part 2: optimal car driver's seat and optimal driver's spinal model. *Journal of Manipulative Physiol Ther.* 2000;23:37-47.

5. Makhsous M, et al. Sitting with adjustable ischial and back supports: biomechanical changes. *Spine.* 2003;28:1113-21.

6. Harrison DD, et al. Sitting biomechanics part 1: review of the literature. *Journal of Manipulative Physiol Ther.* 1999;22:594-609.

7. Nidorf D. Proctalgia fugax. *American Family Physician.* 1995;52:2238-2240.

8. Ger G. Evaluation and treatment of chronic intractable rectal pain—a frustrating endeavor. *Diseases of the Colon and Rectum.* 1993;36:139-145.

9. Babb R. Proctalgia fugax. *Postgraduate Medicine.* 1996;99:263-264.

10. Morris L. Use of high-voltage pulsed galvanic stimulation for patients with levator ani syndrome. *Physical Therapy.* 1987;67:1522-1525.

CHAPTER 10
PROLO YOUR ANKLE AND FOOT PAIN AWAY!

1. Mann R. Pain in the foot. *Postgraduate Medicine.* 1987;82:154-174.

2. Mankin H. Localization of tritiated thymidine in articular cartilage of rabbits inhibits growth in immature cartilage. *Journal of Bone and Joint Surgery.* 1962;44A:682.

3. Karr S. Subcalcaneal heel pain. *Orthopedic Clinics of North America.* 1994;25:161-175.

4. Hauser RA, et al. Dextrose Prolotherapy with human growth hormone to treat chronic first metatarsophalangeal joint pain. *The Foot and Ankle Online Journal.* 2012:5(9):1.

5. Merriman J. Presentation at the Hackett Foundation Prolotherapy meeting, Indianapolis, IN, October 1995.

6. Hauser RA, et al. A retrospective observational study on Hackett-Hemwall dextrose Prolotherapy for unresolved foot and toe pain at an outpatient charity clinic in rural Illinois. *Journal of Prolotherapy.* 2011;3(1):543-551

7. Kirvela O. Treatment of painful neuromas with neurolytic blockade. *Pain.* 1990;41:161-165.

8. Benedetti R. Clinical results of simultaneous adjacent interdigital neurectomy in the foot. *Foot and Ankle International.* 1996;17:264-268.

9. Hauser RA, et al. Dextrose Prolotherapy treatment for unresolved "Morton's neuroma" pain. *The Foot and Ankle Online Journal.* 2012:5(6):1.

10. Deese J. Compressive neuropathies of the lower extremity. *Journal of Musculoskeletal Medicine.* 1988; November: 68-91

11. Hollinshead W. *Functional Anatomy of the Limb and Back.* Fifth Edition. Philadelphia, PA: W.B. Saunders, pp. 316-338.

12. Trevino S. Management of acute and chronic lateral ligament injuries of the ankle. *Orthopedic Clinics of North America.* 1994;25:1-16.

13. Hauser RA, et al. Dextrose Prolotherapy injections for chronic ankle pain. *Practical Pain Management.* Jan-Feb 2010;10(1):70-76.

CHAPTER 11
PROLO YOUR ELBOW, WRIST, AND HAND PAIN AWAY!

1. Armstrong T. Upper-extremity pain in the workplace—role of usage in causality in clinical concepts. From *Regional Musculoskeletal Illness.* Grune and Straton, Inc., 1987, pp. 333-354.

2. Dominguez R, et al. *Total Body Training.* East Dundee, IL: Moving Force Systems, 1982, pp. 33-37.

3. Bucci L. *Nutrition Applied to Injury Rehabilitation and Sports Medicine.* Boca Raton, FL: CRC Press, 1995, pp. 167-176.

4. Hauser R, et al. Hackett-Hemwall Dextrose Prolotherapy for unresolved elbow pain. *Practical Pain Management.* Oct 2009;9(6):14-26.

5. Cooney W. Anatomy and mechanics of carpal instability. *Surgical Rounds for Orthopedics.* 1989, pp. 5-24.

6. Ibid.

7. Kozin S. Injuries to the perilunar carpus. *Orthopaedic Review.* 1992;21:435-448.

8. Hauser R, et al. Dextrose Prolotherapy for unresolved wrist pain. *Practical Pain Management.* Nov-Dec 2009;9(9):72-89.

9. Waters P. Unusual arthritic disorders in the hand: part one. *Surgical Rounds for Orthopaedics.* 1990, pp. 15-20.

10. Laseter G. Management of the stiff hand: a practical approach. *Orthopedic Clinics of North America.* 1983;14:749-765.

11. Hauser R, et al. A retrospective observational study on Hackett-Hemwall dextrose Prolotherapy for unresolved hand and finger pain at an outpatient charity clinic in rural Illinois. *Journal of Prolotherapy.* 2010;2(4):480-486.

12. Hauser RA, et al. Treatment of basal thumb osteoarthritis: a retrospective study of dextrose prolotherapy injections as an alternative treatment. *Journal of Prolotherapy.* 2013;5:e913-e921.

13. Fleming B, et al. Ligament injury, reconstruction and osteoarthritis. *Curr Opin Orthop.* 2005;16:354-362.

14. Frank C. Ligament structure, physiology and function. *Journal of Musculoskeletal and Neuronal Interactions*. 2004;4:199-201.

15. Connell D. MR imaging of thumb carpometacarpal joint ligament injuries. *Journal of Hand Surgery*. 2004;29:46-54.

CHAPTER 12

PROLO YOUR CHEST AND RIB PAIN AWAY!

1. Tietze A. Uber eine eigenartige hafung ion fallen mit dystrophie der rippenknorpel. *Berl. Klin. Wchnschr.* 1921;58:829.

2. Rawlings M. The "rib syndrome." *Diseases of the Chest.* 1962;41:432-441.

3. Davies-Colley R. Slipping rib. *British Medical Journal*. 1922;1(3194):432.

4. McBeath A. The rib-tip syndrome. *Journal of Bone and Joint Surgery*. 1975;57A:795-797.

5. Holmes J. A study of the slipping-rib cartilage syndrome. *New England Journal of Medicine*. 1941; 224:928-932.

6. Kelly TR. Thoracic outlet syndrome: Current concepts of treatment. *Annals of Surgery*. 1979; 190(5):657-662.

7. Phull P. Management of cervical pain. In Rehabilitation Medicine. Delisa, J. (ed.), Philadelphia, PA: Lippincott Publisher, 1988, pp. 761-764.

CHAPTER 13

PROLO YOUR ARTHRITIS PAIN AWAY!

1. Abhishek A, et al. Diagnosis and clinical presentation of osteoarthritis. *Rheum Dis Clin N Am*. 2013;39(1):45–66.

2. Woldin B, et al. Pain in osteoarthritis: can Prolotherapy help? *The Pain Practitioner*. 2014;24(3):16-22.

3. Hauser RA, et al. Ligament injury and healing: a review of current clinical diagnostics and therapeutics. *Open Rehab J*. 2012;5:48-66.

4. McGonagle D, et al. Heberden's nodes and what Heberden could not see: the pivotal role of ligaments in the pathogenesis of early nodal osteoarthritis and beyond. *Rheumatology*. 2008;47(9):1278-85.

5. Brandt KD, et al. Yet more evidence that osteoarthritis in not a cartilage disease. *Ann Rheum Dis*. 2006;65:1261-4.

6. Blalock D, et al. Joint instability and osteoarthritis. *Clin Med Insights Arthritis Musculoskelet Disord*. 2015;8:15–23.

7. Fleming BC, et al. Ligament injury, reconstruction and osteoarthritis. *Curr Opin Orthop*. 2005 Oct;16(5):354–362.

8. Simon D, et al. The relationship between anterior cruciate ligament injury and osteoarthritis of the knee. *Advances in Orthopedics*. 2015; Article ID 928301, 11 pages. doi:10.1155/2015/928301

9. Christie R. The medical uses of proteolytic enzymes. From *Topics in Enzyme and Fermentation Biotechnology*. Chichester, England: Ellis Horwood Ltd., 1980, pp. 25.

10. Jakich A, et al. Prolotherapy saved me from bilateral knee replacements! *JOP*. 2009;1(1):29-31.

11. Fujiwara A, et al. The effect of disc degeneration and facet joint osteoarthritis on the segmental flexibility of the lumbar spine. *Spine*. 2000;25(23):3036–3044.

12. An HS, et al. Intervertebral disc degeneration: biological and biomechanical factors. *Journal of Orthopaedic Science*. 2006 Sep;11(5):541–552.

13. Topol GA, et al. Chondrogenic effect of intra-articular hypertonic dextrose (Prolotherapy) in severe knee osteoarthritis. *PM R*. 2016 Apr 4. pii: S1934-1482(16)30054-5.

14. Hauser RA. The regeneration of articular cartilage with Prolotherapy. *Journal of Prolotherapy*. 2009;1(1):39-44.

15. Hauser RA, et al. Standard clinical X-ray studies document cartilage regeneration in five degenerated knees after Prolotherapy. *Journal of Prolotherapy*. 2009;1:22-28.

16. D'Lima DD, et al. Human chondrocyte apoptosis in response to mechanical injury. *Osteoarthritis Cartilage*. 2001 Nov;9(8):712-9.

17. Hembree WC, et al. Viability and apoptosis of human chondrocytes in osteochondral fragments following joint trauma. *J Bone Joint Surg Br*. 2007 Oct;89(10):1388-95.

18. Dang AC, et al. Chondrocyte apoptosis after simulated intraarticular fracture: a comparison of histologic detection methods. *Clin Orthop Relat Res.* 2009 Jul;467(7):1877-84. doi: 10.1007/s11999-009-0829-3.

19. Smith RL, et al. Pressure and shear differentially alter human articular chondrocyte metabolism: a review. *Clin Orthop Relat Res.* 2004 Oct;(427 Suppl):S89-95.

20. Lane Smith R, et al. Effects of shear stress on articular chondrocyte metabolism. *Biorheology.* 2000;37(1-2):95-107.

CHAPTER 14

PROLO YOUR SPORTS INJURIES AWAY!

1. Laros,G. Influence of physical activity on ligament insertions in the knees of dogs. *Journal of Bone and Joint Surgery.* 1971;53:275.

2. Hunter L. *Rehabilitation of the Injured Knee.* St. Louis, MO: C.V. Mosby, 1984.

3. Arnoczky S. Meniscal degeneration due to knee instability: an experimental study in the dog. *Trans. Orthop. Res. Soc.* 1979;4:79.

4. Tipton C. The influence of physical activity on ligaments and tendons. *Med. Sci. Sports.* 1975;7:165.

5. Woo S. Effect of immobilization and exercise on strength characteristics of bone-medial collateral ligament-bone complex. *Am. Soc. Mech. Eng. Symp.* 1979;32:62.

6. Noyes F. Biomechanics of anterior cruciate ligament failure: an analysis of strain rate sensitivity and mechanism of failure in primates. *Journal of Bone and Joint Surgery.* 1974;56A:236.

7. Noyes F. Biomechanics of ligament failure: an analysis of immobilization, exercise and reconditioning effects in primates. *Journal of Bone and Joint Surgery.* 1974;56A:1406.

8. Akeson W. Immobility effects on synovial joints: the pathomechanics of joint contracture. *Biorheology.* 1980;17:95.

9. Bleakley CM, et al. Cooling an acute muscle injury: can basic scientific theory translate into the clinical setting? *Br J Sports Med.* 2012;46:296-298.

10. Tseng CY, et al. Topical cooling (icing) delays recovery from eccentric exercise-induced muscle damage. *J Strength and Conditioning Research.* 2013 May;27(5):1354-1361.

11. Ho SS, et al. The effect of ice on blood flow and bone metabolism in knees. *Am J Sports Med.* 1994 Jul-Aug;22(4):537-40.

12. van den Bekerom MP, et al. What is the evidence for rest, ice, compression, and elevation therapy in the treatment of ankle sprains in adults? *J Athl Train.* 2012 Jul-Aug;47(4):435-43.

13. Ho SS. Comparison of various icing times in decreasing bone metabolism and blood flow in the knee. *American Journal of Sports Medicine.* 1990;18:376-378.

14. Wrenn R. An experimental study of the effect of cortisone on the healing process and tensile strength of tendons. *Journal of Bone and Joint Surgery.* 1954;36A:588-601.

15. Truhan A. Corticosteroids: a review with emphasis on complications of prolonged systemic therapy. *Annals of Allergy.* 1989;62:375-390.

16. Roenigk R. *Dermatologic Surgery.* Marcel Dekker, Inc., p. 155.

17. Davis G. Adverse effects of corticosteroids. *Systemic Clinical Dermatology.* 1986;4(1):161-169.

18. Gogia P. Hydrocortisone and exercise effects on articular cartilage in rats. *Archives of Physical Medicine and Rehabilitation.* 1993;74:463-467.

19. Chandler GN. Deleterious effect of intra-articular hydrocortisone. *Lancet.* 1958;2:661-663.

20. Peterson L. *Sports Injuries: Their Prevention and Treatment.* Chicago, IL: Year Book Medical, 1986, pp.18-63.

21. Lockhart R. *Anatomy of the Human Body.* Second Edition. Philadelphia, PA: J.B. Lippincott, 1969; pp. 144.

22. International Anatomical Nomenclature Committee: Nomina Anatomica. Excerpta Medical Foundation, Amersterdam, 1966; pp. 38-43.

CHAPTER 15
PROLO YOUR KID'S INJURIES AWAY!

1. Brukner P. *Clinical Sports Medicine.* New York City, NY: McGraw-Hill Book Company, 1995, pp. 521-540.

2. Ehrlich M. Sports injuries in children and the clumsy child. *Pediatric Clinics of North America.* 1992;39:443.

3. Barkley K. Child and adolescent athletes. In Baker C (ed.) *The Hughston Clinic Sports Medicine Book.* Baltimore, MD: William and Wilkins; 1995, pp. 87-93.

4. Palmoski M. Running inhibits the reversal of atrophic changes in canine knee cartilage after removal of a long leg case. *Arthritis and Rheumatism.* 1981;24:1329-1337.

5. Zernicke R. Endurance training. In Sports Medicine: *The School-age Athlete.* Reider B. (ed.) Philadelphia PA: W.B,. Saunders, 1996, pp. 3-18.

6. Noyes F. Biomechanics of ligament failure. II. An analysis of immobilization, exercise, and reconditioning effects in primates. *Journal of Bone and Joint Surgery.* 1974;56A:1406-1418.

7. Kocher MS, et al. Management of osteochondritis dissecans of the knee: current concepts review. *American Journal of Sports Medicine.* 2006;34:1181-1191.

8. Aichroth P. Osteochondritis dissecans of the knee: a clinical survey. *Journal of Bone and Joint Surgery British.* 1971;53:440-447.

9. Campbell CJ, et al. Osteochondritis dissecans: the question of etiology. *Journal of Trauma.* 1966;6:201-221.

10. Hauser RA. Prolotherapy as an alternative treatment for osteochondritis dissecans: two cases of young baseball players. *Journal of Prolotherapy.* 2011;3(1):568-571.

11. Kidd R. Recent developments in the understanding of Osgood-Schlatter disease: a literature review. *Journal of Orthopaedic Medicine.* 1993;15:59-63.

12. Topol G, et al. Hyperosmolar dextrose injection for recalcitrant Osgood-Schlatter disease. *Pediatrics.* 2011;128(5):e1-e8.

13. Lysens R. The predictability of sports injuries. *Sports Meidicne.* 1984;1:6-10.

14. Goldberg B. Pre-participation sports assessment-an objective evaluation. *Pediatrics.* 1980;66:736-745.

15. Nicholas J. Risk factors, sports medicine and the orthopedic system: an overview. *Sports Medicine.* 1976;3:243-259.

16. Keller C. The medical aspects of soccer injury epidemiology. *American Journal of Sports Medicine.* 1987;15:230-237.

17. Crosby E. Recurrent dislocation of the patella. Relation of treatment to osteoarthritis. *Journal of Bone and Joint Surgery.* 1976;58:9-13.

18. Hughstone J. Subluxation of the patella. *Journal of Bone and Joint Surgery.* 1968;50:1003-1026.

CHAPTER 16
PROLO YOUR NERVE PAINS AWAY!

1. Dilley A, Lynn B. Quantitative in vivo studies of median nerve sliding in response to wrist, elbow, shoulder and neck movements. *Clin Biomech (Bristol Avon).* 2003;18:899-907.

2. Liao C, Zhang W. Surgical decompression of painful diabetic peripheral neuropathy: the role of pain distribution. *PLoS One.* 2014;9:e109827.

3. Aktan IA, Ucerler H, Uygur M. Dimensions of the anterior tarsal tunnel and features of the deep peroneal nerve in relation to clinical application. *Surg Radiol Anat.* 2007;29:527-30.

4. Pacek CA, Tang J, Goitz RJ. Morphological analysis of the carpal tunnel. *Hand.* 2010; 5:77-81.

5. Sutton JJ, Werner FW, Basu N. Morphology of the cubital tunnel: an anatomical and biomechanical study with implications for treatment of ulnar nerve compression. 56th Annual meeting of the orthopaedic research society. Poster 1776.

6. Mogk JP, Keir PJ. Wrist and carpal tunnel size and shape measurements: effects of posture. *Clin Biomech.* 2008; 23:1112-20.

7. Barker AR, Rosson GD, Dellon AL. Pressure changes in the medial and lateral plantar and tarsal tunnels related to ankle position: a cadaver study. *Foot Ankle Int.* 2007; 28:250-4.

8. Gelberman RH, Yamaguchi K. Changes in interstitial pressure and cross-sectional area of the cubial tunnel and of the ulnar nerve with flexion of the elbow. An experimental study in human cadaver. *J Bone Joint Surg Am.* 1998; 80:492-501.

9. Lyftogt J. Subcutaneous prolotherapy for Achilles tendinopathy. *Australia's Musculoskeletal Medicine Journal.* 2007; 12:107-109.

10. Lyftogt J. Prolotherapy for recalcitrant lumbago. *Australia's Musculoskeletal Journal.* 2008; 13:18-20.

11. Lyftogt J. Subcutaneous prolotherapy treatment of refractory knee, shoulder and lateral elbow pain. *Australia's Musculoskeletal Medicine journal.* 2007; 12:110-112.

12. Hackett GS. Ligament uninhibited reversible antidromic vasodilation in brochiogenic pathophysiologic disease. *Lancet.* 1966; 86:398-404.

13. Hackett GS. Ligament relaxation and osteoarthritis, loose jointed versus close jointed. *Rheumatism.* 1959; 15:28-33.

14. Hackett GS, Huang TC, Raftery A. Prolotherapy for headache. Pain in the head and neck and neuritis. *Headache.* 1962; 2:3-11.

15. Hackett GS, Huang TC. Prolotherapy for sciatica from weak pelvic ligaments and bone dystrophy. *Clinical Medicine.* 1961; 8:2301-2316.

16. Hackett GS. Uninhibited reversible antidromic vasodilation in pathophysiological diseases: arteriosclerosis, carcinogenesis, neuritis and osteoporosis. *Angiology.* 1966; 17:2-8.

CHAPTER 17
CONNECTIVE TISSUE DEFICIENCY CONDITIONS

1. Grahme R. Joint hypermobility syndrome pain. *Current Pain Headache Rep.* 2009;13:427-433.

2. Grahme R. Joint hypermobility and genetic collagen disorders: are they related? *Archives Dis Child.* 1999;80:188-192.

3. Kowitz R. *Osteoarthritis.* Second Edition. Philadelphia, PA: W.B. Saunders, 1992.

4. Ross J, et al. Joint hypermobility syndrome. *British Medical Journal.* 2011;342c:c7167. Available at: http://www.bmj.com/content/342/bmj.c7167.full.

5. Grahame R, et al. Joint hypermobility syndrome is a highly prevalent in general rheumatology clinics, its occurrence and clinical presentation being gender, age and race-related. *Annals of Rheumatic Diseases.* 2006;54:515-523.

6. Grahame R, et al. British consultant rheumatologists; perceptions about the hypermobility syndrome: a national survey. *Rheumatology (Oxford).* 2001;40:559-562.

7. Pacey V, et al. Generalized joint hypermobility and risk of lower limb joint injury during sport: a systematic review with meta- analysis. *American Journal of Sports Medicine.* 2010;38:1487-1497.

8. Lotz JC, et al. Innervation, inflammation, and hypermobility may characterize pathologic disc degeneration: review of animal model data. *Journal of Bone and Joint Surgery Am.* 2006;88S:76-82.

9. Collinge R, et al. Hypermobility, injury rate and rehabilitation in a professional football squad-a preliminary study. *Physical Therapy and Sports.* 2009;10:91-96.

10. De Coster PJ, et al. Generalized joint hypermobility and temporomandibular disorders: inherited connective tissue disease as a model with maximum expression. *Journal of Orofacial Pain.* 19:47-54.

11. Peyron JG. Clinical features of osteoarthritis, diffuse idiopathic skeletal hyperostosis, and hypermobility syndromes. *Current Opinions of Rheumatology.* 1991;3:653-661.

12. Davies AN, et al. Joint hypermobility syndrome in childhood. A not so benign multisystem disorder? *Rheumatology (Oxford)*. 2005;44:744-750.

13. Engelbert RH, et al. Exercise tolerance in children and adolescents with musculoskeletal pain in joint mobility and joint hypermobility syndrome. *Pediatrics*. 2006;118:e690-696.

14. Bendik EM, et al. Joint hypermobility syndrome: a common clinical disorder associated with migraine in women. *Cephalalgia*. 2011 Apr;31(5):603-13.

15. Beighton P, et al. Articular mobility in an African population. *Annals of Rheumatic Diseases*. 1973;32:413-418.

16. Grahame R. The revised (Brighton 1998) criteria for the diagnosis of benign joint hypermobility syndrome. *Journal of Rheumatology*. 2000;27:1777-1779.

17. Russek LN. Examination and treatment of a patient with hypermobility syndrome. *Physical Therapy*. 2000;80:386-398.

18. Hollister DW. Heritable disorders of connective tissue: Ehlers-Danlos syndrome. *Pediatric Clinics of North America*. 1978;25:575- 591.

19. Callewaert B, et al. Ehlers-Danlos syndromes and Marfan syndrome. *Best Pract Res Clin Rheumatol*. 2008;22:165-189.

20. Bravo JF. Ehlers-Danlos syndrome, with special emphasis in the joint hypermobility syndrome. *Rev Med Chil*. 2009;137:1488-1497.

21. Byers PH. Ehlers-Danlos syndrome: recent advances and current understanding of the clinical and genetic heterogeneity. *J Invest Dermatol*. 1994;103(5 Suppl):47S-52S.

22. Oderich GS, et al. The spectrum, management and clinical outcome of Ehlers-Danlos syndrome type IV: a 30-year experience. *Journal of Vascular Surgery*. 2005;42:98-106.

23. Savasta S, et al. Ehlers-Danlos syndrome and neurological features: a review. *Childs Nerv Syst*. 2010: August 10 epub PMID: 20697718. Available at: http://www.ncbi.nlm.nih.gov/ pubmed/20697718.

24. Voermans NC, et al. Neuromuscular involvement in various types of Ehlers-Danlos syndrome. *Annals of Neurology*. 2009;65:687-697.

25. Voermans NC, et al. Pain in Ehlers-Danlos syndrome is common, severe, and associated with functional impairment. *Journal of Pain and Symptom Management*. 2010;40:370-378.

26. Wheaton M, et al. The ligament injury connection to osteoarthritis. *Journal of Prolotherapy*. 2010;2:294-304.

27. Bierma-Zeinstra SM. Risk factors and prognostic factors of hip and knee osteoarthritis. *Nature Clinical Practice, Rheumatology*. 2007;3:78-85.

28. Kirk JA, et al. The hypermobility syndrome-musculoskeletal complaints associated with generalized joint hypermobility. *Annals of Rheumatic Diseases*. 1967;26:419-425.

29. Gordon K, et al. The case for utilizing Prolotherapy as a promising stand-alone or adjunctive treatment for Over-Manipulation syndrome. *Journal of Applied Research*. 2013;13(1):1-28.

30. Scott MW, et al. Injury analysis of impacts between a cage-type propeller guard and submerged head. *Safe Journal*. 1994;24:13-23.

31. Jaumard NV, et al. Spinal facet joint biomechanics and mechanotransduction in normal, injury and degenerative conditions. *Journal of Biomechanical Engineering*. 2011;133 doi:10.1115/1.4004493.

32. Winkelstein BA, et al. The cervical facet capsule and its role in whiplash injury: a biomechanical investigation. *Spine*. 2000;25:1238-1246.

33. Yoganandan N, et al. Geometric and mechanical properties of human cervical spine ligaments. *Journal of Biomechanical Investigation*. 2000;122:623-629.

34. Quinn KP, et al. Cervical facet capsular ligament yield defines the threshold for injury and persistent joint-mediated neck pain. *Journal of Biomechanics*. 2007;40:2299-2306.

35. Ivancic PC, et al. Whiplash causes increased laxity of cervical capsular ligament. *Clinical Biomechanics*. 2008;23:159-165.

36. DeVries NA, et al. Biomechanical analysis of the intact and destabilized sheep cervical spine. *Spine*. 2012;37:E957-63.

37. Oxland TR, et al. An anatomic basis for spinal instability: a procine trauma model. *Journal of Orthopaedic Research*. 1991;9:452-462.

38. Goel VK, et al. An in-vitro study of the kinematics of the normal, injured and stabilized cervical spine. *Journal of Biomechanics*. 1984;17:363-76.

39. Bogduk N, et al. Biomechanics of the cervical spine part 3: minor injuries. *Clinical Biomechanics*. 2001;16:267-75.

40. Stemper BD, et al. Effects of abnormal posture on capsular ligament elongations in a computational model subjected to whiplash loading. *Journal of Biomechanics*. 2005;38:1313-23.

41. Yunnus, M. Primary fibromyalgia syndrome and myofascial pain syndrome: clinical features and muscle pathology. *Archives of Physical Medicine and Rehabilitation*. 1988;69:451-454.

42. Pillemer, S. *The Fibromyalgia Syndrome*. The Harworth Medical Press, Inc., 1994.

43. Moldofsky, H. Induction of neurasthenic musculoskeletal pain syndrome by selective sleep stage deprivation. *Psychosomatic Medicine*. 1976;38:35.

44. Reeves, K. Treatment of consecutive severe fibromyalgia patients with Prolotherapy. *Journal of Orthopaedic Medicine*. 1994; 16:84-89.

45. Travell, J. *Myofascial Pain and Dysfunction*. Baltimore, MD: Williams and Wilkins, 1983, pp. 103-164.

46. Fishbain D. Male and female chronic pain patients categorized by DSM-III psychiatric diagnostic criteria. *Pain*. 1986;26:181-197.

47. Gerwin R. A study of 96 subjects examined both for fibromyalgia and myofascial pain (Abstract). *Journal of Musculoskeletal Pain*. 1995;3:121.

48. Simons D, et al. *Myofascial Pain and Dysfunction: The Trigger Point Manual*. Volume 1. Baltimore, MD: Williams and Wilkins, 1999; pp. 1-94.

49. Sola A. Incidence of hypersensitive areas in posterior shoulder muscles. *American Journal of Physical Medicine*. 1955;34:585-590.

50. Frohlich, D. Piriformis syndrom: eine haufige differentialdiagnose des lumboglutaalen schmerzes (Piriformis syndrome: a frequent item in the differential diagnosis of lumbogluteal pain). *Manuelle Medizin*. 1995;33:7-10.

51. Travell J. Pain and disability of the shoulder and arm: treatment by intramuscular infiltration with procaine hydrochloride. *Journal of the American Medical Association*. 1942;120:417-422.

52. Travell J. Myofascial pain syndromes: mysteries of the history. In *Advances in Pain Research and Therapy: Myofascial Pain and Fibromyalgia*, Volume 17. Edited by Fricton, J. New York, NY: Raven Press, 1990; pp. 129-137.

53. Travell J. and Rinzler S. The myofascial genesis of pain. *Postgraduate Medicine*. 1952;11:425-434.

54. Simons D, et al. *Myofascial Pain and Dysfunction: The Trigger Point Manual*. Volume 1. Baltimore, MD: Williams and Wilkins, 1999; pp. 94-177.

55. Hong C. Difference in pain relief after trigger point injections in myofascial pain patients with and without fibromyalgia. *Archives of Physical Medicine and Rehabilitation*. 1996; 77:1161-1166.

56. Caro XJ, et al. The role and importance of small fiber neuropathy in fibromyalgia pain. *Curr Pain Headache Rep*. 2015;19:55.

57. Cazzato D, et al. Small fiber neuropathy is a common feature of Ehlers-Danlos syndromes. *Neurology*. 2016;87:155-9.

58. Grigoriou E, et al. Postural Orthostatic Tachycardia Syndrome (POTS): association with Ehler-Danlos syndrome and orthoepaedic considerations. *Clinical Orthopaedics and Related Research*. Feb 2015;473(2): 722-728.

59. Levine TD, et al. Routine use of punch biopsy to diagnose small fiber neuropathy in fibromyalgia patients. *Clin Rheumatology*. 2015;34:413-417.

60. Giannoccaro MP, et al. Small nerve fiber involvement in patients referred for fibromyalgia. *Muscle Nerve.* 2014;49:757-759.

61. Uceyler N, et al. Small fibre pathology in patients with fibromyalgia syndrome. *Brain.* 2013;136:1857-1867.

62. Caro XJ, et al. Evidence of abnormal epidermal nerve fiber density in fibromyalgia: clinical and immunologic implications. *Arthritis Rheumatol.* 2014;66:1945-54.

63. Oaklander AL, et al. Objective evidence that small-fiber polyneuropathy underlies some illnesses currently labeled as fibromyalgia. *Pain.* 2013;154:2310-2316.

64. Singer W, et al. Prospective evaluation of somatic and autonomic small fibers in selected autonomic neuropathies. *Neurology.* 2004;62:612-618.

CHAPTER 18

WHY YOU DON'T HEAL

1. Sibinga N. Opioid peptides and opioid receptors in cells of the immune system. *Annu. Rev. Immunol.* 1988;6:219-249.

2. Bryant H. Role of adrenal cortical activation in the immunosuppressive effects of chronic morphine treatment. *Endocrinology.* 1991;128:3253-3258.

3. Pellis N. Suppression of the induction of delayed hypersensitivity in rats by repetitive morphine treatments. *Experimental Neurology.* 1986;93:92-97.

4. Lopez M. Spleen and thymus cells subsets modified by long-term morphine administration and murine AIDS. *International Journal of Immunopharmacology.* 1993;15:909-918.

5. Sei Y. Morphine-induced thymic hypoplasia is glucocorticoid-dependent. *Journal of Immunology.* 1991;146:194-198.

6. Bryant H. Immunosuppressive effects of chronic morphine treatment in mice. *Life Sciences.* 1987; 41:1731-1738.

7. Bussiere J. Differential effects of morphine and naltrexone on the antibody response in various mouse strains. *Immunotoxicol.* 1992;14:657-673.

8. Hung C. *Proc. Soc. Exp. Biol. Med.* 1973;142:106-111.

9. Nair M. A decreased natural and antibody-dependent cellular cytotoxic activities in intravenous drug abusers. *Clin. Immunol. Immunopathol.* 1986;38:68-78.

10. Eisenstein T. Opioid modulation of immune responses: effects on phagocyte and lymphoid cell populations. *Journal of Neuroimmunology.* 1998;83:36-44.

11. Gilman A. *The Pharmacological Basis of Therapeutics.* Elmsford, NY: Pergamon Press, 1990, p. 486.

12. Gordin K, et al. The case for utilizing Prolotherapy as a promising stand-alone or adjunctive treatment for Over-Manipulation syndrome. *The Journal of Applied Research.* 2013;13(1):1-28.

13. Jacobson E. *You Must Relax.* McGraw-Hill Book Company. New York,1957.

14. Nicolson G. Mycoplasma infections in chronic illnesses: fibromyalgia and chronic fatigue syndromes, Gulf War illness, HIV-AIDS and rheumatoid arthritis. *Medical Sentinel.* 1999;4:172-175.

15. Nicolson G. Diagnosis and treatment of chronic mycoplasmal infections in fibromyalgia and chronic fatigue syndromes: relationship to Gulf War illness. *Biomedical Therapy.* 1998;16:266-271.

16. Steere A. Musculoskeletal manifestations of Lyme disease. *American Journal of Medicine.* 1995; 98:4A-45S.

17. Tortorice K. Clinical features and treatment of Lyme disease. *Pharmacotherapy.* 1989;9:363-371.

18. *Merriam Webster's Collegiate Dictionary,* Tenth Edition, Springfield, MA: Merriam-Webster, Inc. 1995.

19. Hallesby O. *Temperament and the Christian Faith.* Minneapolis, MN, Augsburg Publishing House, 1962.

20. LaHaye T. *Transformed Temperaments.* Wheaton, IL: Tyndale House Publishers, 1971.

21. LaHaye T. *Spirit-Controlled Temperament.* Wheaton, IL: Tyndale House Publishers, 1966.

22. Littauer F. *Personality Plus.* Grand Rapids, MI: Fleming H. Revell, 1992.

23. Wright H. *A More Excellent Way.* Thomaston, GA: Pleasant Valley Publications, 1999.

24. *How to Resolve Seven Deadly Stresses. A Health Manual for All Nations.* Oak Brook, IL: Institute in Basic Life Principles, Inc., 2008.

CHAPTER 19

PROLOTHERAPY VS. SURGERY

1. Wiesel S. A study of computer-related assisted tomography. The incidence of positive CAT scans in an asymptomatic group of patients. *Spine.* 1984;9:549-551.

2. Verwoerd AJ, et al. Diagnostic accuracy of history taking to assess lumbosacral nerve root compression. *Spine J.* 2014 Sep 1;14(9):2028-37. doi: 10.1016/j.spinee.2013.11.049.

3. Guermazi A, et al. MRI-based semiquantitative scoring of joint pathology in osteoarthritis. *Nat Rev Rheumatol.* Apr;9(4):236-51. doi: 10.1038/nrrheum.2012.223.

4. Porcheret M, et al. Developing a model osteoarthritis consultation: a Delphi consensus exercise. *BMC Musculoskeletal Disorders.* 2013;14:25. DOI: 10.1186/1471-2474-14-25.

5. Maynard J. Morphological and biomechanical effects of sodium morrhuate on tendons. *Journal of Orthopaedic Research.* 1985;3:236-248.

6. Symposium: the role of spine fusion for low back pain. International Society for the Study of the Lumbar Spine. New Orleans, Louisiana, May 27, 1980. *Spine.* 1981;6:277-314.

7. Park P, et al. Adjacent segment disease after lumbar or lumbosacral fusion: review of the literature. *Spine.* 2004;29:1938-1944.

8. Hilibrand AS, et al. Adjacent segment degeneration and adjacent segment disease: the consequences of spinal fusion? *The Spine Journal.* 2004;4:190S-194S.

9. Sears WR, et al. Incidence and prevalence of surgery at segments adjacent to a previous posterior lumbar arthrodesis. *The Spine Journal.* 2011;11:11-20.

10. Hilibrand AS, et al. Radiculopathy and myelopathy at segments adjacent to the site of a previous anterior cervical arthrodesis. *Journal of Bone and Joint Surgery.* 1999;81A:519-528.

11. Turner J. et al. Patient outcomes after lumbar spinal fusions. *Journal of the American Medical Association.* 1992;286:907-910.

12. Schmid A, et al. Results after cartilage shaving studied by electron microscopy. *American Journal of Sports Medicine.* 1987;15:386-387.

13. Allen PR, et al. Late degenerative changes after meniscectomy: factors affecting the knee after operation. *J Bone Joint Surg.* 1984;66-B(5):666-671.

14. Englund M, et al. Patellofemoral osteoarthritis coexistent with tibiofemoral osteoarthritis in a meniscectomy population. *Ann Rheum Dis.* 2005;64:1721-1726.

15. Jackson JP. Degenerative changes in the knee after meniscectomy. *Brit Med J.* 1968;2:525-527.

16. Rangger C. Osteoarthritis after arthroscopic partial meniscectomy. *Am J Sports Med.* 1995;23(2):240-241.

17. Roos H, et al. Knee osteoarthritis after meniscectomy: prevalence of radiographic changes after twenty-one years, compared with matched controls. *Arthritis & Rheumatism.* 1998;41(4):687-693.

18. Raynauld JP, et al. Long term evaluation of disease progression through the quantitative magnetic resonance imaging of symptomatic knee osteoarthritis patients: correlation with clinical symptoms and radiographic changes. *Arthritis Research & Therapy.* 2006;8(1):R21.

19. Wluka A, et al. Knee cartilage loss in symptomatic knee osteoarthritis over 4.5 years. *Arthritis & Research Therapy.* 2006;8(4):R90.

20. Kirkley A, et al. A randomized trial of arthroscopic surgery for osteoarthritis of the knee. *N Engl J Med.* 2008;359:1097–1107.

21. Moseley JB, et al. A controlled trial of arthroscopic surgery for osteoarthritis of the knee. *N Engl J Med*. 2002;347:81–88.

22. Bach B, et al. Arthroscopically assisted anterior cruciate ligament reconstruction using patellar tendon autograft. *Am J of Sports Med*. 1998;26:181-188.

23. Clancy W, et al. Anterior and posterior cruciate ligament reconstruction in rhesus monkeys. *Journal of Bone and Joint Surgery*. 1981;63A:1270-1284.

24. Burns T, et al. Arthroscpic treatment of shoulder impingement in athletes. *American Journal of Sports Med*. 1992;20:13-16.

25. Hauser RA, et al. Journal of Prolotherapy international medical editorial board consensus statement on the use of Prolotherapy for musculoskeletal pain. *JOP*. 2011;3(4):744-764.

26. Trojani C, et al. Causes for failure of ACL reconstruction and influence of meniscectomies after revision. *Knee Surg Sports Traumatol Arthrosc*. 2011 Feb;19(2):196-201.

27. Edwards D. Radiographic changes in the knee after meniscal transplantation. *American J Sports Med*. 1996;24:222-229.

28. Jorgensen U, et al. Long-term follow-up of meniscectomy in athletes. *J Bone Joint Surg*. 1987;69-B(1):80-83.

29. McNicholas MJ, et al. Total meniscectomy in adolescents: a thirty-year follow-up. *J Bone Joint Surg Br*. 2000;82-B(2):217-221.

30. Hoser C, et al. Long-term results of arthroscopic partial lateral meniscectomy in knees without associated damage. *J Bone Joint Surg Br*. 2001;83-B(4):513-516.

31. Tapper EM, et al. Late results after meniscectomy. *J Bone Joint Surg Am*. 1969;51-A(3):517-603.

32. Hauser RA, et al. A retrospective study on dextrose Prolotherapy for unresolved knee pain at an outpatient charity clinic in rural Illinois. *Journal of Prolotherapy*. 2009;1(1):11-21.

33. Hauser RA, et al. The case for utilizing Prolotherapy as first-line treatment for meniscal Pathology. *Journal of Prolotherapy*. 2010;2(3):416-437.

34. Sakellariou VI, et al. Risk assessment for chronic pain and patient satisfaction after total knee arthroplasty. *Orthopedics*. 2016 Jan-Feb;39(1):55-62.

35. American Orthopaedic Society for Sports Medicine. Cadaver tissue fails nearly 25% of the time in young ACL reconstructions. *ScienceDaily*. 12 July 2008. Available at: www.sciencedaily.com/releases/2008/07/080710070813.htm. Accessed Sept 26, 2016.

36. McCarthy M, et al. Long term follow up of pediatric ACL reconstruction in New York state high rates of subsequent ACL reconstruction. *The Orthopaedic Journal of Sports Medicine*. Jul 2015;3(7)(suppl 2). DOI: 10.1177/2325967115S00129

37. Wright RW, et al. Ipsilateral graft and contralateral ACL Rupture at five years or more following ACL reconstruction. *Journal of Bone and Joint Surgery*. 2011;93:1159-1165.

38. Ardern CL, et al. Return to pre-injury level of competitive sports after anterior cruciate ligament reconstruction surgery: Two-thirds of patients have not returned by 12 months after surgery. *Am J Sports Med*. 2011; 39(3):538-5438.

39. McCullough KA, et al. Return to high school- and college-level football after anterior cruciate ligament reconstruction: a Multicenter Orthopaedic Outcomes Network (MOON) cohort study. *Am J Sports Med*. 2012 Nov;40(11):2523-9.

40. Frank CB, et al. Abnormality of the contralateral ligament after injuries of the medial collateral ligament. An experimental study in rabbits. *Journal of Bone and Joint Surgery America*. 1994;76:403-412.

41. Samitier G, et al. Failure of anterior cruciate ligament reconstruction. *Arch Bone Jt Surg*. 2015 Oct; 3(4): 220–240.

42. Getelman MH, et al. Revision ACL reconstruction: autograft versus allograft. *Arthroscopy*. 1995;11(1):378.

43. Howell SM. Autogenous graft choices in ACL reconstruction. *Current Opinion in Orthopaedics*. 2001;12:149-155.

44. Harner CD, et al. Evaluation and treatment of recurrent instability after anterior cruciate ligament reconstruction. *J Bone Joint Surg Am.* 2000;82:1652-1664.

45. Zaltz I. The biomechanical case for labral debridement. *Clin Orthop Relat Res.* 2012;470;3398-3405.

46. Greaves LL, et al. Effect of acetabular labral tears, repair and resection on hip cartilage strain: a 7T MR study. *J Biomech.* 2010;43:858-863.

47. Hauser RA. The acceleration of articular cartilage degeneration in osteoarthritis by nonsteroidal anti-inflammatory drugs. *Journal of Prolotherapy.* 2010;2:305-322.

48. Hauser RA, et al. Prolotherapy as an alternative to surgery: a prospective pilot study of 34 patients from a private medical practice. *Journal of Prolotherapy.* 2010;(2)1:272-281.

49. Perez R, Pragt E, Geurts J, Zuurmond W, Patijn J, Van Kleef M. Treatment of patients with complex regional pain syndrome type 1 with mannitol: A prospective, randomized, placebo-controlled, double blind study. *The Journal of Pain.* Volume 9, Number 8(august)2008: pp.678-686.

50. Reuben S. Preventing the development of complex regional pain syndrome after surgery. *Anesthesiology.* 2004;101:1215-1224.

51. Rowbotham M. Pharmacologic management of complex regional pain syndrome. *Clin J Pain.* 2006; 22:425-429.

52. Blake H. Strain and psychological distress among informal supporters of reflex sympathetic dystrophy patients. *Disabil Rehabil.* 2000;22(18):827-832.

53. Birklein F, et al. Neurological findings in complex regional pain syndromes-analysis of 145 cases. *Acta Neurologica Scandinavica.* 2000;101:262-269.

54. Allen G, et al. Epidemiology of complex regional pain syndrome: a retrospective chart review of 134 patients. *Pain.* 1999;80:539-544.

55. Stanton-Hicks MD, et al. An updated interdisciplinary clinical pathway for CRPS: Report of an expert panel. *Pain Practice* (2002). Volume 2, Number 1, 1-16.

56. Duman I, et al. Reflex sympathetic dystrophy: a retrospective epidemiological study of 168 patients. *Clin Rheumatol.* 2008; 26:1433-1437.

57. Pak TJ, et al. Reflex sympathetic dystrophy: Review of 140 cases. *Minn Med.* 1970;53:507-512.

58. Small E. Reflex sympathetic dystrophy: Reflections from a clinician. *Adolesc Med.* 2007;18: 221-225.

59. Reuben S, et al. The incidence of complex regional pain syndrome after fasciectomy for Dupuytren's contracture: A prospective observational study of four anesthetic techniques. *Anesth Analg.* 2006;102; 499-503.

CHAPTER 20
PROLOTHERAPY VS. OTHER POPULAR TREATMENTS

1. The American Academy of Pain Medicine. AAPM Facts and Figures on Pain. http://www.painmed.org/patientcenter/facts_on_pain.aspx. Accessed Oct 6, 2016.

2. Agel J, et al. Anterior cruciate ligament injury patterns among collegiate men and women. *J Athl Train.* 1999;34:86-92.

3. Hauser RA, et al. Ligament injury and healing: a review of current clinical diagnostics and therapeutics. *The Open Rehabilitation Journal.* 2013;6:1-20.

4. Frank C, et al. Collagen fibril diameters in the healing adult rabbit medial collateral ligament. *Connect Tissue Res.* 1993;27:251-63.

5. Peloso P, et al. Medicinal and injection therapies for mechanical neck disorders (Review) *Cochrane Database Syst Rev.* 2007;3:CD000319. (PubMed)

6. Peloso PM, et al. Pharmacological interventions including medical injectins for neck pain: an overview as part of the ICON Project. *Open Orthop J.* 2013; 7:473-493.

7. Gross AR, et al. Physician-delivered injection therapies for mechanical neck disorders: a systematic review update (non-oral, non-intravenous pharmacological interventions for neck pain). *Open Orthop J.* 2013; 7:562-581.

8. Manchikanti L, et al. Utilization of interventional techniques in managing chronic pain in the Medicare population: analysis of growth patterns from 2000 to 2011. *Pain Physician.* 2012;15:e969-e982.

9. Amon C, et al. Assessment: use of epidural steroid injections to treat radicular lumbosacral pain: report of the Therapeutics and Technology Assessment Subcommittee of the American Academy of Neurology. 2007;6:68-723-9.

10. Apkarian AV, et al. Towards a theory of chronic pain. *Prog Neurobiol.* 2009;87:81-97.

11. Atlas SJ, et al. Evaluating and managing actue low back pain in the primary care setting. *J Gen Intern Med.* 2001;16:120-131.

12. Deyo RA, et al Lumar spine films in primary care: current use and effects of selective ordering criteria. *J Gen Intern Med.* 1986;1:20-5.

13. Jensen MC, et al. Magnetic resonance imaging of the lumbar spine in people without back pain. *N Engl J Med.* 1994; 331:69-73.

14. Boden SD, et al. Abnormal magnetic resonance scans of the cervical spine in asymptomatic subjects. A prospective investigation. *J Bone Joint Surg Am.* 1990;72:1178-84.

15. Hackett G. Joint stabilization. *American Journal of Surgery.* 1955;89:968-973.

16. Hackett G. Referred pain from low back ligament disability. *AMA Archives of Surgery.* 1956; 73:878-883.

17. Hackett G. *Ligament and Tendon Relaxation Treated by Prolotherapy.* First Edition. Springfield, IL: Charles C. Thomas, 1956.

18. Hackett G. *Ligament and Tendon Relaxation Treated by Prolotherapy.* Third Edition. Springfield, IL: Charles C. Thomas, 1958.

19. Jaeger B. Double-blind controlled study of different myofascial trigger point injection techniques (Abstract). *Pain.* 1987;4:S292.

20. Hackett G. Low back pain. *British Journal of Physical Medicine.* 1956;19:25-35.

21. Klinghardt D. Neural Therapy. *Townsend Letter for Doctors and Patients.* July 1995, pp. 96-98.

22. Dosch P. *Facts About Neural Therapy.* First English Edition. Heidelberg, Germany: Haug Publishers, 1985, pp. 25-30.

23. Dosch P. *Manual of Neural Therapy.* First English Edition. Heidelberg, Germany: Haug Publishers, 1984, pp. 74-77.

24. Dosch P. *Illustrated Atlas of the Techniques of Neural Therapy with Local Anesthetics.* First English Edition. Heidelberg, Germany: Haug Publishers, 1985.

CHAPTER 21
THE EVOLUTION OF PROLOTHERAPY

1. Hauser R, Hauser M. *Prolo Your Sports Injuries Away!* Oak Park, IL, Beulah Land Press, 2001.

2. Hackett G. *Ligament and Tendon Relaxation Treated By Prolotherapy.* Third Edition. Springfield, IL: Charles C. Thomas, 1958.

3. Hackett G. Joint stabilization: An experimental, histologic study with comments on the clinical application in ligament proliferation. *American Journal of Surgery.* 1955;89:968-973.

4. Hackett G. Back pain following trauma and disease—Prolotherapy. *Military Medicine.* 1961; July: 517-525.

5. Hackett G. Prolotherapy in whiplash and low back pain. *Postgraduate Medicine.* 1960; February: 214-219.

6. Hackett G. Low back pain. *The British Journal of Physical Medicine.* 1956;19:25-35.

7. Hackett G. Prolotherapy for headache. *Headache.* 1962; April: 3-11.

8. Kayfetz D, et al. Whiplash injury and other ligamentous headache—its management with Prolotherapy. *Headache.* 1963;3:1-8.

9. Hackett G. Referred pain from low back ligament disability. *AMA Archives of Surgery.* 1956; 73:878-883.

10. Hackett G. Referred pain and sciatica in low back diagnosis. *Journal of the American Medical Association.* 1957;163:183.

11. Hackett G. Prolotherapy for sciatica from weak pelvic ligaments and bone dystrophy. *Clinical Medicine.* 1961; Volume 8, Number 12.

12. Hackett G. Shearing injury to the sacroiliac joint. *Journal of the International College of Surgeons.* 1954;22:631-642.

13. Schneider R. Fatality after injection of sclerosing agent to precipitate fibro-osseous proliferation. *Journal of the American Medical Association.* 1959;170:1768-1772.

14. An abstract of a poster presentation (poster #49) at the 59th Annual Assembly of the American Academy of Physical Medicine and Rehabilitation printed in the Archives of Physical Medicine and Rehabilitation.

15. Kim M. Myofascial trigger point therapy: comparison of dextrose, water, saline, and lidocaine. *Archives of Physical Medicine and Rehabilitation.* 1997;78:1028.

16. Shallenberger F. Prolozone(R) Pain Therapy. Available at: www.antiagingmedicine.com/treatments/prolozone-therapy.

17. Shallenberger F. Prolozone – regenerating joints and eliminating pain. *Journal of Prolotherapy.* 2011;630-638.

18. Sanseverino E. Knee joint disorders treated by oxygen-ozone therapy. *Europa Medicophysica.* 1989;3:163-170.

19. Wong R. Ozonoterapia analgesica. *Revista CENIC Ciencias Biologicas.* 1989;20:143-150.

20. Siemsen C. The use of ozone in orthopedics in Proceedings: Ozone in Medicine, 12th World Congress of the International Ozone Association (Zurich: International Ozone Association, 1995),125-130.

21. Ceballos A, et al. Tratamiento de la osteoarthritis con ozono. *Revista CENIC Ciencias Biologicas.* 1989;20:15-153.

22. Escarpanter J, et al. Resultados terapeuticos en la osteoarthritis de la rodilla con infiltraciones de ozona. *Rev Cubana Invest Biomed.* 1997;16:124-132.

23. Al-Jaziri A. Pain killing effect of ozone-oxygen injection on spine and joint osteoarthritis. *Saudi Medical Journal.* 2008;29:553-557.

24. Paoloni M. Intramuscular oxygen-ozone therapy in the treatment of acute back pain with lumbar disc herniation-a multicenter, randomized, double-blind, clinical trial of active and simulated lumbar paravertebral injection. *Spine.* 2009;34:1337-1344.

25. Bonetti M. Intraformainal O2-O3 versus periradicular steroidal infiltrations in lower back pain: randomized controlled study. *American Journal of Neuroradiology.* 2005;26:996-1000.

26. Viebahn R. *The Use of Ozone in Medicine. Second Edition.* Heidelberg, Germany: Karl F. Haug Publishers; 1994.

27. Rilling S, et al. *Praxis der Ozon-Sauerstoff-Therapie.* Heidelberg, Germany: Auflage, Verlag Fur Medizin Dr. Ewald Fischer; 1990.

28. Washuttl J, et al. Biochemische Aspekte der Ozon-Sauerstoff-Therapie ArsMedici. 1986;5:194-199.

29. Lyftogt J. Subcutaneous Prolotherapy treatment of refractory knee, shoulder and lateral elbow pain. *Australasian Musculoskeletal Medicine Journal.* 2007;12:110-112.

30. Lyftogt J. Subcutaneous Prolotherapy for Achilles tendinopathy: The best solution? Australian *Musculoskeletal Medicine Journal.* 2007;12:107-109.

31. Reeves K. Prolotherapy: Basic science, clinical studies, and technique. *Pain Procedures in Clinical Practice.* Second Edition. Edited by Lennard T. Philadelphia PA: Hanley and Belfus, Inc., 2000, pp. 172-189.

32. Lyftogt J. Prolotherapy for recalcitrant lumbago. *Australasian Musculoskeletal Medicine Journal.* 2008;13:18-20.

33. Caterina M, et al. The capsaicin receptor: a heat-activated ion channel in the pain pathway. *Nature.* 1997;389:816-824.

34. Hackett G. Ligament uninhibited reversible antidromic vasodilation in brochiogenic patholophysiologic disease. *Lancet.* 1966;86:398-404.

35. Hackett G. Ligament relaxation and osteoarthritis, loose jointed versus close jointed. *Rheumatism.* 1959;15:28-33.

CHAPTER 22
PROLOTHERAPY PROVIDES RESULTS

1. Liu, Y. An in situ study of the influence of a sclerosing solution in rabbits' medial collateral ligaments and its junction strength. *Connective Tissue Research.* 1983;11:95-102.

2. Maynard, J. Morphological and biochemical effects of sodium morrhuate on tendons. Journal of Orthopaedic Research. 1985;3:236-248.

3. Hackett G. *Ligament and Tendon Relaxation Treated by Prolotherapy.* Third Edition. Springfield, IL: Charles C. Thomas, 1958, p. 5.

4. Hackett G. Referred pain and sciatica in diagnosis of low back disability. *Journal of the American Medical Association.* 1957;163:183-185.

5. Hackett G. Joint stabilization: an experimental, histological study with comments on the clinical application in ligament proliferation. *American Journal of Surgery.* 1955;89:968-973.

6. Hackett G. Referred pain from low back ligament disability. *AMA Archives of Surgery.* 73:878-883, November 1956.

7. Klein R. Proliferant injections for low back pain: histologic changes of injected ligaments and objective measures of lumbar spine mobility before and after treatment. *Journal of Neurology, Orthopedic Medicine and Surgery.* 1989;10:141-144.

8. Interview with Thomas Dorman, MD. *Nutrition and Healing.* 1994, pp. 5-6.

9. Dorman T. Treatment for spinal pain arising in ligaments using Prolotherapy: a retrospective study. *Journal of Orthopaedic Medicine.* 1991;13(1):13-19.

10. Ongley M, Dorman T, et al. Ligament instability of knees: a new approach to treatment. *Manual Medicine.* 1988;3:152-154.

11. Klein R. A randomized double-blind trial of dextrose-glycerine-phenol injections for chronic, low back pain. *Journal of Spinal Disorders.* 1993;6:23-33.

12. Ongley M. A new approach to the treatment of chronic low back pain. *Lancet.* 1987;2:143-146.

13. Reeves KD. Prolotherapy: present and future applications in soft-tissue pain and disability. *Physical Medicine and Rehabilitation Clinics of North America.* 1995;6:917-925.

14. Reeves KD. Technique of Prolotherapy. *Physiatric Procedures.* Edited by Lennard, T. Philadelphia, PA: Hanley and Belfus, Inc., 1995 pp. 57-70.

15. Reeves KD. Prolotherapy: Basic science, clinical studies, and technique. *Pain Procedures in Clinical Practice.* Second Edition, Edited by Lennard, T. Philadelphia, PA: Hanley and Belfus, Inc., 2000, pp. 172-189.

16. Reeves KD, et al. Prolotherapy: Regenerative injection therapy. In: Waldman SD (ed): *Pain Management.* Philadelphia; Saunders (Elsevier), 2nd ed; 2011:1027-1044.

17. Reeves KD, et al. Evidence-based regenerative injection therapy (Prolotherapy) in sports medicine. In Seidenberg PH, Beutler PI. (Eds). *The Sports Medicine Resource Manual.* Saunders (Elsevier); 2008:611-619.

18. Reeves KD, et al. Randomized, prospective double-blind placebo-controlled study of dextrose Prolotherapy for knee osteoarthritis with or without ACL laxity. *Alternative Therapies.* 2000;6:68-79.

19. Reeves KD, et al. Randomized, prospective, placebo-controlled double-blind study of dextrose Prolotherapy for osteoarthritic thumb and finger joints: evidence of clinical efficacy. *Journal of Alternative and Complementary Medicine.* 2000;6:311-320.

20. Reeves KD. Treatment of consecutive severe fibromyalgia patients with Prolotherapy. *Journal of Orthopaedic Medicine.* 1994;16(3):84-89.

21. Reeves KD. Long-term effects of dextrose Prolotherapy for anterior cruciate ligament laxity. *Alternative Ther Health Med.* May-Jun 2003;9(3):58-62.

22. Topol GA, et al. Regenerative injection of elite athletes with career-altering chronic groin pain who fail conservative treatment: a consecutive case series. *Am J Phys Med Rehabil.* 2008;87(11):890-902.

23. Topol GA, et al. Efficacy of dextrose Prolotherapy in elite male kicking-sport athletes with chronic groin pain. *Archives Phys Med Rehabil.* 2005;86:697-702.

24. Topol GA, et al. Chondrogenic effect of intra-articular hypertonic-dextrose (Prolotherapy) in severe knee osteoarthritis. *PM R.* 2016; April. doi: 10.1016/j.pmrj.2016.03.008.

25. Topol GA, et al. Hyperosmolar dextrose injection for recalcitrant Osgood-Schlatter disease. *Pediatrics.* 2011 Nov;128(5):e1121-8.

26. Rabago D, et al. Dextrose prolotherapy for knee osteoarthritis: a randomized controlled trial. *Ann Fam Med.* 2013 May-Jun;11(3):229-37. doi: 10.1370/afm.1504.

27. Hauser R, et al. Dextrose Prolotherapy injections for chronic ankle pain. *Practical Pain Management.* 2010;70-76.

28. Hauser R, et al. Dextrose Prolotherapy for unresolved low back pain: a retrospective case series study. *Journal of Prolotherapy.* 2009;1(3):145-155.

29. Hauser R, et al. Hackett-Hemwall dextrose Prolotherapy for unresolved elbow pain. *Practical Pain Management.* 2009;October:14-26.

30. Hauser R, et al. A retrospective observational study on Hackett-Hemwall dextrose Prolotherapy for unresolved foot and toe pain at an outpatient charity clinic in rural Illinois. *Journal of Prolotherapy.* 2011;3(1):543-551.

31. Hauser R, et al. A retrospective observational study on Hackett-Hemwall dextrose Prolotherapy for unresolved hand and finger pain at an outpatient charity clinic in rural Illinois. *Journal of Prolotherapy.* 2010;2(4):480-486.

32. Hauser R, et al. A retrospective study on Hackett-Hemwall dextrose Prolotherapy for chronic hip pain at an outpatient charity in rural Illinois. *Journal of Prolotherapy.* 2009;1(2):76-88.

33. Hauser R, et al. A retrospective study on dextrose Prolotherapy for unresolved knee pain at an outpatient charity clinic in rural Illinois. *Journal of Prolotherapy.* 2009;1(1):11-21.

34. Hauser R, et al. Dextrose Prolotherapy for unresolved neck pain. *Practical Pain Management.* 2007;October:56-69.

35. Hauser R, et al. A retrospective study on Hackett-Hemwall dextrose Prolotherapy for chronic shoulder pain at an outpatient charity clinic in rural Illinois. *Journal of Prolotherapy.* 2009;1(4):205-216.

36. Hauser R, et al. Dextrose Prolotherapy and pain of chronic TMJ dysfunction. *Practical Pain Management.* 2007;Nov/Dec:49-55.

37. Hauser R, et al. Dextrose Prolotherapy for unresolved wrist pain. *Practical Pain Management.* 2009;November/December:72-89.

38. Hauser RA, et al. Prolotherapy: a non-invasive approach to lesions of the glenoid labrum; a non-controlled questionnaire based study. *The Open Rehabilitation Journal.* 2013;6:69-76.

39. Hauser RA, et al. Regenerative injection therapy (Prolotherapy) for hip labrum lesions: rationale and retrospective study. *The Open Rehabilitation Journal.* 2013;6:59-68.

40. Hauser RA, et al. Outcomes of Prolotherapy in chondromalacia patella patients: improvements in pain level and function. *Clinical Medicine Insights: Arthritis and Musculoskeletal Disorders.* 2014;7:13-20 doi: 10.4137/CMAMD.S13098.

41. Hauser RA, et al. The case for utilizing Prolotherapy as first-line treatment for meniscal pathology: a retrospective study shows prolotherapy is effective in the treatment of mri-documented meniscal tears and degeneration. *Journal of Prolotherapy.* 2010;2(3):416-437.

42. Hauser RA, et al. Standard clinical x-ray studies document cartilage regeneration in five degenerated knees after prolotherapy. *Journal of Prolotherapy.* 2009;1(1):22-28.

43. Hauser RA. The regeneration of articular cartilage with Prolotherapy. *Journal of Prolotherapy.* 2009;1(1):39-44.

44. Hauser RA, et al. Ligament injury and healing: an overview of current clinical concepts. *Journal of Prolotherapy.* 2011;3(4)836-846.

45. Hauser RA, et al. Ligament injury and healing: a review of current clinical diagnostics and therapeutics. *The Open Rehabilitation Journal.* 2013;6:1-20.

46. Hauser RA, et al. Structural basis of joint instability as cause for chronic musculoskeletal pain and its successful treatment with regenerative injection therapy (Prolotherapy.) *The Open Pain Journal.* 2014;7:9-22.

47. Hauser RA, et al. Chronic neck pain: making the connection between capsular ligament laxity and cervical instability. *The Open Orthopaedics Journal.* 2014;8:326-345.

48. Hauser RA, et al. Upper cervical instability of traumatic origin treated with dextrose Prolotherapy: a case report. *Journal of Prolotherapy.* 2015;7:e932-e935.

49. Hauser RA, et al. Cervical instability as a cause of Barré-Lieou Syndrome and definitive treatment with Prolotherapy: a case series. *European Journal of Preventive Medicine.* 2015;3(5):155-166.

50. Hauser RA, et al. The biology of Prolotherapy and its application in clinical cervical spine instability and chronic neck pain: a retrospective study. *European Journal of Preventive Medicine.* Vol. 3, No. 4, 2015, pp. 85-102. doi: 10.11648/j.ejpm.20150304.1.

51. Hauser RA. Prolotherapy of the arcuate ligament of the knee. *Journal of Prolotherapy.* 2011;3(2):662-663.

52. Hauser RA, et al. Direct bone marrow injections for avascular necrosis of the talus: a case report. *Journal of Prolotherapy.* 2012;4:e891-894.

53. Hauser RA, et al. Treatment of basal thumb osteoarthritis: a retrospective study of dextrose Prolotherapy injections as an alternative treatment. *Journal of Prolotherapy.* 2013;5:e913-e921.

54. Hauser RA, et al. Regenerative injection therapy with whole bone marrow aspirate for degenerative joint disease: a case series. *Clinical Medicine Insights: Arthritis and Musculoskeletal Disorders.* 2013;6:65-71.

55. Hauser RA, et al. Rationale for using direct bone marrow aspirate as a proliferant for regenerative injection therapy (Prolotherapy). *The Open Stem Cell Journal.* 2013;4:7-14.

56. Hauser RA, et al. Treating osteoarthritic joints using dextrose Prolotherapy and direct bone marrow aspirate injection therapy: patient-reported outcomes. *The Open Arthritis Journal.* 2013;6:6-14.

57. Hauser RA, et al. Dextrose Prolotherapy with human growth hormone to treat chronic first metatarsophalangeal joint pain. *The Foot and Ankle Online Journal.* 2012:5(9):1.

58. Hauser RA, et al. The use of Prolotherapy in the treatment of chronic overuse shoulder and neck pain, neurogenic pain and hip degeneration in an incomplete C4-C5 spinal cord injury patient. *Journal of Prolotherapy.* 2009;1(3):166-171.

59. Hauser RA, et al. The theoretical basis for and treatment of complex regional pain syndrome with Prolotherapy. *Journal of Prolotherapy.* 2010;2(2):356-370.

60. Hauser RA, et al. Dextrose Prolotherapy for recurring headache and migraine pain. *Practical Pain Management.* 2009;9(5):58-65.

61. Hauser RA, et al. Treatment of joint hypermobility syndrome, including ehlers-danlos syndrome, with Hackett-Hemwall Prolotherapy. *Journal of Prolotherapy.* 2011;3(2):612-629.

62. Hauser RA, et al. Dextrose Prolotherapy treatment for unresolved "Morton's Neuroma" pain. *The Foot and Ankle Online Journal.* 2012:5(6):1.

63. Hauser RA, et al. Non-operative treatment of cervical radiculopathy: a three part article from the approach of a physiatrist, chiropractor, and physical therapist. *Journal of Prolotherapy.* 2009;1(4):217-231.

64. Hauser RA, et al. Pain in osteoarthritis: can Prolotherapy help? *The Pain Practitioner.* 2014;9:16-22.

65. Hauser RA. Prolotherapy as an alternative treatment for osteochondritis dissecans: two cases of young baseball players. *Journal of Prolotherapy.* 2011;3(1):568-571.

66. Gordin K, et al. The case for utilizing Prolotherapy as a promising stand-alone or adjunctive treatment for over-manipulation syndrome. *Journal of Applied Research.* 2013;13(1):1-28.

67. Hauser RA, et al. Platelet rich plasma Prolotherapy as first-line treatment for meniscal pathology. *Practical Pain Management.* Jul-Aug 2010;10(6):53-75.

68. Hauser RA, et al. Prolotherapy as an alternative to surgery: a prospective pilot study on 34 patients from a private medical practice. *Journal of Prolotherapy.* 2010;2(1):272-281.

69. Hauser RA, et al. Evidence-based use of dextrose Prolotherapy for musculoskeletal pain a system review. *Journal of Prolotherapy.* 2011;3(4)765-789.

70. Hauser RA, et al. A systematic review of dextrose Prolotherapy of chronic musculoskeletal pain. *Clinical Medicine Insights: Arthritis and Musculoskeletal Disorders.* 2016;9:139-159.

71. Hauser RA, et al. Journal of Prolotherapy medical editorial board consensus statement for the use of Prolotherapy for musculoskeletal pain. *Journal of Prolotherapy.* 2011;3(4)744-764.

72. Kim J. The effect of Prolotherapy for osteoarthritis of the knee. *Journal of the Korean Academy of Rehabilitation Medicine.* 2002;26:445-448.

73. Kim J. Effects of Prolotherapy on knee joint pain due to ligament laxity. *The Journal of the Korean Pain Society.* 2004;17:47-50.

74. Miller M, et al. Treatment of painful advanced internal lumbar disc derangement with intradiscal injection of hypertonic dextrose. *Pain Physician.* 2006;9:115-121.

75. Hooper R, et al. Prospective case series of litigants and non-litigants with chronic spinal pain treated with dextrose Prolotherapy. *International Musculoskeletal Medicine Journal.* 2011;33:15-20.

76. Klein R, et al. Proliferant injections for low back pain: histologic changes of injected ligaments and objective measurements of lumbar spine mobility before and after treatment. *Journal of Neurology, Orthopedic Medicine and Surgery.* 1989;10:141-144.

77. Dagenais S, et al. Intraligamentous injection of sclerosing solutions (Prolotherapy) for spinal pain: a critical review of literature. *Journal of Spine.* 2005;5:310-3128.

78. Daganais S, et al. Evidence-informed management of chronic low back pain with Prolotherapy. *Journal of Spine.* 2008;8:203-212.

79. Hooper R, et al. Retrospective case series on patients with chronic spinal pain treated with dextrose Prolotherapy. *Journal of Alternative and Complementary Medicine.* 2004;10:670-674.

80. Gabbi A, et al. Biological approaches for cartilage repair. *Journal of Knee Surgery.* 2009;22:36-44.

81. Richter W. Mesenchymal stem cells and cartilage in situ regeneration. *Journal of Internal Medicine.* 2009;266:390-405.

82. Richter W. Cell-based cartilage repair: illusion or solution for osteoarthritis. *Current Opinions in Rheumatology.* 2007;19:451-456.

83. Bruder S, et al. Mesenchymal stem cells in bone development, bone repair, and skeletal regeneration therapy. *Journal of Cell Biochemistry.* 1994;56:283-294.

84. Lee K, et al. Injectable mesenchymal stem cell therapy for large cartilage defects-a porcine model. *Stem Cells.* 2007;25:2964-2971.

85. Wakitani S, et al. Repair of articular cartilage defects in the patella-femoral joint with autologous bone marrow mesenchymal cell transplantations: three case reports involving nine defects in five knees. *Journal of Tissue Engineering & Regenerative Medicine.* 2007;1:74-79.

86. Hooper R, et al. Case series on chronic whiplash related neck pain treated with intraarticular 88. zygapophysial joint regeneration injection therapy. *Pain Physician.* 2007;10:313-318.

87. Centeno C, et al. Fluoroscopically guided cervical Prolotherapy for instability with blinded pre and post radiographic reading. *Pain Physician.* 2005;8:67-72.

88. Jo D, et al. The effects of Prolotherapy on shoulder pain. *Korean Journal of Anesthesiology.* 2004;46:589-592.

89. Kim W, et al. A randomized controlled trial of intra-articular Prolotherapy versus steroid injection for sacroiliac joint pain. *Journal of Alternative and Complementary Medicine.* 2010;16:1285-1290.

90. Ryan M, et al. Sonographically guided intratendinous injections of hyperosmolar dextrose/lidocaine: a pilot study for the treatment of chronic plantar fasciitis. *British Journal of Sports Medicine.* 2009;43:303-306.

91. Lyftogt J. Subcutaneous Prolotherapy for Achilles tendinopathy: The best solution? *Australasian Musculoskeletal Medicine Journal.* 2007;12:107-109.

92. Sampson S, et al. Platelet rich plasma injection grafts for musculoskeletal injuries: a review. *Current Review of Musculoskeletal Medicine.* 2008;1:165-174.

93. Reeves KD. Prolotherapy: injection of growth factors or growth factor production stimulants to growth normal cells or tissue. In Waldman SD (ed): *Pain Management.* Philadelphia, Elsevier, 2006, pp. 1106-1127.

94. Martinez-Zapata M, et al. Efficacy and safety of autologous plasma rich in platelets for tissue regeneration: a systematic review. *Transfusion.* 2009;49:44-56.

95. Creaney L, et al. Growth factor delivery methods of sports injuries: the state of play. *British Journal of Sports Medicine.* 2008;42:314-320.

96. Sanchez M, et al. Platelet-rich therapies in treatment of orthopaedic sport injuries. *Sports Medicine.* 2009;39:345-354.

97. Mishra A, et al. Treatment of chronic elbow tendinosis with buffered platelet rich plasma. *American Journal of Sports Medicine.* 2006;10(10):1-5.

98. Maxwell N, et al. Sonographically guided intratendinous injection of hyperosmolar dextrose to treatment chronic tendinosis of the Achilles tendon: a pilot study. *American Journal of Roentgenology.* 2007;189:W215-220.

99. Scarpone M, et al. The efficacy of Prolotherapy for lateral epicondylosis: a pilot study. *Clinical Journal of Sports Medicine.* 2008;18:248-254.

100. James S, et al. Ultrasound guided dry needling and autologous blood injection for patellar tendinosis. *British Journal of Sports Medicine.* 2007;8:518-521.

101. Edwards S, et al. Autologous blood injections for refractory lateral epicondylitis. *Am J Hand Surg.* 2003;28(2):272-8.

102. Smith R, et al. Abnormal microvascular responses in lateral epicondylitis. *Br J Rheum.* 1994;33:1166-1168.

103. Jobe F, et al. Lateral and medial epicondylitis of the elbow. *J Am Acad Orthop Surg.* 1994;2:1-8.

104. Hamilton P. The prevalence of humeral epicondylitis: a survey in general practice. *J R Coll Gen Pract.* 1986;36:464-465.

105. Labelle H, et al. Lack of scientific evidence for the treatment of lateral epicondylitis of the elbow. *J Bone Joint Surg Br.* 74:646-651 1992.

106. Karli D, et al. Platelet rich plasma for hamstring tears. *Practical Pain Management.* 2010;June:9-15.

107. Hammond J, et al. Use of autologous platelet-rich plasma to treat muscle strain injuries. *The American Journal of Sports Medicine.* 2009;37:1135-1143.

108. Park J, et al. Ultrasonographic findings of healing of torn tendon in the patients with lateral epicondylitis after Prolotherapy. *Journal of the Korean Society of Medical Ultrasound.* 2003;22:177-183.

109. Linetsky F, et al. Pain management with regenerative injection therapy. In: Boswell MV, Cole BE(eds.) *Weiner's pain management: a practical guide.* 7th ed. Boca Raton, FL: CRC Press; 2006;939-965.

110. Curtin M, et al. The effectiveness of Prolotherapy in the management of recalcitrant medial tibial stress syndrome: a pilot study. *British Journal of Sports Medicine.* 2011;45e1. doi:10.1136/bjsm.2010.081554.8.

111. Lazzara M. The non-surgical repair of a complete Achilles tendon rupture by Prolotherapy: biological reconstruction. A case report. *J Orthopaedic Med.* 2005;27:128-132.

112. Grote W, et al. Repair of a complete anterior cruciate tear using Prolotherapy: a case report. *International Musculoskeletal Medicine.* 2009;1:31(4):159-165.

113. Hall M, et al. Platelet-rich plasma:current concepts and application in sports medicine. *Journal of the American Academy of Orthopedic Surgeons.* 2009;17:602-608.

114. Hackett G. Back pain following trauma and disease – Prolotherapy. *Military Medicine.* 1961;July:517-525.

115. Hackett G. Prolotherapy in whiplash and low back pain. *Postgraduate Medicine.* 1960;February:214-219.

116. Reeves KD. Sweet Relief: Prolotherapy targets sprains and strains. *Biomechanics.* 2004;9:24-35.

117. Kim M, et al. Comparison on treatment effects of dextrose water, saline, and lidocaine for trigger point injections. *Journal of the Korean Academy of Rehabilitation Medicine.* 1997;21:967-973.

118. Reeves KD. Prolotherapy for patients with musculoskeletal disorders. *Journal of Musculoskeletal Medicine.* 2002;390-301.

119. Hakala R, et al. The use of Prolotherapy for temporomandibular joint dysfunction. *Journal of Prolotherapy.* 2010;2(3):439-446.

120. Kayfetz D, et al. Whiplash injury and other ligamentous headache-its management with Prolotherapy. *Headache.* 1963;3:21-28.

121. Myers A. Prolotherapy treatment of low back pain and sciatica. *Bulletin of the Hospital for Joint Diseases.* 1961;22:1-10.

122. Hackett G. Prolotherapy for sciatica from weak pelvic ligaments and bone dystrophy. *Clinical Medicine.* 1961;8:2301-2316.

123. Hackett G. Prolotherapy for headache. *Headache.* 1962;1:3-11.

124. Hemwall G. Barré-Lieou syndrome. *Journal of Orthopedic Medicine (UK).* 1989;11:79-81.

125. Kayfetz D. Occipito-cervical (whiplash) injuries treated by Prolotherapy. *Medical Trial Technical Quarterly.* 1963;June:9-29.

126. Oh J, et al. Sequential effects of high glucose on meningeal cell transforming growth factor-beta 1 and fibronectin synthesis. *Kidney International.* 1998;54:1872-1878.

127. Hackett G, et al. Prolotherapy for headache. Pain in the head and neck, and neuritis. *Headache.* 1962;2:20-28.

128. Hirschberg G, et al. Treatment of the chronic iliolumbar syndrome by infiltration of the iliolumbar ligament. *The Western Journal of Medicine.* 1982;136:372-374.

129. Kim B, et al. The effect of Prolotherapy for the chronic pain of musculoskeletal system. *The Journal of the Korean Academy of Rehabilitation Medicine.* 2001;25:128-133.

130. Kim S, et al. Effects of Prolotherapy on chronic musculoskeletal disease. *The Korean Journal of Pain.* 2002;15:121-125.

131. Khan S, et al. Dextrose Prolotherapy for recalcitrant coccygodynia. *Journal of Orthopaedic Surgery.* 2008;16:27-29.

132. Lyftogt J. Chronic exertional compartment syndrome and Prolotherapy. *Australasian Musculoskeletal Medicine Journal.* 2006;11:83-85.

133. Jo D, et al. The effects of Prolotherapy on the lumbar nucleus pulposus. *Journal of the Korean Pain Society.* 2003;16:68-72.

134. Foye P. Dextrose Prolotherapy for recalcitrant coccygodynia fractures. *Journal of Orthopedic Surgeon (Hong Kong).* 2008;16:27-29.

135. Hechtman K. Platelet-rich plasma injection reduces pain in patients with recalcitrant epicondylitis. *Orthopaedics.* 2011;34:92-99.

136. Tsatsos G, et al. Prolotherapy in the treatment of foot problems. *Journal of the Podiatric Medical Association*. 2002;92:36-368.

137. Kirk J, et al. The hypermobility syndrome-musculoskeletal complaints associated with generalized joint hypermobility. *Annals of Rheumatic Diseases*. 1967;26:419-425.

138. Ohgi S, et al. Glucose modulates growth of gingival fibroblasts and periodontal ligament cells: correlation with expression of basic fibroblast growth factor. *Journal of Periodontal Research*. 1996;31:579-588.

139. Lee C. Prolotherapy. *The Journal of the Korean Pain Society*. 2004;Dec:17S:94-98.

140. Hernigou P, et al. The use of percutaneous autologous bone marrow transplantation in nonunion and avascular necrosis of bone. *Journal of Bone and Joint Surgery British*. 2005;87:896-902.

141. McLain R, et al. Aspiration of osteoprogenitor cells for augmenting spinal fusion: comparison of progenitor cell concentrations from the vertebral body and iliac crest. *Journal of Bone and Joint Surgery America*. 2005;87:2655-2661.

142. Muscler G, et al. Aspiration to obtain osteoblast progenitor cells from human bone marrow: the influence of aspiration volume. *Journal of Bone and Joint Surgery*. 1997;70A:1699-1709.

143. Gedney E. The hypermobile joint: further reports on the injection method. Read before *Osteopathic Clinical Society of Pennsylvania*, February 13, 1938.

144. Caplan A, et al. Mesenchymal stem cells and tissue repair. In: *The Anterior Cruciate Ligament: Current and Future Concepts*. Ed. By DW Jackson. New York, Raven press, 1993, p. 405-417.

145. Hackett G. Ligament relaxation and osteoarthritis, loose jointed versus close jointed. *Rheumatism*. 1959;15:28-33.

146. Lyftogt J. Subcutaneous Prolotherapy treatment of refractory knee, shoulder and lateral elbow pain. *Australasian Musculoskeletal Medicine Journal*. 2007;12:110-112.

147. Lyftogt J. Prolotherapy for recalcitrant lumbago. *Australasian Musculoskeletal Medicine Journal*. 2008;13:18-20.

148. Schultz L. A treatment of subluxation of the temporomandibular joint. *JAMA*. 1937;109:1032-1035.

149. Schultz L. Twenty years' experience in treating hypermobility of the temporomandibular joints. *American Journal of Surgery*. Vol. 92, December 1956.

150. Refai H, et al. The efficacy of dextrose Prolotherapy for temporomandibular joint hypermobility: a preliminary prospective, randomized, double-blind, placebo-controlled clinical trial. *Journal of Oral Maxillofacial Surgery*. 2011;July 12: (Epub ahead of print).

151. Lee C, et al. Clinical experience of Prolotherapy for chronic musculoskeletal disease. *The Journal of The Korean Pain Society*. 2001;14:114-117.

152. Distel L, et al. Prolotherapy: a clinical review of its role in treating chronic musculoskeletal pain. *Physical Medicine and Rehabilitation*. 2011;3(6Suppl):S78-81.

153. Gedney E. Disc Syndrome. *Osteopathic Profession*. September 1951;11-15,38-46.

154. Gedney E. Use of sclerosing solution may change therapy in vertebral disc problems. *Osteopathic Profession*. April 1952; 11-13,34,38-39.

155. Hackett G. Joint stabilization: an experimental, histological study with comments on the clinical application in ligament proliferation. *American Journal of Surgery*. 1955;89:968-973.

156. Merriman J. Prolotherapy versus operative fusion in the treatment of joint instability of the spine and pelvis. *Journal of the International College of Surgeons*. 1964;42:150-159.

157. Wilkinson H. Injection therapy for enthesopathies casing axial spine pain and the "failed back syndrome": a single blinded, randomized and cross-over study. *Pain Physician*. 2005;8:167-173.

158. Marx R, et al. Platelet rich plasma (PRP): a primer. *Practical Pain Management*. March 2008;8(2):46-47.

159. Watson J, et al. Treatment of chronic low-back pain: a 1-year or greater follow-up. *Journal of Alternative and Complementary Medicine.* 2010;16:951-958.

160. Misra A, et al. Treatment of tendon and muscle using platelet-rich plasma. *Clinics in Sports Medicine.* 2009;28:113-125.

161. Sanchez M, et al. Comparison of surgically repaired Achilles tendon tears using platelet-rich fibrin matrices. *American Journal of Sports Medicine.* 2007;35:245-251.

162. de Mos M, et al. Can platelet-rich plasma enhance tendon repair? A cell culture study. *American Journal of Sports Medicine.* 2008;36:1171-1178.

163. Gedney E. Progress report on use of sclerosing solutions in low back syndromes. *The Osteopathic Profession.* 1954;August:18-21,40-44.

164. Gedney E. The application of sclerotherapy in spondylolisthesis and spondylolysis. *The Osteopathic Profession.* 1964;September:66-69,102-105.

165. Hackett G. Joint stabilization through induced ligament sclerosis. *Ohio State Medical Journal.* 1953;49:877-884.

166. Leedy R. Analysis of 50 low back cases 6 years after treatment by joint ligament sclerotherapy. *Osteopathic Medicine.* 1976;6:15-22.

167. Weibrich G. Effect of platelet concentration in platelet rich plasma on peri-implant bone regeneration. *Bone.* 2004;34:665-671.

168. Fleming J, et al. Bone cells and matrices in orthopedic tissue engineering. *Orthopaedic Clinics of North America.* 2000;31:357-274.

169. Hernigou P, et al. Treatment of osteonecrosis with autlogous bone marrow grafting. *Clincal Orthopaedic and Related Research.* 2002;405:14-23.

170. Lee E, et al. The potential of stem cells in orthopaedic surgery. *Journal of Bone and Joint Surgery.* 2006;88:841-851.

171. Kuroda R, et al. Treatment of a full-thickness articular cartilage defect in the femoral condyle of an athlete with autlogous bone-marrow stromal cells. *Osteoarthritis and Cartilage.* 2006;15:226-231.

172. Chang T, et al. Repair of a large full-thickness articular cartilage defects by transplantation of autologous uncultured bone-marrow-derived mononuclear cells. *Journal of Orthopaedic Research.* 2008;18-26.

173. Wakitani W, et al. Human autogous culture expanded bone marrow mesenchymal cell transplantation for repair of cartilage defects in osteoarthritic knees. *Osteoarthritis and Cartilage.* 2002;10:199-206.

174. Hui J, et al. Review article: stem cell therapy in orthopaedic surgery: current status and ethical considerations. *Malaysian Orthopaedic Journal.* 2009;3:4-12.

175. Wakitani W, et al. Autlogous bone marrow stroma cell transplantation for repair of full-thickness articular cartilage defects in human patellae: two case reports. *Cell Transplantation.* 2004;13:595-600.

176. Quarto R, et al. Repair of large bone defects with the use of autlogous bone marrow stroma. cells. *New England Journal of Medicine.* 2001;344:385-386.

177. Eslamian F. Therapeutic effects of prolotherapy with intra-articular dextrose injection in patients with moderate knee osteoarthritis: a single-arm study with 6 months follow up. *Ther Adv Musculoskelet Dis.* 2015 Apr;7(2):35-44.

178. Jacks A, et al. Lumbosacral Prolotherapy: a before-and-after study in an NHS setting. *International Musculoskeletal Medicine.* 2012;34(1):7-12.

CHAPTER 23

ANSWERS TO COMMON QUESTIONS ABOUT PROLOTHERAPY

1. Meyers A. Prolotherapy treatment of low back pain and sciatica. *Bulletin of the Hospital for Joint Disease.* 1961;22:1.

2. Bland J. *Disorders of the Cervical Spine.* Philadelphia, PA: W.B. Saunders, 1987.

3. Butler D. Biomechanics of ligaments and tendons. *Exercise and Sports Scientific Review.* 1975;6:125.

4. Tipton C. Influence of immobilization, training, exogenous hormones, and surgical repair of knee ligaments from hypophysectomized rats. *American Journal of Physiology.* 1971;221:1114.

5. Nachemson A. Some mechanical properties of the third human lumbar interlaminar ligament. *Journal of Biomechanics.* 1968;1:211.

6. Akeson W. The connective tissue response to immobility: an accelerated aging response. *Experimental Gerontology.* 1968;3:239.

7. Travell J. *Myofascial Pain and Dysfunction.* Baltimore, M.D.: Williams and Wilkins, 1983, pp. 103-164.

8. Schumacher H. *Primer on the Rheumatic Diseases.* Tenth Edition. Atlanta, GA: Arthritis Foundation, 1993, pp. 8-11.

9. Ballard, W. Biochemical aspects of aging and degeneration in the invertebral disc. *Contemporary Orthopedics.* 1992;24:453-458.

10. Jacobs R. Pathogenesis of idiopathic scoliosis. Chicago, IL: *Scoliosis Research Society,* 1984, pp. 107-118.

11. Crowninsheild R. The strength and failure characteristics of rat medial collateral ligaments. *Journal of Trauma.* 1976;16:99.

12. Tipton C. Response of adrenalectomized rats to exercise. *Endocrinology.* 1972;91:573.

13. Tipton C. Response of thyroidectomized rats to training. *American Journal of Physiology.* 1972;215:1137.

14. Bucci L. *Nutrition Applied to Injury Rehabilitation and Sports Medicine.* Boca Raton, FL: CRC Press, 1995, pp. 167-176.

15. Batmanghelidj F. *Your Body's Many Cries for Water.* Second Edition. Falls Church, VA: Global Health Solutions, Inc., 1996, pp. 8-11.

16. Welbourne T. Increased plasma bicarbonate and growth hormone after an oral glutamine load. *American Journal of Clinical Nutrition.* 1995; pp. 1058-1061.

17. Hurson M. Metabolic effects of arginine in a healthy elderly population. *Journal of Parenteral and Enteral Nutrition.* 1995; pp. 227-230.

18. Dominguez R, et al. *Total Body Training.* East Dundee, IL: Moving Force Systems, 1982; pp. 33-37.

19. McGaw W. The effect of tension on collagen remodeling by fibroblasts: a sterological ultrastructural study. *Connective Tissue Research.* 1986;14:229-235.

20. Bucci L. *Nutrition Applied to Injury Rehabilitation and Sports Medicine.* Boca Raton, FL: CRC Press, 1995, pp. 167-176.

21. Woo S. Injury and repair of the musculoskeletal soft tissues. *American Academy of Orthopaedic Surgeons.* 1987.

22. Mankin H. Localization of tritiated thymidine in articular cartilage of rabbits inhibits growth in immature cartilage. *Journal of Bone and Joint Surgery.* 1962;44A:682.

23. Butler D. Biomechanics of ligaments and tendons. *Exercise and Sports Scientific Review.* 1975;6:125.

24. Brandt K. Should osteoarthritis be treated with nonsteroidal anti-inflammatory drugs? *Rheumatic Disease Clinics of North America.* 1993;19:697-712.

25. Brandt K. The effects of salicylates and other nonsteroidal anti-inflammatory drugs on articular cartilage. *American Journal of Medicine.* 1984;77:65-69.

26. Obeid G. Effect of ibuprofen on the healing and remodeling of bone and articular cartilage in the rabbit temporomandibular joint. *Journal of Oral and Maxillofacial Surgeons.* 1992, pp. 843-850.

27. Dupont M. The efficacy of anti-inflammatory medication in the treatment of the acutely sprained ankle. *American Journal of Sports Medicine.* 1987;15:41-45.

28. Newman N. Acetabular bone destruction related to nonsteroidal anti-inflammatory drugs. *Lancet.* 1985; July 6:11-13.

29. Serup J, et al. Salicylate arthropathy: accelerated coxarthrosis during long-term treatment with acetylsalicylic acid. *Praxis.* 1981;70:359.

30. Ronningen H et al. Indomethacin treatment in osteoarthritis of the hip joint. *Acta Ortho. Scand.* 1979;50:169-174.

31. Newman N. Acetabular bone destruction related to nonsteroidal anti-inflammatory drugs. *Lancet.* 185; July 6:11-13.

32. Serup J, et al. Salicylate arthropathy: accelerated coxarthrosis during long-term treatment with acetylsalicylic acid. *Praxis.* 1981;70:359.

CHAPTER 24

MAXIMIZE YOUR
PROLOTHERAPY POTENTIAL

1. Adams R and Victor M. (eds.), *Principles of Neurology.* Fourth Edition. St. Louis, MO: McGraw Hill, 1989, pp. 737-738.

2. Guyer D. The long-range prognosis of arachnoiditis. *Spine.* 1989;14:1332-1341.

3. Hoffman G. Spinal arachnoiditis—what is the clinical spectrum? *Spine.* 1983;8:538-540.

INDEX

OTHER BOOKS BY ROSS & MARION HAUSER

- *Joint Instability*
  The Missing Diagnosis
  ©2017

- *The Hauser Diet®*
  A Fresh Look At Healthy Living
  ©2007

- *Prolotherapy*
  An Alternative to Knee Surgery
  ©2004

- *Treating Cancer with Insulin Potentiation Therapy*
  ©2002

- *Prolo Your Sports Injuries Away!*
  Curing Sports Injuries and Enhancing Athletic Performance with Prolotherapy
  ©2001

- *Prolo Your Arthritis Pain Away!*
  Curing Disabling and Disfiguring Arthritis Pain with Prolotherapy
  ©2000

- *Prolo Your Back Pain Away!*
  Curing Chronic Back Pain with Prolotherapy
  ©2000

- *Prolo Your Headache and Neck Pain Away!*
  Curing Migraines and Chronic Neck Pain with Prolotherapy
  ©2000

- *Prolo Your Fibromyalgia Pain Away!*
  Curing Disabling Body Pain with Prolotherapy
  ©2000

RESEARCH BY THE CARING MEDICAL TEAM

Our team is continuously striving to add to the published results and research on Prolotherapy, Cellular Prolotherapy, and other pain treatments. To check out our research papers, please visit CaringMedical.com/prolotherapy-research/, or contact our office. ∎

Purchasing Information:
Sorridi Business Consulting
715 Lake Street, Suite 600
Oak Park, Illinois 60301
www.amazon.com

Got Pain?
Get Prolo!

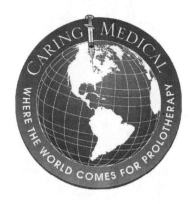

Contact us and become a patient:

Caring Medical Regenerative Medicine Clinics

CHICAGOLAND OFFICE
715 Lake Street Suite 600
Oak Park, IL 60301
Phone: **708-628-5217**

SOUTHWEST FLORIDA OFFICE
9738 Commerce Center Ct.
Fort Myers, FL 33908
Phone: **239-303-4308**

E-mail: **info@caringmedical.com**
Website: **www.caringmedical.com**
Fax: **855-779-1950**

www.facebook.com/caringmedical
www.twitter.com/caringmedical
www.youtube.com/user/caringmedical
www.caringmedical.com/prolotherapy-news

We look forward to connecting with you and helping you get back the active lifestyle you desire! Our offices have been blessed to treat patients who travel to us from all around the world. We are happy to review your case if you are considering a trip to our office. Contact us to tell us more about your case and together we can determine if you sound like a good Prolotherapy candidate.